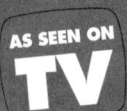
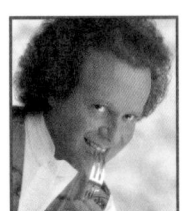
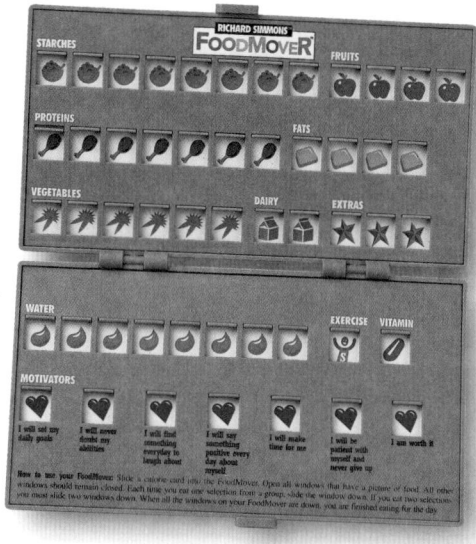
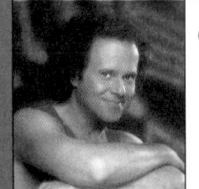

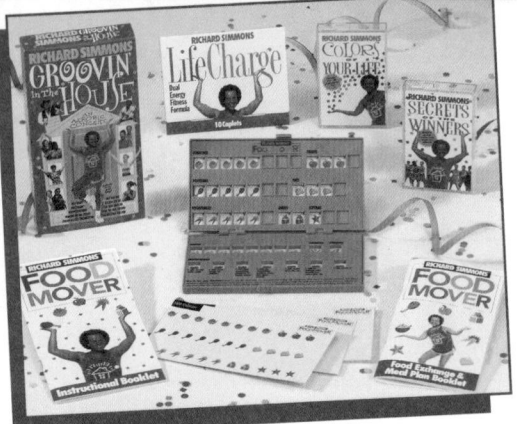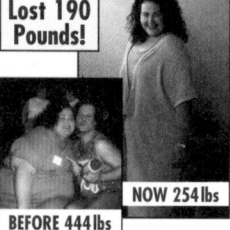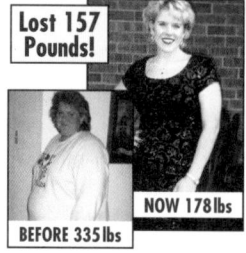

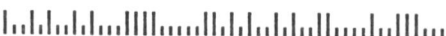

Still Hungry—
After All These Years

Still Hungry—
After All These Years

My Story

Richard Simmons

GT Publishing • New York

Produced by Richard Simmons,
Jenifer Catalano, David Ricketts, and Barbara Marks

Published by GT Publishing Corporation
16 East 40th Street, New York, NY 10016

Library of Congress Catalog Card Number: 99-073299
ISBN: 1-57719-356-3

Printed in the United States of America

2 4 6 8 10 9 7 5 3 1

First Printing

DESIGNED BY BARBARA MARKS

The names of some individuals and places as well as conversations
may have been changed or altered to protect individuals' privacy.

All photographs, other than noted, are from the private collection of the author.

Endpaper photo credits:
Richard looking in mirror: Robert Blakeman; Richard with his Dalmatians: Harry Benson;
Richard with bags of mail: Michael Maron.

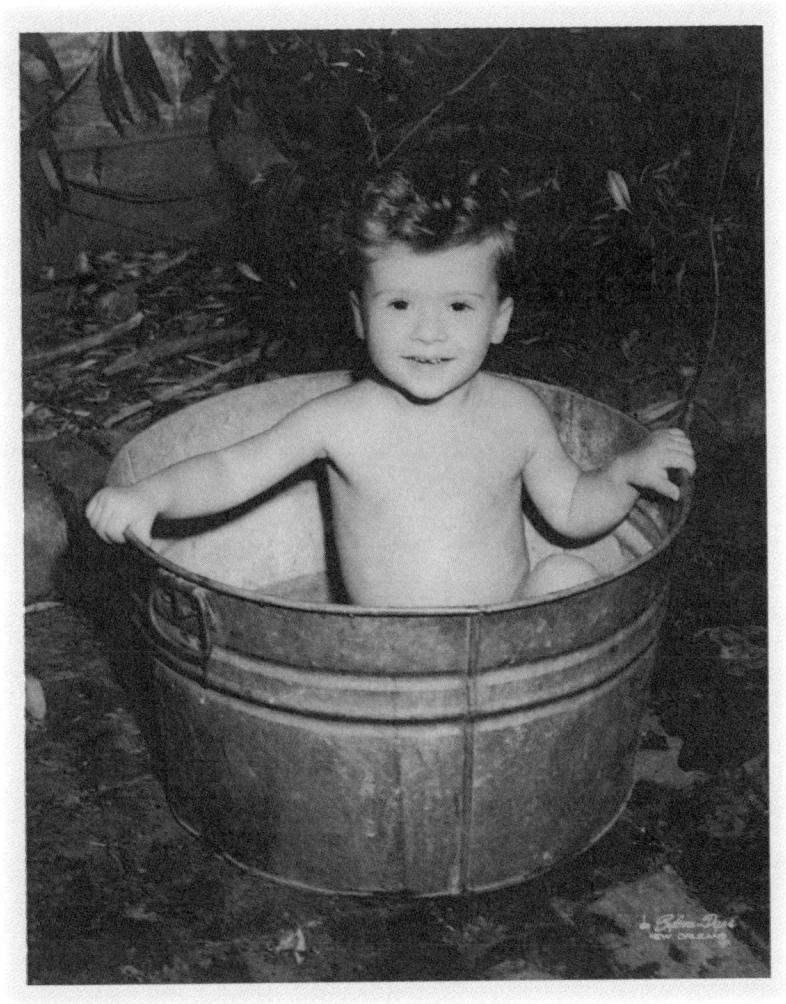

My first centerfold

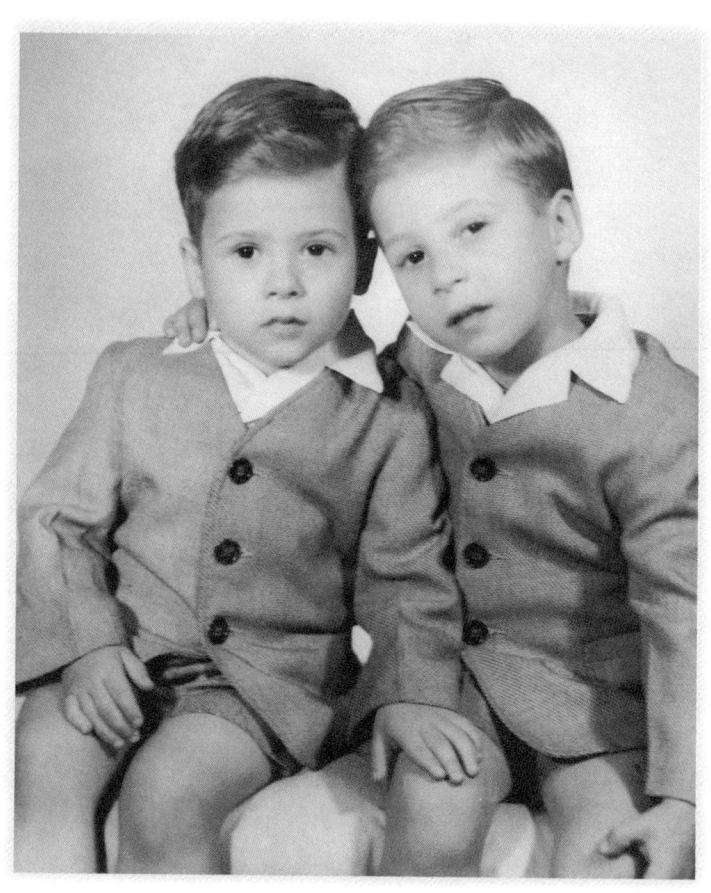

Me and Lenny

The Promise

"Hello? Lenny? It's me. It's your favorite brother calling."

"Dicky, you're my *only* brother. What's new?"

"Did I tell you I'm working on another book?"

"Oh. You're doing another book. What is it? A salad book? Is it a casserole book? I just loved your other two."

"No, no. It's not a cookbook. I'm fifty now, you know. So, I'm doing my autobiography."

Click.

Had Lenny really hung up on me? I hit the redial button. "Lenny, what happened? We got disconnected. Please, just listen to me. So I was saying, I'm doing a story about me and my relationship with food." And then I mumbled very fast, with my hand over the receiver, "And I'm going to include a little bit about mother and dad and you. Okay. And so anyway . . . "

"Wait! Wait! Dicky? Promise me that I'll see everything that goes into this book—before it's printed."

"Lenny! Listen to me. This is *my* autobiography. If you want to write your own, then write your own!"

"No. I don't want to write my own. I just want to make sure everything you have in yours is right."

"Okay. Don't worry. It'll be just the way I remember it."

"The way you remember it? Oh, no! Then I'll *really* want to read every word."

"Okay, Lenny. I promise I'll check everything with you."

"Promise?"

"Yes. I promise. I love you."

"No! You didn't say it like you meant it."

"I *promise!*"

"Dicky, I love you, too. Bye."

$* \atop * *$

The Visit

For seventeen years now I've stayed in the same room at the Omni Royal Orleans Hotel in New Orleans. From the tall, small-paned balcony windows, I can look out onto my past.

Down the street is the praline store where I used to work in grade school and on into high school. Across the street is the bar where Napoleon was offered refuge in 1814. And if I lean out to the right, I can just make out the steps of 926 St. Louis Street. It's the house where I grew up as a child with my mother and father—Shirley and Leonard—and my older brother, Lenny.

I'm back in New Orleans, my hometown. It's a city so full of food and music. All our neighbors were exotic dancers and musicians who worked two blocks away on Bourbon Street. When I went to sleep at night as a little kid, I could hear them playing the music from the clubs—it was my lullaby. I had quite a beginning.

I'm here to visit my mother, Shirley. I used to come home at least once a month. Now, I'm here more often. To be honest, she hasn't been doing well. She's homebound now, and every time I see her, she becomes more of a shadow. Once an adult, twice a child. It's hard for me to face all this.

At dusk, I leave the hotel and travel through the French quarter, past places that bring back lots of memories of my growing up in the Vieux Carré, which literally means "Old Square." It's a ten-minute ride to where Shirley lives. I find her in her room, lying in bed. She is sleeping peacefully next to Brent, her twelve-year-old Dalmatian. He never lets her out of his sight. The two of them even go into the bathroom together. Instead of waking her, I take her hand and kiss it, holding on tightly. She looks so small and fragile, a delicate china doll. She is eighty-seven pounds—and for the first time, her age matches her weight.

I sit quietly and look around. My brother and I fill this room, in pictures and framed clippings, going all the way back to when we were babies. I don't think my mother ever threw anything out. There are some pictures of my father and Shirley, too. But my mother was clearly devoted to her two boys.

In the corner, an old-fashioned fan spins noisily. The base is black and made of heavy metal, and the thick blades push lots of air around. They don't make 'em like that anymore. From the day my father brought it home and repaired the broken cord over fifty years ago, that fan has been turning, cooling us on hot Louisiana nights. If only that fan could talk, oh the stories it would tell!

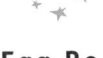

Egg Roll

*I*t was the summer of 1948 and New Orleans was hot, one of the hottest summers anybody could remember. The big black fan was whirling, and Shirley, in her capri pants and loose, pink cotton smock, was sitting in front of it, trying to cool off. Her legs rested on the fringed ottoman. Being eight and a half months pregnant in humid, sticky Louisiana was not fun.

Shirley had given birth to her first son, Lenny Jr.—my older brother—only twenty months earlier, on the thirtieth of October. Then it had been cool. But now, beads of sweat ran down her forehead. Her thick Russian sable hair was braided from ear to ear and piled high on her head.

One thing was for sure—making dinner was out of the question.

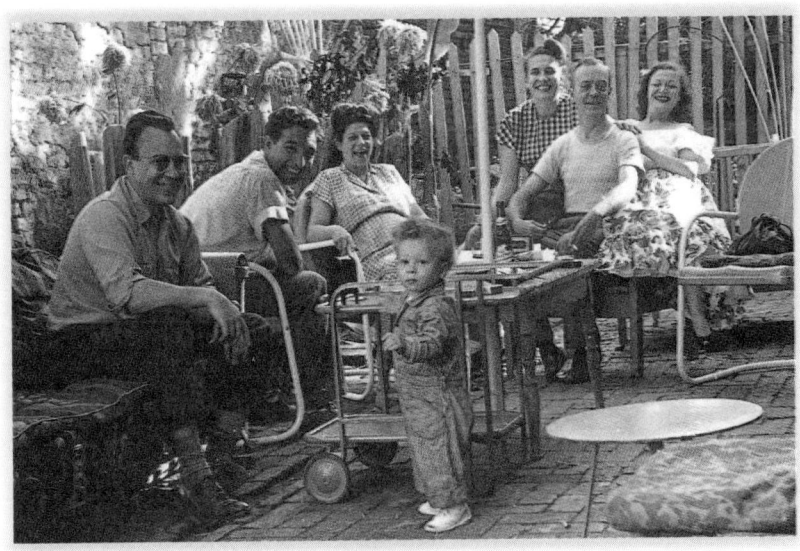

*There's Shirley in the center, visiting with some of the neighbors on the patio
and pregnant with Guess Who.*

There'd be no cooking over a hot stove tonight. Besides, she'd been having the strangest cravings all day. All she could think about now, through the squeaky noise of the spinning fan blades, was a plate of shrimp foo young from Gin's Restaurant—and maybe an egg roll.

Shirley had just put her head back and shut her eyes to rest when the front door opened. Her husband was home.

"Len, let's go out for Chinese food tonight. I think our biscuit in the oven needs an egg roll." That sounded good to Len. He didn't feel like cooking, either.

Shirley, a glamorous woman, never left the house unless she was in full makeup—foundation, eyeliner, lashes, blush, and deep, lush lipstick applied ever so delicately with her retractable lip brush. Applying makeup was no easy task for her these days. Her growing midsection made it difficult for her to get close to her vanity mirror. But still, Shirley always looked like a flawless star from the cover of a movie magazine.

Fifteen minutes later, Shirley was balancing in her four-inch heels, quite an accomplishment for a woman who stood four foot ten and who could no longer see her toes. Holding little Lenny's hand and guided by her handsome husband—a dead ringer for Fred Astaire—Shirley led her family down the street, the three short blocks to Gin's.

Gin's Restaurant served the best Chinese food in the French quarter, and Shirley could hardly wait to get those chopsticks in her hands. She wanted her egg roll. Mr. Gin, the owner, always wore a heavily starched apron that draped all the way to his shoes. He was five feet tall—petite like Shirley—and probably weighed the same as he had when he was fourteen. He greeted every customer with a big smile, always bowing, almost as though his shirt or apron was caught on something. He just looked like Mr. Happiness, smiling and laughing.

"So very good to see you all," Mr. Gin said to Shirley, beaming. "Oh, little Lenny is growing so fast. And, oh, Miss Shirley going to have a big, big baby real soon." Mr. Gin steered them toward a table near the front window.

"Oh, come sit down here, Miss Shirley. What can I bring you—boy or girl?"

Everyone laughed. Leonard answered, "We don't care. Just as long as our baby's healthy—and loves Chinese food. Isn't that right, honey?"

Leonard caught the look on Shirley's face. It was time. The fo

Leonard caught the look on Shirley's face. It was time. The fortune cookie had broken. Shirley was about to give birth.

The room went crazy. Mr. Gin rushed outside to the middle of the street, trying to wave down a cab. Little Lenny started crying loudly. Lenny Sr. panicked, rushing back and forth between the front door and the table where Shirley struggled to get up. And me—I was on my way.

The Checker cab pulled up to the emergency entrance of Touro Infirmary, just a quick five-minute ride from the restaurant. In no time, Shirley was on a gurney, off to the delivery room. In the waiting room, Leonard took off his beige herringbone jacket, folded it up, and made a pillow for Lenny. He then took a Pall Mall out of the pack he always kept in his shirt pocket, and lit up. It was going to be a long night.

As he looked around the waiting room at all the other men, pacing and making baby chitchat, Leonard noticed something right away. Every guy there was about twenty-three or twenty-four, and some even younger. Leonard was fifty-one years old. He froze at the thought of bringing up two boys at the half-century mark of his life. He worried that as he got older he might not be able to keep up with them. And he worried about Shirley. She was thirty-seven, and in 1948, having a baby that late in life was sort of a rarity. After Lenny Jr. was born, the doctors advised Shirley not to have any more children. She had such a tiny frame that another pregnancy at her age could be difficult and maybe dangerous. But they'd both wanted a big family, and a year after having Lenny Jr., Shirley had been overjoyed to discover she was pregnant once again.

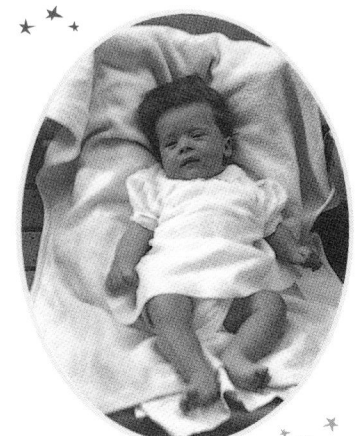

It was a difficult labor. Some pain medication wasn't given properly, and we almost lost Shirley—and, maybe, almost me. My delivery was finally by cesarean, at 11:18 A.M. the following morning, July 12. I weighed 6 pounds, 6½ ounces, and I was a little more than two weeks early.

"God's given you a beautiful, healthy baby boy," the doctor told her. "He's got a full head of curly dark hair. The nurses can't get over it. They've never seen such a mane of hair before."

Oh, come let us . . .
me at three weeks

When Shirley finally brought me home from the hospital, the whole neighborhood did what it knew best. What else? They threw a big pot-luck party! For some reason, there just weren't a lot of kids around the quarter. So when there was a new baby, watch out—it was reason to celebrate. From my very beginning, I knew about parties and food!

I was born nameless—Len and Shirley thought there would be another two weeks to go. They now pondered long and hard about a name for their round, bubbly tot.

"How about Milton, after my older brother?" Leonard suggested. "He's a good man and he's very smart."

So Milton it was, and Milton I am—until years later, when I became Richard, then Dicky, then Richard again.

* ⋆ ⋆

My First Word: "Kitchen"

*N*ine twenty-six St. Louis Street was to be my new home. It was a shotgun house: All the rooms were in a direct line with each other, from front to back. It was like living in a long, long train. That's how they built them in New Orleans back in those days. First, you entered a large hallway that led to a bedroom. Then you passed through the living room, another bedroom, a dining room, breakfast area, kitchen, and finally, the caboose—the bedroom I shared with my brother. Notice I didn't mention the bathroom. You had to go outside for that. There was an outhouse behind a cluster of banana trees in the backyard. Shortly after my birth, my parents had a bathroom added on. I just loved that house. It had been built in the late 1800s, and all the charm was still there: high ceilings with lots of ornate moldings, crystal chandeliers, French doors with beveled glass, a fireplace with a marble mantel in the living room.

But my favorite room, as early as I can remember, was the kitchen. Bet you're not surprised by that! And what a fascinating place it was. Because the kitchen was right next to my room, I could watch the hustle and bustle through the bars of my pigpen—I mean, playpen. Assorted cast-iron skillets hung on nails above the stove. One of the first words I learned was not "mama," not "papa," but "stove." There was always something cooking on those burners, and the house was always full of such wonderful smells.

Long before I started getting teeth, I was using my nose. Near the stove, there was this white shiny object called the icebox. It seemed to be quite the place to go. Len and Shirl opened and closed it, day and night.

My father did practically all the cooking. From my playpen, I could carefully watch the kitchen routine over and over again: First, Len and Shirl would get a few things from one of the shelves in the pantry, and then a few things from the icebox. They'd organize this stuff in a neat little row on the counter near the sink—another word I picked up quickly was "sink."

Then it really began. *Click*—on went the radio, filling the kitchen with music. *Peel, snap, stir*—more kitchen music. There was an old, bright red A&P coffee can on the stove, sitting on a cracked dish. A spoon was stuck in the middle, and whenever they took a skillet off the wall and put it on a burner, two big spoonfuls of this white slippery stuff were plopped into the middle of the pan. It was called lard, and it made everything taste better.

Even before I really understood who Len and Shirley were in my life, I could recognize a pound of bacon at twenty feet. When Leonard unwrapped the package, the strips of bacon looked so weak, so flimsy, so sad—until they hit the frying pan. Then they began swimming and dancing, lacing up at the sides and turning golden brown. Another pan was taken off the wall, and *plop*—a spoonful of lard was thrown in. Sunny-side up eggs were cooking away in their pan. *Plop.* The sausages were tossed in, and bursts of hot grease exploded like fireworks. This happened every morning during my babyhood.

After breakfast was over and the dishes were put away, things got quiet for a while. As I settled down for a nap, it wasn't a lullaby that put me to sleep, but the fragrance of breakfast that lingered everywhere—better than Chanel No. 5.

There was a cuckoo clock above an antique painted cabinet where all the canned goods slept until they were needed. When both hands of the clock were pointed up and that bird sang, I'd wake from my nap and the kitchen would come to life again. It was time for lunch, and I was about to witness a ritual like no other—the making of a sandwich. This event by itself could fill almost an entire book.

Shirley went to the breadbox on the counter where there were two styles of bread—the pre-sliced kind, such as Sunbeam (with the picture of the little girl on the package), and the whole loaves of French bread, pumpernickel, or rye that were bought at Solari's, a gourmet food store in our neighborhood. While Shirley began cutting the loaves and arranging the slices on a platter, Leonard all of a sudden appeared at the icebox. He'd take out lots of jars and bottles: mayonnaise, Dijon mustard, yellow mustard, black olives, green olives stuffed with pimentos, and pickles—gherkins, sweet, sour, dill, and bread-and-butter. I realized then that the icebox was really just a buffet waiting to happen.

Another trip to the shelves of that enchanted appliance and Leonard would come out with these waxy envelopes that were folded and taped, and a fresh head of crisp iceberg lettuce. Then he'd walk over to the windowsill, where the sun was drenching the Creole tomatoes, turning them deep, juicy red. This was one of the first Golden Rules of Food I learned, even before I could speak: Never put a tomato in the fridge—it won't taste like a tomato anymore.

Next, I would hear a ripping sound behind me as Shirley opened a bag of fresh chips. Into a bowl they went. Now it was time to open the mail—the waxed-paper mail. Each flat, white envelope held something wonderful. There was bologna, corned beef, roast beef, and liverwurst, as well as Swiss, Cheddar, and American cheeses—all thinly sliced. These were all arranged on their own platters. The kitchen was turning into an art gallery of food.

But now the real business started. The top of my hair was even with the edge of the table, so I would stand on my tiptoes, straining to see the platters, bowls, and jars.

A stranger peeking through our kitchen window might wonder, How many people were coming to visit? Was it a special occasion? A party? No—it was just another Simmons family lunch.

Each person in my family had their very own special way of making a sandwich.

First, there was my brother Lenny. He wasn't all that interested in food, so he'd casually toss a little mustard or mayo on two slices of bread, slap on a few pieces of meats or cheeses in no particular order, and start eating. That's what his half of our bedroom looked like—tossed together.

When I watched my mother and father create their sandwiches, I began to wonder if maybe Lenny wasn't adopted. I was sure that when I had my chance to make my own sandwich one day, I would create a masterpiece, just like my father.

She'd take little pieces of the roast beef, and she'd give me

I studied Leonard as he carefully spread the mayo on a slice of bread, so artfully and evenly, as if he were painting a fresco. Once, I swore I caught him signing his name at the bottom of a slice of rye. Then he would delicately alternate the cheeses and the luncheon meats, paying close attention to the color scheme and texture. Next, he'd paint another piece of bread with bright yellow splashes of mustard, and always with a clean knife. Then the Creole tomatoes would be sliced and salted—just a little salt. *Waaap!* He'd hit the iceberg lettuce against the side of the sink and easily pull the core from the middle. Slowly, he'd peel off every leaf, then wash and individually dry each one. On the sandwich the leaves would go. What began as just a bunch of flat, lonely ingredients was transformed into something staggering. From where I watched at the edge of the table on my tippytoes, that sandwich with the bottles and jars behind it almost looked like a dazzling new building added to the skyline of New York City. That was how I saw our lunch. I watched my family really having a ball when it came to eating. Eventually, I would spend too much time at the ball!

Shirley would make her own version of Len's sandwich. While my father favored liverwurst and Swiss cheese, my mother laid out the pieces of roast beef and Cheddar. When she was done making her sandwich, she would pick me up and sit me on her lap. She'd take little pieces of the roast beef, and she'd give me a big hug, kiss me, and say, "I love you." Then she'd feed me those pieces, while she gently rocked me. She'd break off a corner of a slice of Cheddar, and she'd kiss me and say, "This is Cheddar cheese, honey." No little jars of beige vegetable mush or pureed meat for me. I got the real thing. It was almost like communion.

Even through the eyes of an infant, this kitchen was an exciting place to be. It was a three-ring circus, and I wanted to be the ringmaster. Occasionally my mother would glance over and catch me watching her doing something wonderful, like stuffing an artichoke the size of my head.

Long before I learned about the ways of the world, through hard knocks and otherwise, I was quickly becoming a food expert. Food was my life, and around it I could feel the flow of love.

Did I tell you there were candy dishes in every room of our house? This was almost as important as the refrigerator, which was the mother lode. Russell Stover was our main supplier. There were chocolate-covered candies, hard candies, and everything else you can imagine. There was even a candy dish in the bathroom that was usually filled with mints. It was like having little surprises everywhere.

* * *

The Love Palace

*Y*ou can see that food was all around me when I was growing up. It was love and food. And where was all this love coming from? From the love palace, of course, or what most people called the grocery store.

When I was old enough to walk, my father would often take me along on his shopping trips. Because we lived in the French quarter, everything was within walking distance. We didn't own a car because we didn't need one. Long ago my mother was involved in a serious car accident, so she had no intention of ever sitting behind the wheel again. And my father never learned how to drive.

After breakfast, my father began to make his grocery list for dinner that evening. He never shopped weekly, but instead picked up groceries every day, just like they do in Europe. Everything had to be fresh.

We would start out at the A&P. The grocery store for me was like an amusement park. My father got a cart and he put Lenny and me in it. I watched as he took out his neatly folded list from his pocket. Up and down the aisles we went, exploring the entire store.

I loved the cereal aisle. It was like going to a toy store. I always made my father read the back of each box out loud so I could tell him what kind of cereal we should get. Would I have to send away for the Captain Midnight decoder ring shown on the back of the box, or would I discover that little treasure inside? My father had so much patience as he read each and every package. While other kids' parents read bedtime stories to their children, I insisted my father do his reading to me in the grocery store.

My other big discovery, besides cereal, was Cracker Jacks. Not only did you get a cute little box with the sailor on it, but when you ripped it open and ate it all, there was always a prize waiting for you at the bottom.

Our next stop was the meat department. My father knew the name of every person at every store where he shopped.

"Hello, Charles," he greeted the butcher. "What have you got that's fresh today?"

Evelyn handed Lenny and me a cookie and told us how cute we

Len had been eyeing the pork chops, but Charles steered him away from them and suggested, "Oh, we've got these delicious lamb chops I've just trimmed, fresh today." While my father inspected them, Charles went over to the meat slicer and cut a little piece of bologna for Lenny and me. We nibbled while Leonard asked Charles to double grind some beef.

"Your two boys are growing so fast," Charles exclaimed, pinching my cheek as he slipped me an extra slice of luncheon meat.

Next, we hit the produce aisle. Almost all the vegetables we ate were fried, and that's how Leonard selected them—could he fry it? Remember, we had that A&P can sitting on the stove at home.

"Oh, look at the ripe eggplant. This will be so delicious in eggplant Parmesan."

My father was a professional shopper, and his knowledge of food was unparalleled. He taught me how to pick the best.

So that was our first stop, the A&P. Now we were off to the French Market, an outdoor food "circus" where restaurant chefs did their shopping. We walked past seafood stalls full of crawfish, soft-shell crabs, oysters, shrimp, all directly off the boats. No purchases today—just looking.

Next stop: Solari's, the gourmet food store I told you about. It was very chic for its time. It had green outdoor carpeting on the floor and background music to soothe the harried shopper. Solari's shipped in food from all over the world. We'd buy saffron for the saffron rice and chocolate from Switzerland. Walking into Solari's was like shopping at Tiffany's, only instead of gold and gems, the aisles were filled with unusual epicurean delights.

And then the best for last, The Four Seasons, a very famous bakery on Royal Street. I loved Evelyn, who worked behind the counter. She helped us pick out our fresh Napoleons—my father's favorite dessert: layers of puff pastry and custard with ripples of chocolate on top. We'd also get fresh fruit tarts: pastry cups filled with rich, creamy custard and decorated with colorful slices of glazed fruits. While we waited our turn, Evelyn handed Lenny and me each a cookie and told us how cute we were. "Here's a *lagniappe*," Evelyn whispered, pinching my cheek. "A little something extra."

Finally, it was time to take our treasures home. My father was extremely organized as he put each item in its own special place, so it could be quickly retrieved when needed. He neatly folded up all the brown bags, which he'd use later to cover Lenny's schoolbooks. And rubber bands and string were put in their own special drawers.

After the kitchen was all neat again, Leonard indulged himself in his usual way. He took the cold coffee from the morning pot, poured it into a glass, added two scoops of vanilla ice cream, then some milk, and stirred it all up. While he sipped his drink, he'd thumb through a cookbook he'd taken down from one of the shelves in the dining room. He drank one of these coffee floats every single day. Never once did he ask Lenny or me if we'd like a sip. This was *his* special treat. I know I would have liked a taste, since there was ice cream in it. As far as I was concerned, you could put ice cream in cod-liver oil and I'd ask for a straw.

Although my father was passionate about food, he was not overweight. Quite the opposite. He was trim and always neatly dressed. He always weighed 145 pounds, regardless of the number of desserts he had at one meal.

Leonard loved to entertain, preferring to cook for others more than for himself. In anything he undertook, he was always thorough. And so it was with food. He studied and experimented, collecting cookbooks as he went. And before long, half the dining room was lined with cookbooks from all over the world. Food became an experience, first for my father and then for all of us. If you couldn't travel to exotic countries, then at least you could eat the food from those places.

Even before the breakfast dishes had been washed and put away, my father would be making plans for dinner, the third and final meal of the day. Breakfast was fun, lunch was casual, but dinner—dinner was sacred. It was a religious experience. My father would plan dinner all day long.

Len insisted on making everything from scratch. That's why he had all those cookbooks. Nothing was canned or frozen. My father would say at breakfast, "Tonight, I think I'll make veal Milanese and we'll have fettuccine Alfredo to go with that." He would also serve an appetizer before the entree. Often it was shrimp remoulade with homemade remoulade sauce, each portion served in its own glass pedestal bowl, with the little shrimp elegantly draped over the side, like a waterfall. After the appetizer, soup would come next (often a gumbo), then salad. An entree would follow, and—it goes without saying—there was always dessert. This was better than a restaurant. Now you can begin to understand why food has always been the major love affair of my life. Like most affairs, though, it was not without its ups and downs. Learning how to control food in my life has always been a struggle.

We almost always ate in the dining room, on a long, long, Last Supper table, very ornate, that could seat ten people. In old New Orleans houses, there are no closets, no built-ins. Things are kept in an armoire, a cabinet, or a sideboard. Our dining room had a crystal chandelier and gorgeous French doors that opened to the patio.

As my father set the table, he'd give me and my brother little jobs to do. I got to help fold the napkins and fill each glass with ice and a long spoon for the iced tea. We had iced tea with every dinner. My father would brew the tea in a blue-and-white ceramic pitcher, then place it in the middle of the table, next to a plate of sliced fresh lemons. That pitcher now sits in my kitchen cupboard. Over the years, it has held more tea than Boston Harbor during the Boston Tea Party.

Meals were punctual. If six o'clock rolled around and you weren't at the table, you'd better have an excuse from a hospital. As far back as I can remember, we always ate to music. My father favored Al Jolson, Mahalia Jackson, Ella Fitzgerald, and Perry Como, all from his wonderful 78 r.p.m. record collection.

We would sit down, say a prayer of thanks, and then the passing of the bowls would begin. But it wasn't as simple as that. You had to have rhythm. The Italian broccoli with slivered garlic and mushrooms came to you from your right, you took some, and then passed it to your left, all in time to the beat of the music. Next came the fettuccine, from right to left; then the veal. We all worked together—it was beautiful, just like synchronized swimmers.

Then Act II: Platters and bowls were passed again, to a different tempo when the record was changed—maybe from a Mahalia Jackson spiritual to a Perry Como ballad. You get the picture. Just a quiet dinner at the Simmons house. This went on until all the platters and bowls were empty and we were full, or a platter had to go back to the kitchen for a refill.

I usually had seconds, and sometimes thirds. Occasionally my father would give me one of his looks, and then he would turn to Shirley and say, "You know, sometimes I think you feed that boy too much."

"No, it's all right," Shirley would answer. "He loves food. He's a growing boy and needs to eat."

"I guess you're right. A little baby fat is okay."

We didn't always have dinner in the formal dining room. On special nights, we'd gather in the living room to eat our dinner off T.V. trays while we watched our favorite shows on the television. Our black-and-white set was the first on the block, and my father was commander of the dials. There was no such thing as a remote control back then, so he'd have to stand up and walk over to the set to change the channel. But there were only three stations, so making a selection wasn't all that difficult.

My mother and I were into the fun shows, like *Variety,* Ed Sullivan, Phil Silvers, Red Skelton, *I Love Lucy.* My brother preferred the dramas. He loved to watch Lassie rescue Timmy from the well each week. My father, on the other hand, loved the game shows. He never missed *I've Got a Secret, To Tell the Truth,* or *What's My Line.* And when *Playhouse 90* was on, no one was allowed to move from their chair.

My really favorite part of television-watching was the commercials. That's when everybody got up and went to the bathroom or got second helpings. Not me. As much as I loved food, I stayed right where I was. I memorized all the jingles in those ads, and then I'd sing them over and over. Ovaltine, Bit-O-Honey, Good & Plenty, Nestle's Quik, and Bosco were part of my routine. Often I would practice them in front of the bathroom mirror. Who would have guessed that this was the early training for my infomercials that I would do more than thirty years later?

After Shirley had washed the dishes and either my brother or I had dried, our T.V. suppers always ended with bowls of ice cream: big scoops of vanilla drizzled with chocolate syrup and topped with maraschino cherries. Of course, extra cherries were always a must for me. Our sundaes had real whipped cream that Len had made from scratch, and no sundae was complete without a little dribble of juice from the cherries across the top and a scattering of finely chopped nuts.

There you have it—a pretty detailed description of the three-squares-a-day at the Simmons house. Whether it was breakfast, lunch, dinner, or dessert, eating at the Simmons household was always a feast—fit for royalty. In fact, my father, who was really quite regal in his manner and dress, came from a much more humble background.

No sundae was complete without a little dribble of juice from

* * *

Leonard

*M*y dad was raised in a very strict, very religious household where proper behavior was expected—no, actually it was enforced by his father, who was a Methodist minister. Born in Norfolk, Virginia, Leonard was the youngest in a family of seven (one of his brothers, my Uncle Milton, was later to play a very important role in my life).

Since Leonard was the baby of the family, he was pampered. In fact, you might even say he was spoiled. So from the very beginning, Leonard was used to getting his own way. If he didn't, he could be real stubborn, and that stubbornness would later get him into trouble.

To make ends meet for his large family, my grandfather—the Reverend Simmons—also worked as a stave maker, constructing wooden barrels. In the family, hard work was expected, and when that didn't put food on the table, somehow the good Lord and the Methodist congregation provided.

However, the Simmons family was not exactly poor, or at least they were not without their resources. The family had one of the first indoor bathtubs on their block. And even back then, my father loved entertaining others. He'd conduct tours of the tub for his friends. He was happiest when he was the center of attention. You also have to remember that he was very good-looking. My brother Lenny thought he resembled Edward VIII, the duke of Windsor, the royal who gave up his throne for Wallis Warfield Simpson. Now I know you can see the family resemblance in me! Right?

My father so wanted a stage career that he began performing when he was eight years old, around 1911. He replaced the young Eddie Cantor in a group called the Gus Edwards Young Vaudevillians. Singing and dancing were in his blood. He performed with this group until 1917, when he enlisted in the army to fight in the Great War.

When the war was over, Leonard returned to Norfolk, but he was ready to move on. There he was, in the middle of Smithfield Ham country, thinking, What's next? That's when he read about Georgie Jessel, who was going from city to city, holding auditions and looking for new talent. Maybe this was the way out. Well, my father went down to the auditorium and signed up for the audition. When it came his turn, he got up on stage and did a little singing and a little dancing and a little talking—and he won the talent

erries across the top and a scattering of finely chopped nuts.

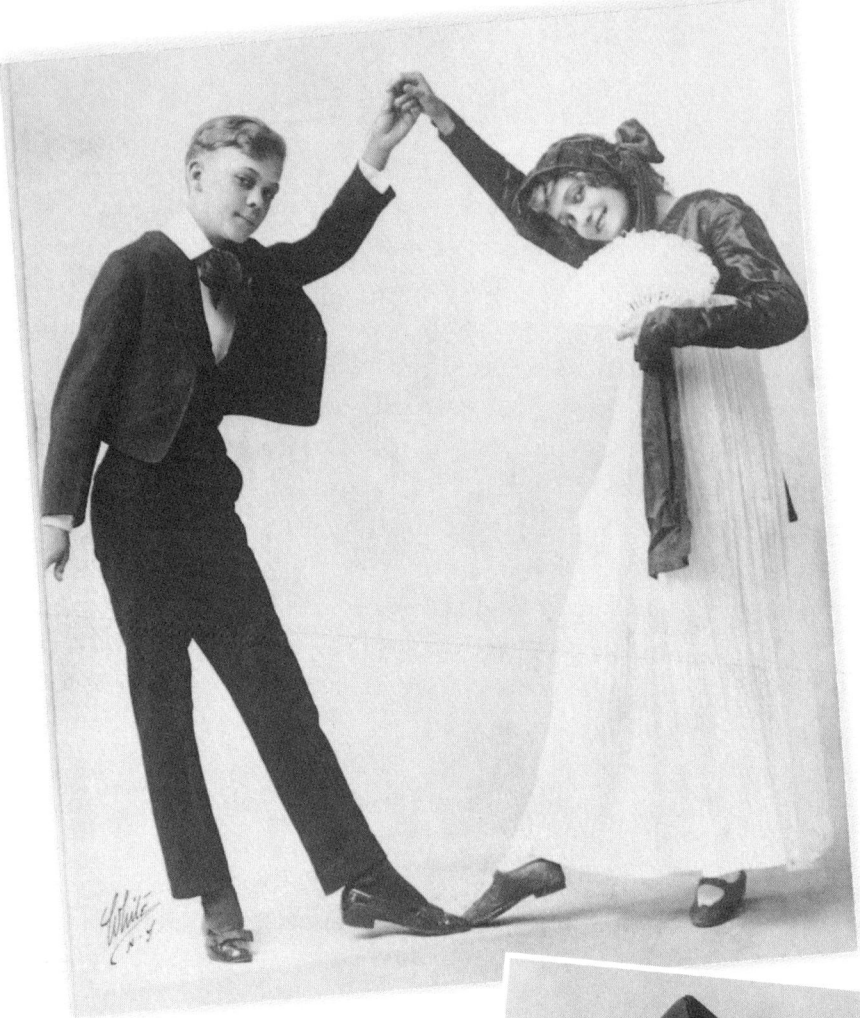

*From vaudeville hoofer
to World War I flier—
my dad, Leonard*

As I got older, I began to notice something unusual during the

show. His family was shocked. Performing on a stage? That was okay for other people, but not for Leonard Simmons. Methodists just didn't do such things. But in Leonard's head, the twister had started. If he could win this talent show, then what might be next? Jessel even gave him the names and addresses of some show-business contacts in New York.

So, my father made his decision. He announced to the family that he was moving to New York City. He was going into show business. They couldn't believe it. How could he do such a thing? How could he go to a place like New York City, full of people with loose morals? And to be in the theater? How could he leave their happy family? They were ashamed. Leonard instantly became the black sheep of the family. But there was no looking back for him. His career was off and running.

During the next several years, Leonard spent time in Los Angeles, working for Paramount Studios and getting bit parts in the new talkies, including a role in *The Student Prince.* He worked with some of the big bands in Chicago, emceeing and doing a little dancing and singing. When Leonard walked out onto the stage, it lit up. Everybody—humans, dogs, cats, anything that breathed—just loved him. Women went gaga over him. At first fans thought he was Fred Astaire—but no. It was Leonard. Well, actually it was Bobby Leonard. That was my father's stage name.

There was one little problem, however. Leonard had a temper. Maybe the better way to say it is that Leonard was used to having his own way. If somebody didn't see eye-to-eye with him, watch out. His glare was infamous. He would never actually say anything critical about a director, or about the other performers. No, that wasn't his style. He would just announce that this show, or this part, wasn't "right" for him. And he would leave.

And so there, in a nutshell, is Leonard's life—well, at least most of it—before Lenny and I arrived on the scene.

⋆

As I got older, I began to notice something unusual during the grocery-shopping trips with my dad. I saw mostly women in the A&P, at the French Market, and in the bakery—women with their kids. There was an elderly man or two, but my father was the only man with kids. Now at this point in my life, I really didn't care who did the shopping, as long as I got

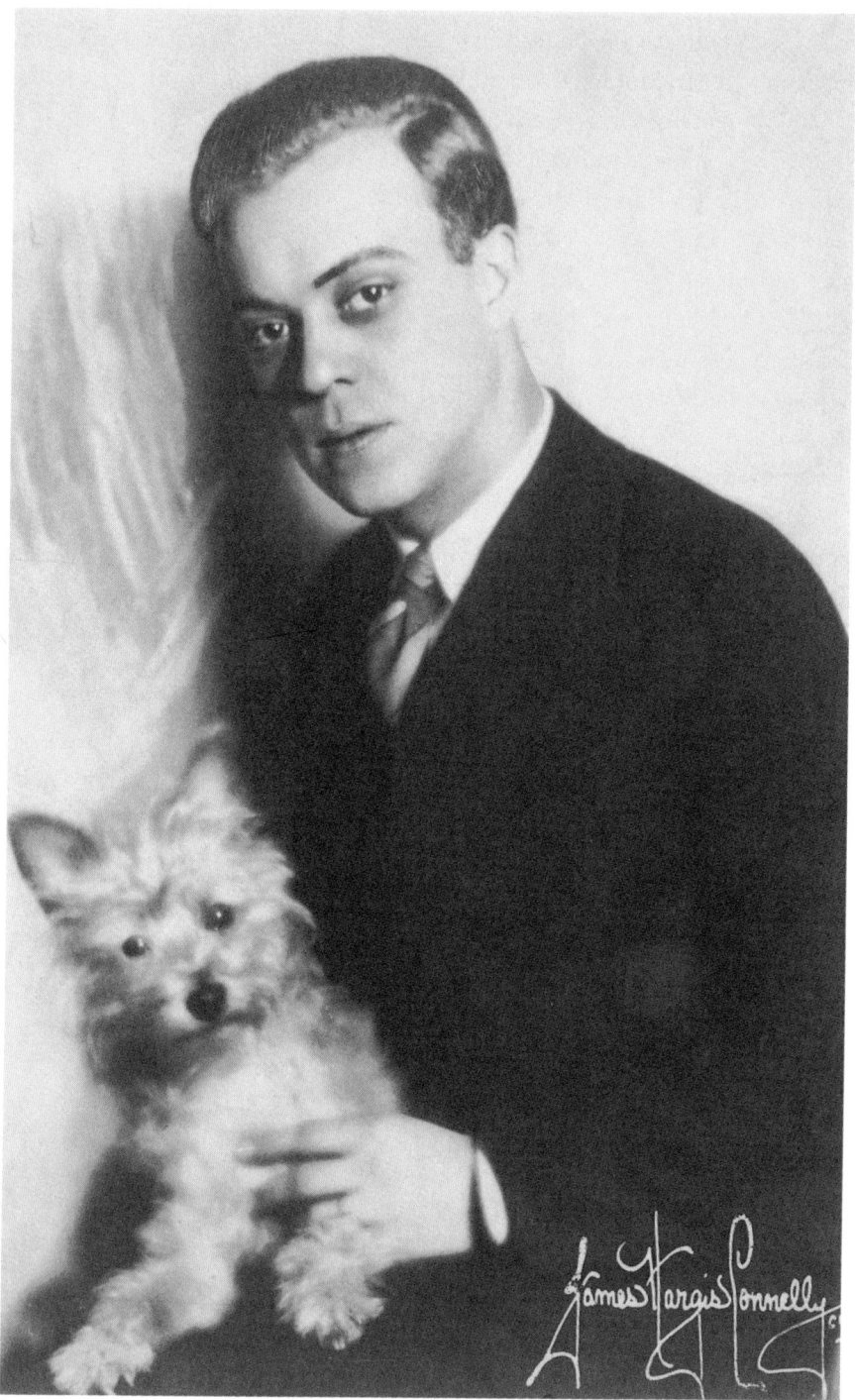

My father's "duke of Windsor" look

My mother, with luggage in hand, seemed to mysteriously disa

to go along. It was only years later that I finally realized that Leonard was the original Mr. Mom. He stayed home, while Shirley was somewhere else. (We also had Victor and Hattie, a black couple who helped around the house, but more about them later.) My mother, with luggage in hand, seemed to mysteriously disappear every so often. Where was she going and what was she doing? I didn't know and, really, I didn't care. I just wanted her home with us.

At such a tender age, it was impossible for me to understand that my mother wasn't exactly sneaking off for relaxing vacations at a spa or country club. She was working to support her family, something she was quite capable of, having done it a good part of her life for her own brothers and sisters. Like my father, Shirley hadn't come from a wealthy background. In fact, her past had been remarkably similar to my father's. Her family had been strict and extremely religious. The type of religion is where their families differed.

* * *

Shirley

Shirley's parents were Russian Jews who arrived in New York City around 1905. When they reached Ellis Island, one of the first things her father, Abraham Wacsatinsky, did was to shorten the family name to Satinsky. That was the fashion then—changing names and shortening them.

The Satinskys, Abraham and Lola, had two little girls. In New York at that time, several diseases were running through the population. Sadly, the girls came down with scarlet fever, and they died a short time later. Devoutly religious, Abraham and Lola relied on their faith to get them through this difficult time.

Devastated and wanting to flee the bad memories of New York, the Satinskys moved to Philadelphia, where their next child, Sadie, was born. Time passed, and Abraham was still not happy. Maybe he didn't feel American enough. So he shortened the family name again—this time to Satin. And he didn't stop there. Their daughter, Sadie, became Shirley—Shirley Satin, my mother.

In Philadelphia, Abraham went into business making potato chips, naming them Shirley's Potato Chips, after his daughter. As Abraham's business grew, so did his family. He began a fruit and vegetable company and had six more children—the last one in 1929.

That was when tragedy struck the family again. Shirley's mother died giving birth to this child, her ninth. Since Shirley was the oldest, she had to quit high school to take care of her six younger brothers and sisters. She was responsible for a lot at a very early age. Her father remarried in 1934, and he and his new wife had one child, Irwin—that's my Uncle Irwin, who now lives in New Jersey.

Since there was a new wife in the house to help take care of the kids, Shirley could finally be more on her own. Always self-reliant, she managed to get a job modeling shoes, stockings, and gloves at Gimbel's in Philadelphia. She was quite a looker—petite and with a very attractive gymnast's body. After getting a peek at the glamorous "outside" world, she decided that maybe it was now time to do a little more with her life—more than just living at home and modeling. But what could she do? Well, she really loved ballet and dance and gymnastics. So why not try to turn these into some kind of career?

Shirley made her decision. She announced to her family that she was moving to New York City to find her star. She wanted to dance and perform. Sound familiar? It was Leonard's story all over again. Can you believe this? Well, the Satins couldn't. Their little girl, leaving Philadelphia to go to New York City, to show off her legs? The shame of it all. They said no. But Shirley said yes, and there was no talking her out of it. She became the "blue sheep" of her family—of course that's not as bad as being the black sheep, as Leonard had been.

⋆ ⋆ ⋆

The Meeting

ow the story really gets juicy. At the same time this was all happening to Shirley, Leonard had moved back to New York City. In Manhattan there were lots of boardinghouses that took in young men and women all wanting to become George Raft, William Holden, Joan Crawford, or Vivien Leigh. Leonard moved into one of these places while he tried to find theater work.

A couple of hundred miles south, in Philadelphia, Shirley had packed

Their little girl, leaving Philadelphia to go to New York City,

her trunks, bought her train ticket for New York, and a few days later—you guessed it—moved into the same boardinghouse. It had to be fate.

And if this wasn't enough of a coincidence, Shirley had a girlfriend who told her about a guy she just had to meet, who lived upstairs. He was so much fun, so good-looking, an emcee, and a real man on the rise. Shirley figured that she had nothing to lose. She was new in town and wanting to meet people, so she agreed.

Here's the picture. Shirley was very teeny, very much in love with the ballet, and very quiet. Leonard, who was fourteen years older, was very clever, very Cole Porter-ish,

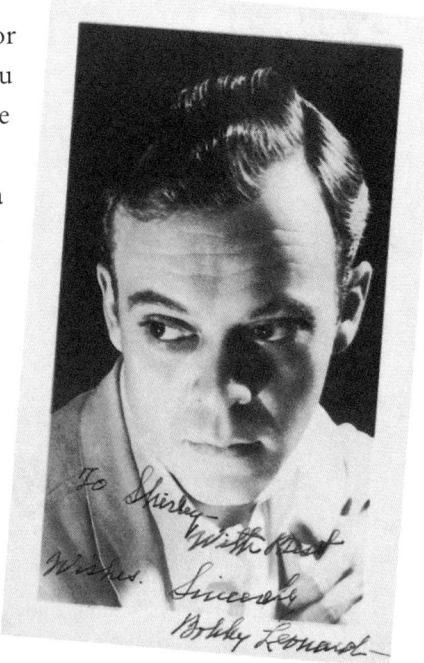

Dad's professional head shot, and guess who got the first copy?

very gregarious, and a very natty dresser. His shirt was freshly ironed, the cuff links shined, and his shoestrings were exactly the same length and perfectly tied. My father, if nothing else, was always meticulous.

When the meeting ended, pleasantly enough, Shirley went right back to her friend and warned, "Oh please! Do me a favor. Don't ever book my dates for me again."

Shirley didn't take well to Leonard at all. He was just a little too much to handle. (And you wonder where I get it from!?) She really wanted to focus on her own career. She could see that Leonard had a huge ego that would require a lot of attention. She just didn't see how a relationship with him was going to work. But I've often thought, although my mom would never admit it, that from that very first meeting, she was kind of attracted to him because he was so charismatic and so good-looking. Leonard, on the other hand, was quite smitten from the very first moment and made no effort to hide it. Shirley reminded him of Rita Hayworth: fiery and fun, and with a great laugh. He wanted to see her again, immediately. He kept asking her out, and she kept saying no, keeping her distance.

w off her legs? The shame of it all. They said no. But Shirley

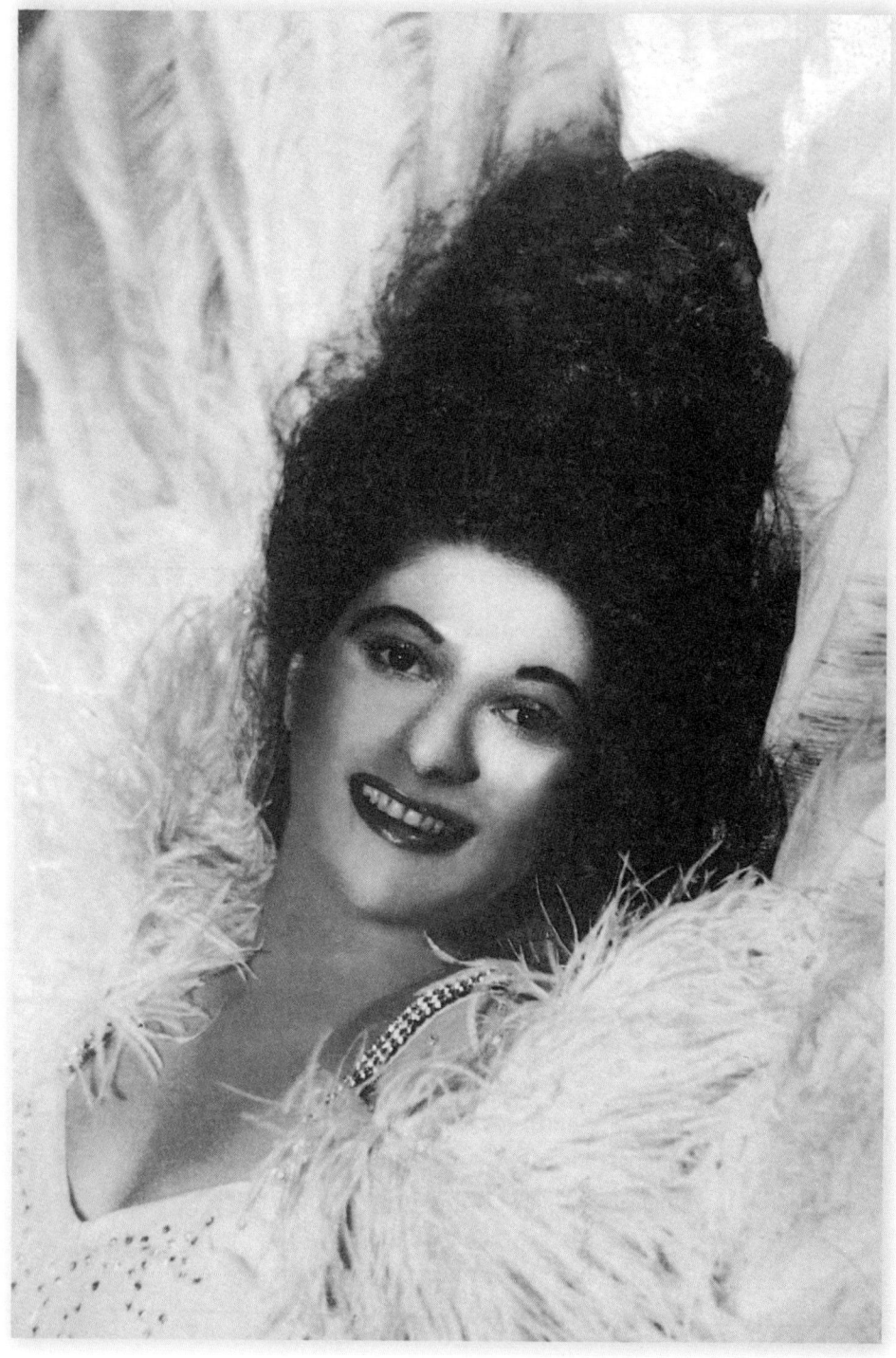

My glamorous mother—feathers optional

"Quick, Shirley. Learn the routine! You're on in an hour!" We

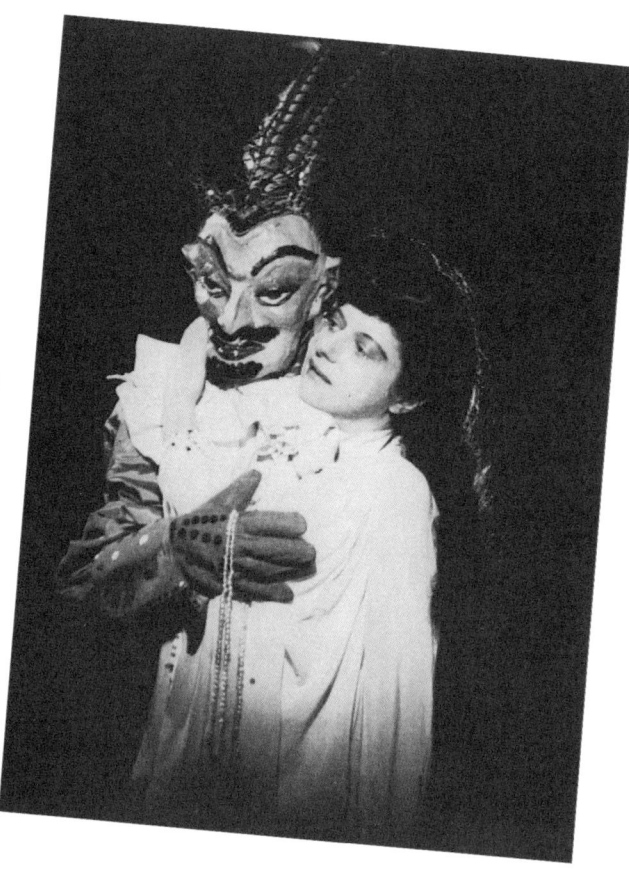

Shirley choreographed all her own numbers, including the crowd-pleasing "The Devil and the Lady."

When Shirley first started working the clubs in New York City, she danced, waited tables, and did whatever else she could to earn money. She traveled the club circuit as well. Her career as a solo artist began one night—I'm not sure exactly where the club was—when the lead fan dancer was stricken with an attack of appendicitis. Panic!

The owner of the club shouted, "Quick, Shirley. Learn the routine! You're on in an hour!" Well! Shirley was like Lucy Ricardo. She'd try anything. So she put on a flesh-colored leotard, and grabbed the fans. Remember, she was only four foot ten, so one of those fans covered her entire body! She learned the dance and went on. The audience loved her. She was a feathered piece of dancing bisque.

As Shirley started getting more and more bookings as a fan dancer, she began to rewrite her act, choreographing a dance called "The Devil and the Lady." The act consisted of the two of them: Her, dressed in an elegant chiffon evening gown, and him, an outrageous papier-mâché Devil's head that fit cleverly over her hand, draped in yards of fabric. A small spotlight would hit that menacing Devil's face, and then it would move over to my mother's. As the spot got bigger, the act began: the devil dancing with my mother as if they were two real people! The club would go wild. The audience leapt to their feet, giving Nancy Lee a standing ovation. Nancy Lee? That was my mother's stage name. To this day, I have no idea where that name came from.

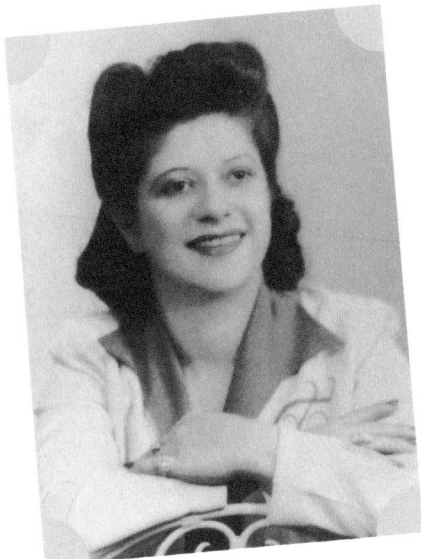
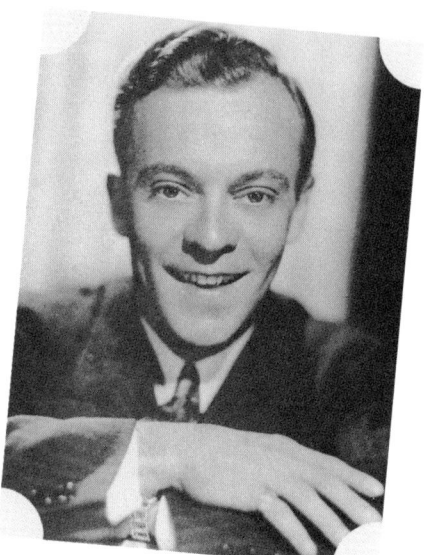

Star-Crossed Lovers

Love Story

By chance, as time went on, Shirley and Leonard got some of the same bookings—sometimes for the same show, sometimes at different clubs but in the same city. Before long, they planned it so that they traveled together. Their friendship blossomed into a romance, and in 1938 they got married in Philadelphia.

One day in 1939, Len came back to the boardinghouse with the news that he'd gotten a two-week emcee job in New Orleans at a club called Pete

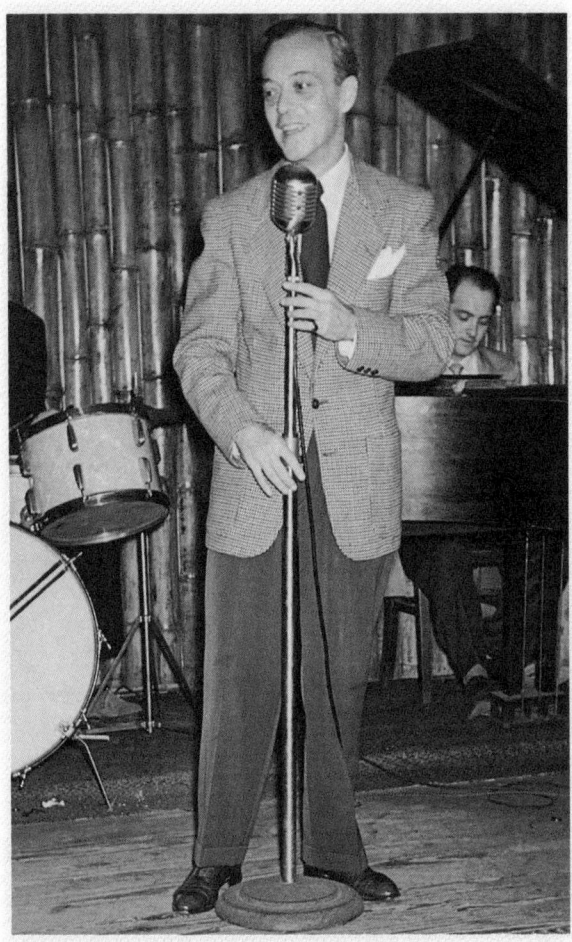

Leonard was such a charmer as the Master of Ceremonies.

Fountain's on Bourbon Street. Shirley, with no job at the moment, went with him to the Big Easy. And what was to be a two-week engagement became the rest of their lives.

The run in New Orleans was going fine, until all of a sudden, Shirley got sick—it was malaria country. Both of their careers had to be put on hold. It took Shirley about a year to recover, and during that time, Leonard turned down offer after offer to travel to other cities to emcee. He stayed in New Orleans to take care of his wife. To make ends meet, he took odd jobs at the different clubs on Bourbon Street—Gungadin, the 500 Club, and Pete Fountain's. His charm worked as usual. He got to be well known about town and people liked him.

But a funny thing happened. Another love affair blossomed—Shirley and Leonard both fell madly in love with New Orleans. They loved the French quarter, they loved the atmosphere, they loved the history, they loved the people. They made many friends, and when Shirley was finally healthy and allowed to travel again, she and Leonard decided to stay right where they were.

So it was destiny that brought my parents together, and destiny that made New Orleans their home.

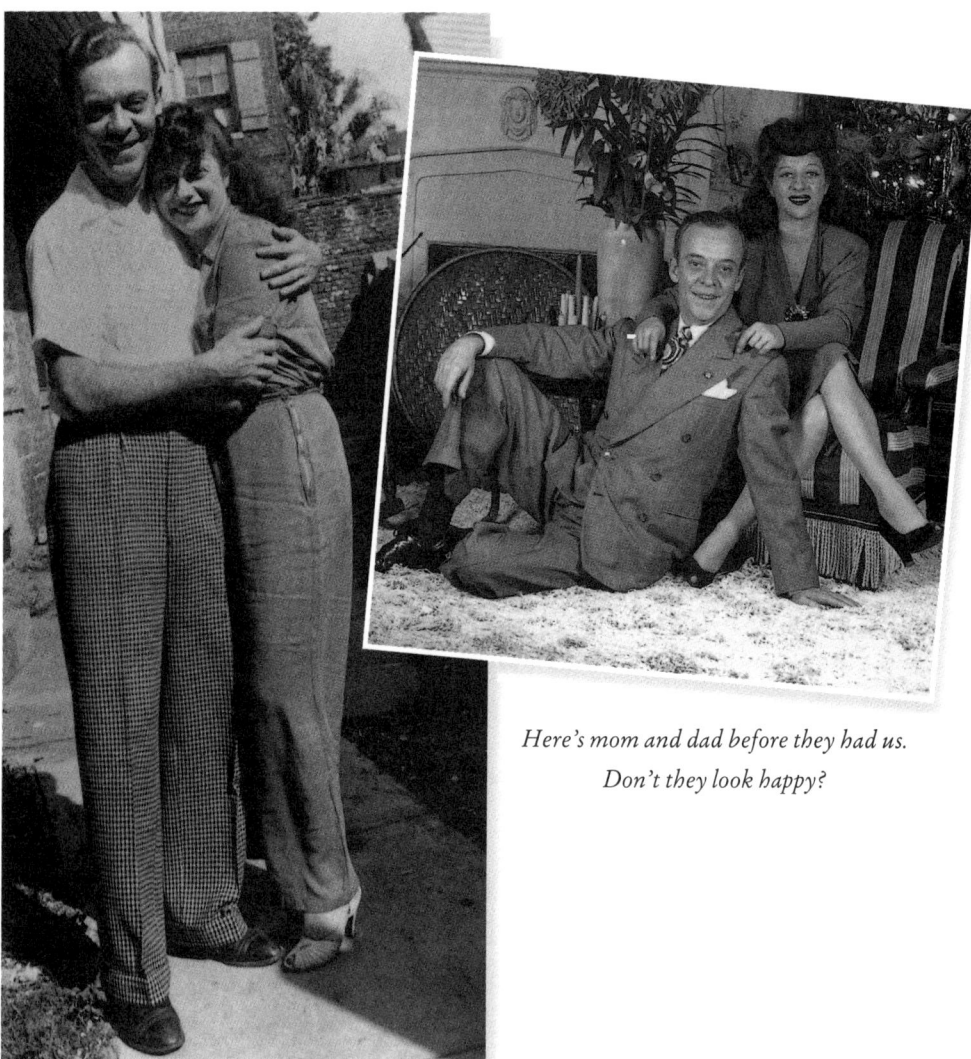

Here's mom and dad before they had us.
Don't they look happy?

* * *

One Big Happy Family?

ntil I was three or four years old, Shirley continued traveling the club circuit. Whenever she left 926 St. Louis Street, the scene was always the same. Lenny and I had no idea Mom was a performer. All I knew about was the bacon frying for breakfast, the sandwiches at noon, and our fancy dinners. I didn't know anything about our family history. I never saw any relatives. As far as I knew, we didn't have any relatives. I didn't know where Shirley went, but when the steamer trunks and hat-boxes came out, I just panicked, and, boy, did I cry. And then Shirley would start to cry. She hated to leave her babies, but she needed to earn the money. Sometimes she'd be gone for weeks, other times just for a weekend. When she came home, she'd drop her bags and pull out new toys for us. This always made her homecoming special, because I always got gifts. But best of all, I got my mother back and we were a family again.

At this point, I began to cause trouble, real trouble. Since I was very devoted to my mother, her leaving all the time really upset me. After the packing of the bags had become a routine in our lives, I created a chant. "Why do you have to go, why do you have to go . . . " My father got very annoyed with me. He didn't know how to explain to me why mom was leaving—it was a secret. When I flew into these rebellious tantrums, he saw in me himself as a child. And we all know how upsetting that can some-times be, seeing ourselves in our own worst moments.

The cab would pull up, and it would be just me and my mother at our front gate. It was a scene, a definite scene. The cab pulled away with Shirley waving in the back seat, and I would just scream. (I've never been subtle.) Leonard, who was now fifty-four, had no clue how to handle me. He had always been the spoiled one, doted on by all his beloved sisters and aunts. So while he knew how to *be* spoiled, he certainly had no idea how to han-dle a child of his own who could be difficult. He had two sons—Lenny, who went with the flow and was practically perfect, and then there was me. Enough said?

While my mother was away, we would fight, my father and I. He treated me like an adult, and that's how I acted. He always had the last word, but as I got older, I thought I should have it—the last word. And when I tried to one-up him, I was punished. This happened a lot when my mother was away. His method of punishment was perfect—he just ignored you. It was the Punishment of Silence. Very effective for a child who craves attention. You didn't exist. He didn't do your laundry, he didn't set a place at the table for you—Milton doesn't live here anymore.

And as if this weren't enough, my father was the master of both "the look" and "the word." Remember, he *was* an actor with a Shakespearean background, and, unbeknownst to him, he was to become my drama coach as I grew up. Much of my theatrics I owe to him, in a subtle way. His look was intense—it was like Bela Lugosi, staring you right in the eye. He had a short fuse, and if it went off, his words could be like daggers, cloaked in the most incredible vocabulary. His temper had style. Rather than being afraid of him, I wanted to see that temper in action and explore how I could twist it. So, I'd push, just to get him going. It was when I didn't answer his questions directly that our battles became like the duels in *Romeo and Juliet,* or scenes from *The Tempest.*

For instance, if Leonard couldn't find the cheese he was looking for in the refrigerator, he would ask, "Milton?"

"Yes, Daddy?"

"Where's the cheese?"

"I guess it's in the refrigerator."

"What do you mean you guess it's in the refrigerator?"

"Well, it's in the cheese drawer."

"You little mouse! You just come in here and find it."

I would begin an elaborate search, all the while knowing there was no cheese. I had polished it off already.

And then he would say, "Why can't you just say you ate the cheese?"

"Because that would just be too easy."

"Go to your room!" That was his second-favorite form of punishment—Banishment to Your Room.

When Shirley came home from being on the road, Leonard was waiting there, ready to tell her what a horrible week he'd had with me, and how difficult I had been. And then it would start between the two of them, and she would often be subjected to the Punishment of Silence, especially if she sided with me or laughed at my funny antics. However, he never sent her to her room—it was hard to do that to your own wife. This scene was

He   w a s   t o   b e c o m e   m y   d r a m a   c o a c h   a s   I   g r e w   u p .   M u c h   o f   m y   t

repeated many times as my mother continued to travel with her Devil. She had one devil on the road, and a little one at home.

During the stretches when Shirley was in New Orleans, she would work in the clubs on Bourbon Street, hostessing in places like the 500 Club. I liked these times. Again, I didn't quite know what she was doing when she got herself all dressed up and went out alone, but I sure did enjoy her being home.

The Agreement

Actually, there was an explanation behind my parents' behavior, but it was kept a secret from Lenny and me. My parents had decided that Leonard would stay home and take care of the boys, while Shirley continued to make a good living working the club circuit. How they came to that decision is sort of complicated.

The day Shirley found out she was pregnant with my brother Lenny, she came home, sat Leonard down, and made the announcement. Of course they had both wanted a family, so they were overjoyed. But it was becoming obvious that their first plan for their life together, Plan Number One, was not working. Seeing their names on theater marquees with big klieg lights sweeping through the night sky—that was not happening, at least not for Leonard. So my father came up with Plan Number Two, and that plan meant raising a family. My father wanted everything perfect, so he decided to erase the past. He had seen what show business could do to kids—it could turn them into little wisecrackers who were not nice to be around. So, definitely not—there would be nothing "show-business" in our family. Leonard would create a brand-new home. It was almost like the movie *Invasion of the Body Snatchers.* These pods opened up and there were all these brand-new people, without a past. That was going to be the whole Simmons family. We would be the perfect *Ozzie and Harriet* family, all created from scratch by my father. And my parents would give us the kind of supportive life they never had. Leonard should have been recruited by the F.B.I. to work in its witness-protection program, where he could have created new identities for all kinds of people.

So all the show-business stuff had to go. In the middle of my parents'

s I owe to him, in a subtle way. His look was intense—it was

conversation about Shirley being pregnant, Leonard jumped up and started racing around the house, pulling out drawers and opening closets and grabbing photo albums, 8×10 publicity glossies of my mother and father in different cities, head shots, and all the other stuff that was part of their show-business past.

Shirley looked up and said, "What are you doing? Where you going with all that?"

"Out to the backyard and burn all this. We're starting clean. I'm getting everything out of the house that says 'show biz.'" This bonfire was not to be discussed—my father made all the decisions in his house. His arms full of photographs and lots of other memories, Leonard headed out through the back door, out past the banana trees and into the far corner of the backyard. He crumpled up some newspaper and tucked in small sticks of wood. He lit the paper. My mother watched him from the kitchen window as he tore apart albums and tossed the pages into the fire.

With the fire still raging, he strode back into the house, not saying a word. He walked right past my mother and into the bathroom, shutting the door. While he was cleaning up, Shirley quickly went out into the yard, picked up a stick, and poked through the fire. She managed to salvage some of the photos. I can picture what she must have looked like, standing there in a smart little dress and high heels, poking through the bonfire of their lives. She came back into the house. Quickly she trimmed the burnt edges from the photos and then hid them away, never saying a word again about the whole affair. So that's how I came to have no family history. And that's why some of the early pictures of my parents in this book are so special, because my mother salvaged them from the flames.

Shortly after my brother Lenny was born, Shirley and Leonard had another talk and arrived at another top-secret decision. Shirley was the breadwinner in the family—that was clear. Since her career as a fan dancer was still going full-tilt, she would continue on with it. Leonard, on the other hand, would stay at home and take care of the house and the family. Now he wouldn't have to worry about losing jobs because of his "strong personality." That would be less of a problem—but still a problem when it came to raising me.

You have to understand what a major decision this was for my father. For him, the grass had always been greener on the other side of the fence.

He had always thought that eventually he would make it in show business. But that's not the way it turned out. A successful career at anything, other than being Mr. Mom, was just not in the cards for him. It was *Death of a Salesman*, it was *A Chorus Line*, it was *42nd Street*. He would always be the salesman who couldn't quite make it or the chorus boy always in the background. And that wasn't my father—he needed to be center-stage. So maybe staying at home was okay. He would create his own little stage in New Orleans with his wife and family, where he would be the star. So what if my mother stayed in the shadows as the real breadwinner?

So the final results of these two decisions—no family history, and Shirley becomes the shadow breadwinner—were to have a profound effect on the rest of my life. I would struggle with these issues, and it would take many years to resolve them, especially with my father.

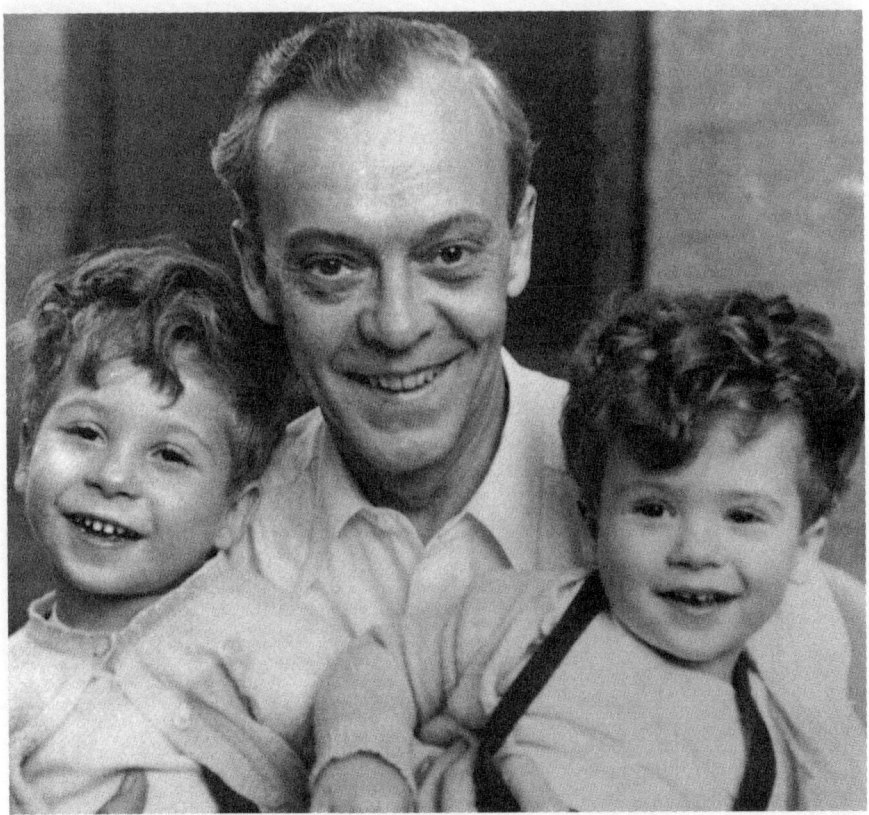

My beaming dad!

he tore apart albums and tossed the pages into the fire. With

* * *

Milton the Menace

*W*hen I was four or five, I discovered something else about my mother. I was in my room next to the kitchen, watching Shirley fix herself a snack, when all of a sudden she doubled up by the sink. I screamed, "What's wrong, Mom?"

"Nothing, honey. Just a little stomach cramp." She managed to get herself over to the icebox, where she took out a carton of milk and poured herself a glass. Clutching her stomach, she gulped it down.

No one in our family talked about anything personal in their own lives, so there was no way that I could know that Shirley had a peptic ulcer. Her doctor had told her that her show-business career was fighting her desire to stay home with her family, and that the conflict between Leonard and me was also taking its toll on her.

As things got worse, she was in and out of the hospital a few times, which didn't improve relations between my father and me.

He took me aside and quietly said, "Are you happy? Are you happy now? See what you've done?"

"What have I done?" I asked. "What?"

"What have you done? You've made your mother sick. You gave her a peptic ulcer. It's all your fault."

"My fault? It's not my fault. What about Lenny? Couldn't Lenny have given her the peptic ulcer? Is my name on it?"

"No. It's not Lenny. It's you. I'll spell it out for you: M-I-L-T-O-N. You aggravate her all the time."

"Aggravate her? How could I do that? I love my mother."

"She sees you fighting with me all the time, and this really upsets her. So, are you happy now?"

But then, I would get to the point where I just couldn't let him get away with it. I'd turn to him and say, "You know what the real problem here is? It's you. If you got a job, then mom wouldn't have to work. She could stay home and get better. It's not my fault—it's yours!" Silence. At least I got the last word. It was truly the last word, since by then Leonard was not speaking to me. And then the Banishment to Your Room. When I got both punishments, I knew I had really crossed the line.

I spent so much time in my room that I had my own little stas

I could be mischievous, no doubt about that. For instance, on Easter mornings, Lenny and I would wake up and, like magic, there would be these two huge, beautifully wrapped Easter baskets, just waiting for us. Well, there was some Easter candy I liked, and some I didn't. I definitely hated those bright yellow, marshmallow chicken things. I knew they were from a different planet. And I hated black jelly beans. I don't know who ever thought them up.

One Easter morning, to make sure I got what I wanted, I snuck out of bed an hour early and rearranged the baskets. In my basket were all the things I loved: see-through eggs, chocolate candies, and so on. My brother's basket—you guessed it—was filled with yellow chickens and black jelly beans. Back to bed I went.

Well, a little later, my brother and I got up and ran to the dining room. Lenny was s-o-o-o excited. My father was there waiting for us. He gave me that look of his and said, "Looks like the Easter bunny came and rearranged things."

"What?" I asked. He just turned and walked away.

"Whaaat?" I asked again. It was quiet. The silent treatment had begun. Lenny and I got dressed, and mom walked us to mass. When we got home, the table was set for three: Mommy, Daddy, and Lenny. My father didn't even look at me. I tried to sit down, and he warned, "Don't even try it."

And then it started, the argument.

My mother would say, "Leonard . . . "

"This is between him and me. Don't get involved, all right? You don't think he does any wrong. You think he's just perfect. He's your little baby."

I guess I was beginning to understand the relationship between my mom and dad. It didn't take much to figure it out. When I was in high school, I remember a time when I was sitting quietly on the couch in the living room watching television, and I turned to my father and said, "The butcher, the baker, the candlestick maker—which one are you?" He was none of them. A little stinker, wasn't I.

I spent so much time in my room that I had my own little stash of food on a shelf in the corner, so I would always be prepared for the long sieges.

After a banishment, my father would finally break the silence by saying something like, "Go get the newspaper." Then it would be a new play: We'd go from *The Bad Seed* to *Our Town*. Suddenly I was the good child again.

One time when I was in grammar school, after having been banished to my room once too often, I finally decided to really push it to the limit.

I announced, "I'm leaving. I'm packing my bags, and I'm just leaving. I want to see more of the world than just my room. This is no way to live."

"Oh, okay. Here. Let me help you pack." Leonard got the luggage out of the closet and put it on my bed.

"First, get out all the clothes you want to take. Where do you want to start? Underwear or socks first?"

"I want to start first with the shirts. Then we'll do the underwear and socks."

It was our own little play, my father's and mine.

My father's method of punishment never changed, but it definitely escalated when I tried to call his bluff. If I threatened to leave, he opened the door. I could never win.

* ⭐ *

Wheezing . . .

When I was three years old, I developed a health problem: asthma, which lasted into my twenties. Back then, lots of people thought asthma was only an emotional thing—that it was just a scheme for getting your way. My father subscribed to that school of thought. He was totally convinced that my asthma was all made up. No one else in our family had ever had it. But the truth of the matter was that I was heavy and was living in the South in very damp weather, and my lungs were always filled with mucus. It was a terrible feeling, not being able to take a deep breath.

Every night I had to take my asthma medicine. Then I'd hop into bed, and my father would open an umbrella over me and the bed. He propped it straight up with books, and then draped a sheet over it and set up a vaporizer inside. Even though my father and I had our differences, he loved me dearly, and in his own way, he was always nurturing. While the mist soothed my sinuses, he'd read to me from some of his favorite magazines—*The Reader's Digest* and *National Geographic*—or I'd listen to music. It was my own private little Casbah. The vaporizer had to be refilled three times for these treatments, so my parents would check on me every so often. I lived with a vaporizer, and that's probably why my skin is so beautiful today. (Haven't you noticed?)

As a child, I always carried an inhaler with me, and I was always seeing doctors. Sometimes when kids see so many doctors, they develop a fear of them or they just begin to dislike them. Not me! I wanted to be a doctor—I loved the white coats. And I loved my pediatrician, Dr. Veith.

Dr. Veith was a Jimmy Stewart type, always in a beautifully starched white physician's coat with his name, "Dr. Veith," stitched in red over the breast pocket. He could have stepped right out of a Norman Rockwell painting—very fatherly, but in a way different from my own father, who was very strict. Dr. Veith was much more affectionate. As the years continued on and I developed my serious weight problems, Dr. Veith was always compassionate, in his restrained, doctorly way. I would go into his office and he would hug me, and I'd smell the cigarette smoke on his coat. I adored him because he treated me so well. I had no secrets from him. However, even he was not spared from my pranks. Once, I spied one of his coats on a hook in the examining room. Using a pen and my fanciest handwriting, I added my own "embroidery" to the coat so that it read: "Dr. Veith loves Milton Simmons." I really respected him. He was my doctor all through high school, until he finally told me he couldn't be my doctor anymore. He was, in fact, a pediatrician, and I had outgrown him long ago.

When I first started to visit Dr. Veith, he gave me these little canister inhalers that I would squirt into my mouth to open my breathing passages. It was called Metahaler. I started with a low-dosage inhaler, and as my breathing got more difficult, I had to move on to stronger and stronger ones until I was eventually on the strongest one.

When I got upset about things, my asthma did get worse. What I didn't know then was that food allergies and dairy products were adding to my mucus buildup. And you know me: Mr. Mayonnaise—hello! Sometimes the attacks were so fierce that my parents would have to take me in a cab to Charity Hospital to get me shots. Besides Dr. Veith, I had my own ear-nose-and-throat specialist.

We'd get my prescriptions filled at Walgreen's, but I was becoming so dependent on the inhalers to help me breathe that I was running through the prescriptions very quickly.

I would say to my father, "I need a refill."

And he'd say, "Look at the date."

I'd plead, "Daddy, I'm out of this."

"Look at the date." He was very strict about the asthma medicine.

You know, all my life I heard that *s-s-s-s* sound, the sound of the inhaler. When there was just a teeny bit left, I'd hold the inhaler on its side at the edge of the table and I would get down on all fours. *S-s-s-s . . . s-s-s-s . . . s-s-s-s.* I'd lick the nozzle, trying to get the last drips. Pretty picture, huh? That was the way it was until I could fill the next prescription. If I had a problem with my breathing, I would just have to sit or lie down and calm myself, trying to get my breathing in order. I would also use pepper—coarse black pepper out of the pepper mill—and stuff it up my nose. It worked. I would sneeze, and all this yucky glop would come out. I'd put more pepper in, and I'd sneeze and more would come out. Then I'd do more umbrella time, and if I was lucky, I'd maybe get a few hours of sleep. I would have to do this every day until I got my next little bottle of spray. And that's how I lived, because those were the rules, according to my father.

Well, my father really didn't believe in all this asthma medicine. He secretly thought that my asthma would get better if I weren't such a brat. My dad also tended to be his own doctor. No matter what was wrong with you, he felt that it could be cured with one of the four remedies from his medicine cabinet: Campho-phenique, cod-liver oil, calamine lotion, or Mercurachrome. That's all you needed.

Even though I've painted a really terrible picture about having asthma, there was one great thing about it: I never had to go to physical education—never. I had so many excuses, I always got out of P.E.

The teachers would say, "Do you have a note?"

"A note?! Which one do you want? I've got one for my asthma, my congestion, my watery eyes, my runny nose. Tell me which one you want."

Besides my asthma, I had this foot problem, too—something I was born with. The joint between my ankle and foot didn't work quite right; as a result, my left leg was doing up to about seventy percent of the work of the right leg. So, in addition to my wheezing and coughing, I had this very distinctive waddle walk. My brother walked sort of the same way. In fact, in school he was called Penguin, and I was known as Penguinette. Add foot doctors to my medical entourage.

Occasionally,   I'd   end   up   with   some   strange   stains   on   my   paja

So during those early years in grammar school, it was me and my vaporizer, hiding under the tent in my room. But even then, while I was trying to get the last word, I was also busy getting the last . . . snack. When the rest of the family had finished their eating for the day, there was still one more chance for me. In the quiet of the evening, I would sneak out from under my umbrella and tiptoe into the kitchen. My parents were a couple of rooms away, and my brother was so distracted with trying to get his homework perfect that he didn't notice a thing. There they were in the refrigerator: leftovers! One last slice of cold meat loaf or a piece of Leonard's banana cream pie. Occasionally, I'd end up with some strange stains on my pajamas, but no one seemed to notice. However, my father, who was the keeper of the refrigerator, would spot the empty plate covered with tin foil the next morning and ask, "Who's been eating the meat loaf?"

"Meat loaf? What meat loaf? Are we having meat loaf for breakfast?"

"No, we're not having any meat loaf, because there's none left."

"Oh. I guess someone must have eaten it then."

"That's what I asked. Who ate the meat loaf?"

"Well, I don't like to tell on people. You know that's not my way. But Lenny did it. Lenny ate the meat loaf." Lenny had already left for the library, so I knew I was safe. And since Lenny was so perfect, I figured blaming him for such a little thing would never hurt his halo. It never occurred to me that my father might question Lenny when he got home. I don't know what I was thinking about sometimes.

My mother was standing in the doorway, taking this all in. When my father went back into the living room, my mother walked over to me. She had that look in her eye.

"Why do you do that?"

"Do what, mom?"

"You know what."

"Mom . . . "

"Honey, please. Don't aggravate your father."

"Me—what did I do?"

She knew that I was angry with my father because he stayed home while she had to go to work. This was not the life I wanted. I wanted to be like other families, where the mother stayed home and the father worked.

Even though I tried to hold my tongue for my mother's sake, most of the time it didn't work and I continued to aggravate my father—I couldn't help it. My anger would get the better of me. And all this just made Shirley's health get worse.

* * *

The Switch

Finally, the doctor laid it out for Shirley: Either she change her life-style to reduce the stress, or he would have to operate. So now what? Shirley realized it was time to give up her Devil dance and find work in New Orleans that would keep her home, all the time. She could make that decision, but her problem was Leonard. She didn't want to tell him any of this until she had gotten a job and there could be no turning back. Other-wise, he would say no and blame the whole thing on Guess Who—me. She needed to find work. She had never finished high school, and all she knew about was show business. But she was streetwise and penny-smart.

Running her errands one day, Shirley spotted a Help Wanted sign at Merle Norman, a cosmetics store. Cosmetics were in her blood. She had been doing her own makeup for a long time—she was expert at making herself gorgeous. So without telling anyone, she applied for the job, and she got it! Instead of selling her dance with the Devil, she would now be selling lipsticks and creams and Mira-cal, Merle Norman's famous product for tightening your skin.

That night, after dinner, Shirley matter-of-factly told Leonard she had been thinking about her dancing, and that she had finally decided it was time for a career change. She wanted to spend more time with her boys. So there would be no more working at the clubs, no more working nights, and no more traveling. And, by the way, she said to Leonard, she had a new job, selling cosmetics. Surprisingly, Leonard just sat and listened to all this—and agreed.

Merle Norman was a teeny shop, holding no more than ten people at a time. Combining her theatrical skills and her love of cosmetics, Shirley was terrific. Word quickly got around about this lady who did beautiful make-overs. As always, Shirley's talents did not go unnoticed.

A year or so after she had started working, a well-dressed woman came into the shop one afternoon while Shirley was waiting on ten customers, all at once. During a lull, the woman introduced herself as the cosmetics buyer at Maison Blanche, an elegant upscale Bloomingdale's kind of department store, housed in a grand white mansion. Maison Blanche and D. H. Holmes were the two main department stores in New Orleans. She told Shirley she could use someone like her, someone who had such a gift for getting along with people and making them feel good. She asked Shirley if she would like to work for her. The idea appealed to Shirley very much. Maison Blanche was a wonderful department store, and she would have the chance to work with more customers. So she said yes and made the switch. The Coty cosmetics line—including the dusting powder with the little orange puffs and the twenty-four-hour lipstick—was to become her kingdom.

My mother was now moving grandly forward into her new career, and she was very good at what she did. She would make files on all her customers, keeping track of what they bought and when. When she noticed that someone's supply of Vitamin A-D cream might be getting low, she'd telephone with a gentle reminder. She was always winning the sales contests at the store—trips, fur coats, and money.

* * *

My Black Parents

While my mother was working days, my other set of parents took care of me. Oh—I mentioned them earlier, but I haven't really told you about them. I was very blessed. I had two sets of parents: one white, Leonard and Shirley; and the other black, Victor and Hattie. We were a biracial family. I don't know exactly where Victor and Hattie came from, and I don't know how they met Leonard and Shirley—but I can't remember them not ever being there at 926 St. Louis Street. They were with us until they died, and to this day, I still don't know how we afforded them. We didn't own the house—we paid about fifty dollars a month in rent. But somehow we managed to have this couple working for us.

Victor did repairs around the house and other odd jobs. Hattie did all the washing and ironing. She mopped, vacuumed, and dusted, always with a cigarette dangling from her mouth.

While Shirley was still doing the club circuit, Hattie became like my

she knew about was show business. But she was streetwise and

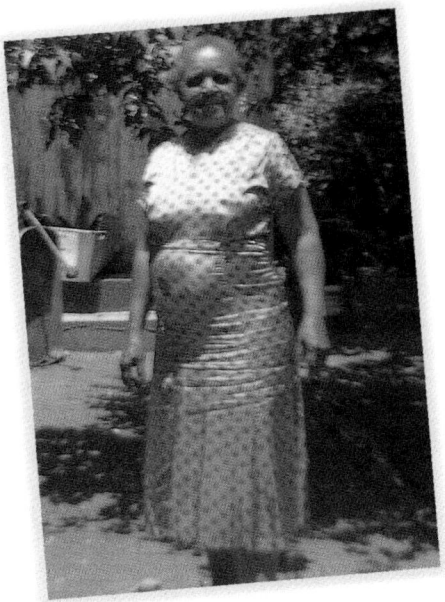

My "second mom"

second mother. And now that Shirley was home but working every day, it was Hattie who would keep an eye on me. When Leonard and I were fighting and I was sent to my room, Hattie would just shake her head and tell me, like my mother did, that I shouldn't aggravate my father. I should try and keep things peaceful at home. But by now, you know that just wasn't my way.

⁺ ✳ ⁺
★

The Renaissance Man

So while my mother was succeeding at her new career at Maison Blanche, it was a different story with Leonard. At age fifty-five, it was difficult for him. He had to find something to do that would keep him busy as well as somehow contribute to his family's well-being. As I look back at him over the years, now that I've gotten past all my anger, I realize he was a wonderfully creative man. And he was always one to help other people. If someone in the neighborhood didn't have enough to eat, he'd invite them over for a meal. If someone needed anything at all, he would find out how to get it for them. That's just the way he was. His strict Methodist background had taught him that charity begins at home. He just loved that idea, and he practiced what he preached.

He eventually decided to take a portion of his day and devote it to charity work. When you're rejected in the big world, you need to hop onto a smaller stage. It really doesn't matter where the stage is, as long as there is an audience. So his new theater was to be the Junior League of New Orleans, where he was the only male volunteer. Mr. Mom was at it again. He worked in the League's thrift shop, receiving the donated items and deciding on how to price them. And what a shop it was! Even though everything in that little store was used, the merchandise was beautiful: furs, furniture, chandeliers, and a hundred other things. Very rich ladies would donate fancy dresses they had worn only once. As had always been the case, Leonard was still being doted on by women. The minute you looked into his eyes, he had you. I think people donated things just to have a chance to see him and say hello. I wonder if people even died on purpose so they could will their things to the shop, and to Leonard.

He also spent hours and hours at the Volunteers of America—doing the same work in their thrift shop—as one of the few men working with that organization, too. Leonard was at it again, center stage. He was the master of ceremonies.

Shirley's wardrobe came from these shops. Everyone knew that my father was married to a wonderful, petite woman, and they would come in and say, "I've got a fur coat your wife will just love." My mother had one chifforobe full of fur coats. Just fur coats, that's it. And there was another one just for the gowns.

My father's wardrobe was even more extensive. His armoires and dressers were filled; you couldn't squeeze in another wire hanger or pair of socks. There were sports coats, vests, shirts, hats, gloves, mufflers, overcoats—and remember, we lived in New Orleans, so it never got that cold. But my father had all these clothes. There were lots and lots of shoes in pristine condition, without a scuff anywhere. With each season, my dad would change all his outfits. When the blue-and-white seersucker suit came out, I knew it was summer. And he also had the beige-and-white seersucker, the linen suit—it was endless. The last thing he did when he dressed was to take a clean handkerchief, give it one spray of the fragrance Vetiver, fold it, and then put it in his back pocket. When I got a whiff of that scent, I knew he was finished and ready to go out.

Our whole house was like a fancy salon out of a Victorian novel. It was an amazing fantasy house. The floors in the house were practically falling in—my father just kept coming home with rugs, and piling them up on top of each other to try and make the floors more stable. Even though nearly all of our furniture was secondhand, including some of the chandeliers and candelabras, the rooms were magical. The living room was full of plush couches and gorgeous end tables, with tall lamps crowned with silk shades. On one wall hung a slave's emancipation paper—the actual piece of paper, pressed between two pieces of glass. (I can't imagine where that came from!) Every inch of our walls was filled with paintings. And every time my father brought home another piece of furniture from the Volunteers of America, Hattie would roll her eyes. She had to dust all this.

My parents had separate bedrooms, for at least as long as I can remember. My mother's room could have been Queen Victoria's boudoir! She

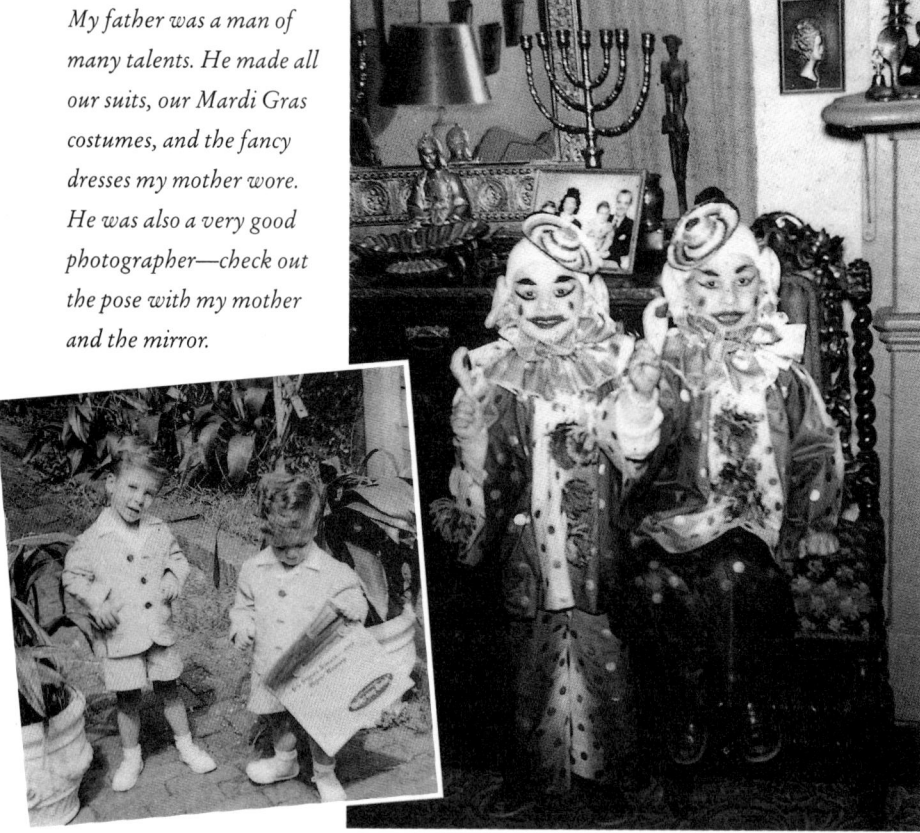

My father was a man of many talents. He made all our suits, our Mardi Gras costumes, and the fancy dresses my mother wore. He was also a very good photographer—check out the pose with my mother and the mirror.

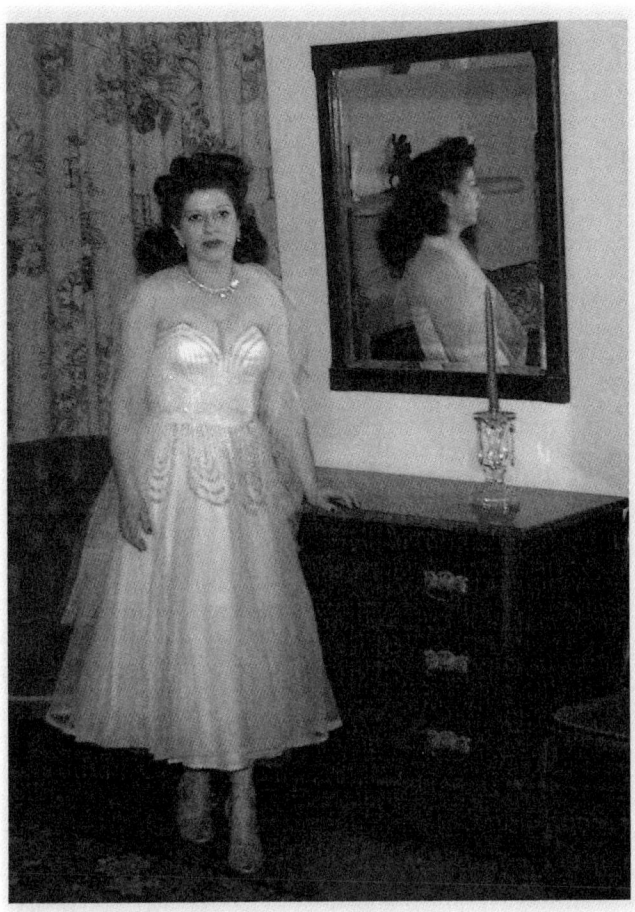

slept in an enormous hand-carved two-poster bed, with lace draping down the sides and billowing out.

My father's bedroom was all done in an Asian style, with lush Persian carpets and an exotic nine-piece bamboo bedroom suite including a mirror, a dresser with gold-bamboo pulls, a grand bed, and a huge wardrobe. And there were silver and ebony boxes everywhere. His bathrobe was very *Teahouse of the August Moon,* and wherever it was hanging, in his bedroom or in the bathroom, we were never to touch it.

Just as my father would change his clothes with the seasons, he would change all the curtains and the bedspreads in the house. For people who really didn't have a lot of money, we did live in a grand style.

I never saw my father not busy. It wasn't that he was compulsive, he just always needed to be doing something, whether it was taking down a chandelier and carefully cleaning it with a vinegar solution, doing electrical work, hanging wallpaper, or painting. And Victor was always there to help him. I'd come home from school one day, and the dining room would be a different color. If a piece of furniture was chipped, Leonard would repair and repaint it. He refinished and reupholstered. That's just the way he was.

He hated waste and disorder. (I'm the same way. You'll never find my dirty clothes thrown about.) Even our garbage was neat. Long before it was fashionable, he tied it up. I mean, it was gift-wrapped. Our garbage man remarked that it was the neatest garbage he had ever seen. Leonard liked order in his life, and if something was even slightly amiss, God protect you. His magazines, his pocket change, his cigarettes, his lighter—they all had to be put in their own specific places. And he saved everything. He saved the ribbon, the bows, and the wrapping paper from gifts.

His change—pennies, nickels, dimes, and quarters—was always neatly stacked on top of his dresser. For Sunday morning mass—Lenny and I would go, but my parents stayed home—Leonard would give us quarters for the collection plate. One Sunday morning, he had forgotten, and he was still sleeping. I tiptoed into his room and went over to the dresser.

My father was a light sleeper. I reached for one of the quarters and accidentally jiggled them.

"Milton, are you near the quarters?" He was a quick one.

And then there were his handkerchiefs. That's where Hattie would drive Leonard crazy. Hattie had cataracts and couldn't see too well. Because of that, she would often iron and fold Leonard's handkerchiefs backwards: the "S" became a "Z." He hated *Zorro* on T.V., so he was always threatening to fire her over this.

His magazines were another whole story. He got tons of them, and he had to read them first before anybody else. The stack was huge: *Look, Life, The Reader's Digest, National Geographic, Saturday Evening Post,* and on and on. If he caught you sneaking a look before he did, you were banned from reading that magazine for at least a week.

My father was an unbelievable reader. Instead of a headboard for his bed, he had neat stacks of books. They almost went to the ceiling. He just devoured books and crossword puzzles.

Every morning he would read the obituaries out loud from the newspaper. Long after I moved away from home, I would call him on the tele-

My father had a secret life. Some days he would just take off

phone, and Leonard would say to me, "Do you remember the man who worked in the candle shop on Bourbon Street when you were a kid?"

"Yeah ..."

Remember he walked with a limp and had a cane?"

"Yeah ... "

"And don't you remember he had two children and four cats?"

"Yeah ... "

"And he lived in that wonderful house?"

"Yeah ... "

"Well, he's dead."

At an early age, he taught me words, taught me spelling, taught me sentences to say, showed me maps of foreign places. I was his apprentice. Leonard taught me everything from making the roux for a good gumbo to sewing up a rip and double knotting the thread so it wouldn't come out. He was a wonderful teacher.

My Father's Secret Life

My father had a secret life. Some days he would just take off in the morning around ten-thirty or eleven o'clock and come back in the afternoon around five, with no groceries or packages or anything else in his hands. He was just a disappearing act. What did he do while he was away all this time? It was very puzzling to busybody me. Was he working for the F.B.I.? Did he have some secret Washington job? Was he a spy stealing Creole recipes for the Russians? I decided it was Sherlock Holmes time.

So one day I tried to follow him. After he was completely dressed as if he were going someplace important—a bow tie, vest, jacket, the handkerchief with the Vetiver, and a hat—out the front door he went. I waited a couple of minutes and then walked after him, keeping my distance. After a block, he turned around. I dodged into a doorway. By the time I slowly stuck my head out to look, he had gone around the corner. This went on for a while, until he stopped in the middle of the street and slowly turned. I was squashed up against a window, but he spotted me.

"Milton, what are you doing? Come here."

"Hi, dad."

"Milton, are you following me?"

"Well . . ."

"You're following me, aren't you?"

"Well, I'm going shopping. And we just happen to be going the same way."

"No, Milton. I know you're following me."

"Okay. I just wanted to see where you were going."

"Go home."

I turned and walked away. But a block farther down the street, I snuck into a doorway and waited until he started on his way. Then I continued to follow him. I wasn't going to give up that easily.

He finally stopped in front of a junk store called Matt's, on Royal Street, right next to the famous cornstalk cast-iron fence, a fence that looked like stalks of corn growing, intertwined with morning glories. There were four chairs out in front of Matt's, and three men were sitting there, just talking away. One of them, of course, was Matt. They all said hello to each other, and Leonard sat down in the empty chair. So this is where Leonard spent some of his secret time. The store was full of all kinds of junk: used comic books, beat-up serving trays, tiny figurines. In the window there was a fish bowl full of water, with little toys stuck in the sand in the bottom—but no fish. A sign said, "$5 a fish." The men sat there and talked and laughed and whispered to each other. People walking by would stop and greet my father. He knew everybody.

After a bit, Leonard got up, shook the hands of the other men, and continued on his walk. I followed him for three blocks. He stopped at a store called The Old Town Praline Shop. A woman name Miss Glen ran the place. My father stood there for a while, talking with her and laughing and carrying on. Remember, my father was a ladies' man. As people stopped to buy pralines, my dad would greet them and talk and smile. I stood there in a doorway, watching all this. So this was how my father spent his time while my mother worked. I got very angry. I had seen enough. I turned around and walked home. I never followed him again.

This is how my parents lived their lives—very separately. Shirley worked from eight in the morning until she took off her high heels at six in the evening, so she didn't see a great deal of my father. And my father roamed all over the French quarter during the day. Everybody in the quarter loved him. When we walked down the street, everyone said hello to him—he was the unofficial Mayor of the Vieux Carré, its Goodwill Ambassador. On the other hand, it was only those women who bought cosmetics at Maison Blanche who recognized my mother.

Although my father was friendly and affectionate with practically everybody in town, we saw none of this at home. That was the paradox of our family. There was no open display of affection between my parents, at least in front of me. I was beginning to see why maybe they had separate bedrooms. My father came from a strict family; and while my mother had the same sort of background, she was much more touchy-feely than my dad. My brother took after my father, both of them not liking to be hugged or kissed. Not me. I took after Shirley. I was always hugging and kissing her, lying in her lap and wrapping myself around her shoulders like an ermine stole.

I was getting more and more angry about the situation between my parents. And because I was more like my mom, I sided with her. As always, it was Leonard's show. Even though Shirley was the breadwinner, she would quietly turn her paycheck over to Leonard. But there was nothing ever said about this: Shirley, the invisible breadwinner.

The Big Easy

So while I was trying to figure out the relationship between my mother and father, I was growing up in the most amazing neighborhood: the French quarter. This was a place where you didn't have to lock your doors; it was a place where everybody knew everybody else. It was almost like the T.V. show *Cheers*, but without the Boston accent—we had our own accent. Dauphine and then Bourbon were only a couple of blocks from St. Louis Street. You could walk everywhere.

Practically all of our neighbors worked in the jazz clubs and dance halls on Bourbon Street. It was funny—I never heard the word "stripper" as a kid, even though we had a few living in an apartment house next door to us. We called them "exotic dancers." There was Lilli Christine, the cat girl with long blond hair who slithered across the stage. And Rosina, who had an act with two boa constrictors. She would baby-sit for Lenny and me and read

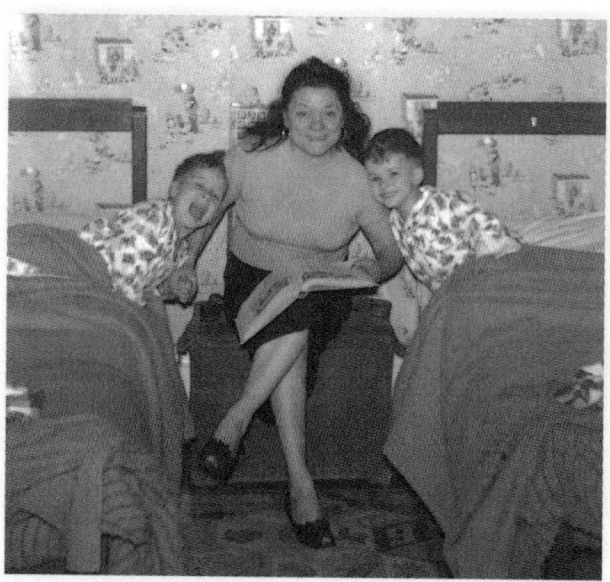

What a baby sitter!

us bedtime stories. There was one hitch, however. She couldn't read. She'd just look at the pictures in the book and make up her own stories. Then there was Alouette, the tassel twirler—and you know where the tassels were. (She's living in Florida now making cute outfits for dancers; I just talked to her on the telephone not too long ago.)

When you strolled through the streets at night in the quarter, you'd pass a man out in front of each club, trying to draw the customers in. A barker—that's what they were called. "Come on in and get a free drink. Come and see our show." Every corner you turned there was a little party—people just hanging out and talking. Everyone was friendly and said hello.

A lot of these people from the quarter would come to our house for dinner—it was very buffet-ish. In fact, it seemed our house was always full of people, almost like the boardinghouse where my parents met.

If the crowds got too big around the dinner table, Hattie would help out. This was especially true on Friday nights. Since we lived in a Catholic neighborhood and were practicing faux Catholics (none of us were baptized Catholics), we followed the rule of Meatless Friday. The streets turned into a neighborhood festival, and the quarter became one big family. Neighbors would make different dishes and you would go from house to house, just eating away. I was in heaven—it was one huge movable feast that covered blocks and blocks. There were platters and bowls of stuffed crabs, fried trout almondine, fried crab legs, red beans and rice, crawfish étouffé, and gumbo. Hattie would take melontons, which look like big green pears, and stuff them with shrimp, crabmeat, bread crumbs, and spices and then bake the whole thing. I loved meatless Fridays.

My father had a friend from the war who was nicknamed Scotty, because he was Scottish. He worked out on the oil rigs in the Gulf for three to four months at a time, and when he came back into town, our house was usually his first stop. If it was Meatless Friday, he'd poke his head in the door and say hello. Every time he stopped to see us, he'd give Lenny and me ten silver dollars each. Then he and Leonard would disappear in a cab. Shirley would call up Ella Mae and Everett, and a couple of her other girlfriends and tell them to come on over. She didn't have many girl-

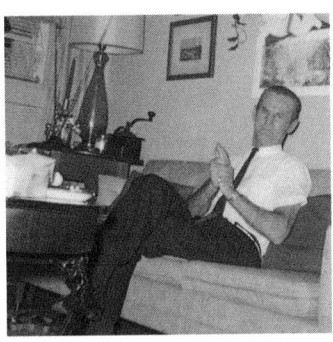

Scotty, my dad's best friend. To me, he was Uncle Scotty.

friends. My mom was not a woman's woman—she was a man's woman. But things were different when Scotty was in town. Shirley and her women friends would spread layers and layers of newspaper all over the dining room table, just in time for Leonard and Scotty to come walking through the door, carrying bags of the most wonderful-smelling food. They'd dump about twenty pounds of crawfish, still steaming, onto the table, along with huge piles of boiled shrimp and boiled crabs. That's why there was so much newspaper on the table, to protect it from the delicious mess. It was like layers of phyllo dough—New Orleans *Times-Picayune* phyllo. There were trays and trays of raw oysters and my father's dipping sauce made with ketchup, horseradish, and his favorite ingredient, Tabasco sauce. He sprinkled Tabasco on everything. He even had special bottles that were labeled, "Made for Leonard Simmons." And there were tubs of potato salad and jambalaya. Coming in the door behind Leonard and Scotty were folks from the neighborhood. The feed was on! Suckin' on crawfish heads and cracking crabs—who cared about hamburgers on Meatless Friday? You were in a city where the lumps of crabmeat were as big as your hand! It was just luscious.

When the feed was over, we all rolled up the newspaper, bent the sides up, and took it out to the trash. You didn't want the smell staying in the house. Shirley would hold our hands under the faucet and squeeze lemon juice all over them. Then she'd smell them, and say, "Here—let me put a little more lemon juice on them. Good. Let's smell. That's better. Now go wash them." That was Friday night at the Simmons house—a celebration with food.

Very often my parents would have friends from out of town come to visit, and they would stay with us. Many of them were actually friends of my parents from their show-business days, or from even earlier times. Even though none of them were actually relatives, my parents referred to them as Aunt and Uncle so-and-so, in an effort to create our instant Simmons family. My favorites were Aunt Blanche and Uncle Carl, who lived in La Mesa, California.

I mean, I knew these people who came to stay were not really relatives, but I called them Aunt or Uncle anyway. I played along, for a time. But sometimes we'd be sitting at the dining room table, eating dinner, and I'd hear a little something about the past. One of my parents would slip, and I would catch it.

"Remember when we played Chicago?" Leonard would ask.

I'd perk up right away and say, "Chicago? What do you mean you played Chicago? Were both you and mom there? Who did you know there?" I just couldn't help myself.

"Stop asking so many questions. I'm talking to your Uncle Carl."

A little later I would hear something about St. Louis.

And I'd start. "St. Louis? What do you mean—mom and you had a great time in St. Louis?" Then my father would give me one of his looks. I knew I was on the edge. If I pressed too much, I was going to be sent you-know-where.

Sometimes when it was just Leonard, Shirley, Lenny, and me at dinner, I would start. I just couldn't help it.

"So, everybody has relatives. Where are mine?"

"They're in other cities," Leonard would answer. "In fact, you saw the card the other day from Aunt Marion."

"No, I didn't. But I want to see her picture. I want to see pictures of all my relatives."

It was a big secret, and I didn't understand it, at all. Were th

That did it. Off to my room I went. It was a big secret, and I didn't understand it, at all. Were these my real parents? Did I have any relatives? Where did I come from? This was the first time I was asking questions, and there were no answers. Everything seemed made up. It was almost like the time I went to East Berlin before the Wall came down. I would go down these streets, and there were the fronts of buildings but with nothing behind them. That was like my life—everything seemed to be a stage set.

* * *

Catholic Khaki

In 1953, by the time I was five, food had already become very important to me. How could it not be, since my earliest memories included a package of bacon and a can of fat on the stove?

Clothing was not important to me, despite the fact that both my mother and father were very fashionable dressers, even though most of the time they were wearing secondhand clothes. My mother usually brought home everyday clothes for Lenny and me from Maison Blanche, and my father handmade all our suits and outfits for special occasions. He even made my mother's gowns. He was a man of many talents, as I've told you before. So up to this point in my life, I had barely set foot in a clothing store.

One morning after our usual breakfast together, Shirley said she had somewhere to take me. I thought we were going to the French Market to see what food the trucks had brought in. I got dressed quickly. There was a good chance that I would get some delicious treats that day.

But that's not where we wound up. Instead, I found myself standing in front of Canal Street Uniform. I knew my first day of school was just around the corner, and I knew I was going to have to get a uniform. I was going to be attending a Catholic elementary school called St. Louis Cathedral, run by the Mothers of the Sacred Heart. They weren't really mothers—they were nuns.

The best schools in our part of town were the parochial schools, and St. Louis Cathedral School was a mere three grocery stores—I mean, three blocks—from my house. It didn't make any difference that my parents weren't Catholic. Remember? Shirley was from a strict Orthodox Jewish household and Leonard was Methodist. No matter—Leonard was sending

Lenny and me to Catholic school, and that was that. Leonard respected the strictness of the nuns—they practiced what he preached, and their style in many ways was similar to his. So he figured the nuns could only do me some good. I'm not sure why he thought that, since his own attempt to be strict with me didn't seem to work.

But the whole thing about Lenny and me going to Catholic school was kind of strange. My parents didn't practice any religion. When I heard church bells, it just meant it was time for dinner. Religion was never talked about in our house, and in fact not much of anything of a personal nature was talked about around the dinner table, unless I started it. Probably had something to do with all those missing relatives. But my parents were religious in their own way, always trying to practice the Golden Rule.

As I've said before, I was growing up faux Catholic. Everybody in our family seemed to have a double life, so why not me? Even though I wasn't baptized Catholic, I went to mass on a regular basis, but I didn't go to confession and I didn't receive communion—you needed to be baptized for that. Saturday was a non-mass day, unless it was a day for a special Saint to whom we needed to say hello. My parents never went to mass with us, and I just couldn't understand that—well, they both did go to my graduations from grammar school and high school. On Sunday morning, my mother would very often be sleeping, so I would turn to my father and say, "Look, why do Lenny and I have to get dressed up every Sunday? Why don't you go to church with us?"

He didn't take too kindly to this. Often he would threaten to send me to my room. Finally, one Sunday morning he just snapped and said, "Look, I'm not Catholic. Your mother's not Catholic. You're going to this school because it's the best and it's only three blocks away."

"Fine. Then let me become Catholic. If I'm doing all this Catholic stuff, and I've got rosaries hanging on my bed, and I have holy cards, why not? Look, Lenny's even an altar boy." And that was very weird, since Lenny wasn't baptized Catholic.

"No, you're not becoming Catholic now. When you become a senior in high school, then you can make that choice as to whether you want to be baptized Catholic. Until then, you do it my way."

Once, after Leonard had helped me learn a prayer from my catechism, he said to me, "See, you just said a prayer. It was the same as being in

She'd think I was sleeping, and I would tiptoe to the door of h

church, but you're home. Wherever you decide to pray, that becomes your own little church. What's important is what you believe. Your mother and I are trying to teach you how to be good to others and good to yourself. That's our religion." That was one of the very rare occasions that my father had a serious talk with me about anything.

Shirley's attitude toward church was the same. My mother, like my father, created her own church. There were nights when she got home late. She'd think I was sleeping, and I would tiptoe to the door of her bedroom, and there she would be—on her knees, praying. Both my parents had their own kind of religion, and just like most things in our family, it was private.

My Catholic grammar school had a simple, but not very pretty, dress code: a uniform consisting of brown shoes, khaki pants, a khaki shirt, a brown belt, and a khaki tie—very World War I and II. Even as a young child, I knew khaki was not my color. In fact, I didn't think it was a color at all—it was as unappealing and dry as the desert. And to this day, I will wear nothing that is khaki.

So there I was, inside Canal Street Uniform. The clerk mumbled and flipped through pants. Each size he gave me was too snug around my waist and legs. Finally, he gave me the biggest boy's size he had, and into the dressing room I went. Somehow I managed to squeeze myself into the pants, dangerously straining the seams. I was sweating in my khaki shirt, and the khaki tie was already in a neat Windsor knot, which my father had taught me how to do. I walked out of the dressing room and turned toward the mirror. I looked like a Vienna sausage with a belt on.

Just as I took a deep breath, the clerk said, "Oh, those are way too tight. You really should go to the Husky Department down in the basement."

I said to Shirley, "You didn't tell me were were getting a dog. Is this a special surprise for me?"

The salesman overheard me and laughed. "No, you don't understand. Husky is a special size in clothing, for boys who are a little bigger than average."

So, Shirley and I went downstairs, and we found the department, between the candy and the pots and pans. A sales clerk walked over, and out came the tape measure. When he measured me, he let out a little gasp. He went over to a rack, pulled out a pair of pants, and handed them to me, pointing to the changing room. I thought, Oh, no, was this going to be another stretch? Well, they fit around the waist, but they were way too long, made for a much taller person, like six foot two. The clerk told my mother they'd have to be altered, substantially. She said we'd take three pairs.

I tried on shirts. My chest was big, but my arms were short, so the sleeves had to be shortened. If I thought this was a humiliating experience, the next stop on our shopping trip became my worst nightmare.

We were at the shoe store. Finally, I was relieved. I may have been hard to fit for pants and shirts, but surely picking a pair of shoes wouldn't pose such a problem. My waistline may have been the wrong size, but I knew my foot size was "average." The shoe clerk marched out of the back room carrying a tower of boxes. Kneeling before me, he took out a pair of stylish loafers from their box and slipped them on my feet. I stood up to get a look in the mirror. It was the strangest thing. The sides of the shoes had widened out, like they were smiling.

"Oh, look at that," the clerk said, "You're pronating."

"He's what?" my mother asked.

"He's pronating. See how he stands with his feet pointed out? He's carrying some extra weight, so his feet are compensating by turning out. Like a duck or a penguin. That's very bad. He should see a doctor." The shoe clerk whisked away all the boxes, and with them went the last shred of my dignity. A minute later, he brought out a pair of shoes that would make me look more like the nuns at school than like the other students.

"These are Stride-Rites. They're the corrective shoe," he pointed out to my mother. Indeed, they were corrective. They had a steel plate inside of them. And on top of that, these orthopedic, Frankenstein things were expensive, which left me no chance to talk my mother into buying both the loafers and the monster shoes.

The night before school was to start, my new uniform laid out nearby, I crawled under my asthma umbrella to think about what I was in for. My brother was in his bed reading *Moby Dick*. I was very nervous about school.

I had gone to a school already, but it didn't really count. It was called La Petite Ecole. It was a tiny school—actually just one class, run by a very rich lady. I went when I was four years old, to learn French. Can you imagine? A finishing school for four-year-olds, and we had no money!

Feeling slightly more than a bit crushed, I came home from m

But grammar school was a whole different experience—a real school.

That night, I asked my brother a million questions. "Lenny, what's school like? What do you do? What are the other kids like? Do you like the nuns? Is it fun?"

Lenny was entering the second grade, so he knew about school.

"Don't worry," he said. "You'll love school. Besides, I'll be there with you." He was very comforting to me, even as a young child.

The next morning, not even the smell of bacon frying could brighten my spirits—and bacon was one of my best friends. I walked out of the house in my khaki uniform, looking like a grocery bag from the A&P, ready to start my first day of school. At least I'd look like everyone else. As my parents walked me to school and led me to my new classroom, my mother started crying just a little bit. Her baby son was growing up. I started crying, too. I guess I've always been sympathetic to other people crying.

All of a sudden, as my mother let go of my hand and nudged me toward my new classmates, I looked around and I was shocked out of my tears. Yes, everyone was dressed in khaki. But unlike me, they were all pencil-thin! The little girls were pencil-thin, with pencil-thin pigtails. The boys were pencil-thin. I didn't look anything like these people! And the first thing I thought of was, Well, somebody better sit these kids down and get them something to eat. They could all use a good meal. I thought about running after my mother and asking her to bring some more lunches, because these kids desperately needed some home cooking.

As I was staring at them, I noticed that they were staring back at me. Suddenly, I felt like I was in an Alfred Hitchcock movie. They started whispering, and there was a little pointing. And that's when I first realized it: I was the one who was different. I was a fat kid.

Feeling slightly more than a bit crushed, I came home from my first day of school and decided it was time to have a serious talk with my parents. Remember, from practically day one, I was very adult-like—someone to be reckoned with. They quickly assured me that I was just blessed with baby fat. Apparently fat babies were a good thing. I was lucky to be so healthy. Besides, my mother had made one of my favorite sandwiches for an after-school snack—fried bologna with mayo on white bread. So my worries about my weight were put off for the moment by a bologna sandwich.

day of school and decided it was time to have a serious talk

In my house, food and love were just about the same thing. My mother used food to comfort me. If my parents loved me and they weren't worried about my weight, why should I be? So what if I really loved food? What could it hurt? Well, my feelings, for one thing.

* ⋆ *

I'm Different . . . I Mean, Special

At school, I quickly became the last one chosen, not just for sports, but for everything. Even Alan, a tiny kid with thick Coke-bottle glasses, was picked before I was. I became determined not to care. What could it matter? I was loved at home and my weight was proof of it.

I didn't totally ignore the situation, however. I did develop a few defenses. One of them was lying, and, I have to say, I came up with some pretty good ones over the years. I had a lot of my classmates believing that my family was well-off because my grandfather owned the Simmons Mattress company. I got a little respect that way. So maybe there was more to me than met the eye—well, there was a lot of me that met the eye. The good thing was that no one could easily prove that grandpa Simmons wasn't the mattress king. Having a mysterious family history was finally paying off.

I also cracked a lot of jokes, mostly about myself, feeling that if I could make fun of myself first, then no one else would feel the need to.

But mostly, I tried to stick to the things I was good at. My father had taken me to museums and art galleries when I was very young, so I knew a lot about painting and drawing and sculpting—I especially loved paintings of food. I was crazy about art class. My art teacher would bring out colorful paints, sticks, cotton balls, and pipe cleaners. We'd spend an hour or two crafting a masterpiece out of those objects, creating something from nothing. I found I was good at working alone from ideas in my head. Then, one of my classmates pointed out that all my art projects had to do with food. I realized it was true. While the other students were making ducks or rabbits, I'd create a hot fudge sundae out of cotton balls, or a plate of spaghetti and meatballs with pipe cleaners and marbles.

The only thing I loved more than art class was the cafeteria. I was always the first in line. I may have been made fun of or laughed at, but my philosophy became, "Sticks and stones may break my bones, but just fix

One day, I finally saw where my father hid the key. I waited f

me a nice piece of roast beef with some mashed potatoes and gravy." I loved the gravy to be level and smooth so it looked almost like a skating rink. When I added salt, my mashed-potato rink looked just like it was covered with ice.

My father would usually walk with me to school. I could see the world around me, but I hadn't had much contact with a lot of people, other than my mother, father, brother, and friends of my parents who came to the house. I was not around kids my own age a lot—I was always surrounded by adults. Going to school, I noticed that everybody else's *mother* brought them. As I settled into the routine at school, classmates and other people started to ask me what my father and mother did. I'd never really had to answer these questions before. I would say, "Well, my mother works and my father stays at home." I heard myself say this, and people would then ask why that was. I didn't know the answer.

So I started to play a little Perry Mason. We'd be sitting around the dining room table, and I'd say, "You know, we were at school today and everybody asked me what my father did." I was very precocious—maybe even a bit obnoxious. Well, maybe a *lot* obnoxious with my dad.

Leonard would say, "I do my volunteer work and lots of other things."

"What does lots of other things mean?"

Well, you know what his answer was.

I made another discovery around this time. My father had this tall, beautiful writing desk in the living room. The top part was a cabinet with two very ornate doors, and in there were some of my father's favorite books. Underneath that was a drop-leaf desk that folded down, but this was always locked. For years I had wondered what could be so important that it had to be locked up. I had to get in there and find out.

One day, I finally saw where my father hid the key. I waited for my chance. Late one afternoon when no one was in the house, I got the key and opened the desk. I found some old pictures of my father and mother from their show-business days—a few he didn't toss into the bonfire in the back-yard. They were some snaps from the past. I had no idea what these pictures were about. Here were more secrets, just like the aunts and uncles who weren't really aunts and uncles. I began to question my entire life. Were Leonard and Shirley really my parents? Was I from an orphanage? Was I from a foreign country? What were they hiding from me?

* * *

Practically every day at St. Louis Cathedral grammar school had its traumatic events. For instance, there was my initiation into bathroom-going. At home, the rule was that when the bathroom door was closed, it was locked and someone was using it. When the door was open, it was yours. And we had a schedule in the morning: Leonard had 60 minutes, Shirley 45 minutes, and Lenny and I, 15 minutes each. I loved my bathroom time, because this is when I could practice my commercials. There was a mirror directly across from the toilet, so I could sit there and rehearse. "Hi. I use Scott tissue because it's so soft."

Well, school was a whole different thing. The bathrooms were the high-quality parochial-school variety: white tiles on the floor and all those sinks lined up along one wall with individual bars of soap (I don't think soap dispensers had been invented yet), and messy towels. Along the other wall was a line of six toilet stalls with light-gray granite partitions. Given our locked-door policy at home, you can understand my reaction to this communal arrangement. Even if I had to do a "onesie," I'd go into a stall and shut the door. I never used the urinals. I didn't have one at home, so why should I use the one at school? Using the stall was much more like home.

At school, I had been singled out by a bully, an older kid. Let's just call him Moose. He singled me out as the boy who stood apart. One day when I was using one of the bathroom stalls, Moose and his gang sneaked into the adjoining stalls and started throwing wet paper towels and cups of water over the top of the partition. I was so scared. My whole young life flashed before my eyes. If I ever got out of this one, I vowed never to get trapped like this again. Well, I did survive, but that was the last time I ever went to the bathroom at school. I even brought my own bar of soap from home and washed my hands in the drinking fountain if they got dirty. If I had to go, I'd hold it in until lunchtime, and then quickly walk home. You couldn't go to the nuns and say, "Sister, let me tell you about this little bathroom problem I have." No, I don't think so. The nuns didn't want to hear any complaining. Plus, I was not going to snitch on my classmates, no matter how awful they might be. My brother snitched on me sometimes, and I didn't like it one bit. Well, this went on for eight years—all through grammar school. And I wasn't the only one who stayed out of the bathrooms. There were a lot of people in the "Hold It In" club.

The nuns were horrified by all my big letters, and they tied n

Another thing about the nuns in the Fifties was that they didn't like people to be left-handed. Everyone should be the same and write with their right hand. Can you believe that? Well, I was born left-handed—God intended me to be that way.

I loved to write. Remember, I was always around grown-ups, so my vocabulary was advanced for my age. My father was always reading to me and he taught me how to write, too. I loved my writing tablets at school. They had those solid navy blue horizontal lines with dotted blue lines in the middle as a guideline for the top of the small letters. Why should any letters be small? Were they being punished? Was it because they were second? Well, I made everything glamorous. I had the prettiest handwriting, with big swooping letters. Very baroque. And I worked at it. If I saw a dramatic "A" in a magazine, I copied it and made it my very own. The nuns were horrified by all my big letters, and they tied my left hand behind me to force me to print right-handed. When they untied me, I went right back to being a lefty.

I told my dad about all of this—the tying my hand around my back. This went too far, even for him. He marched himself down to the school and had a little chat with the nuns. He told them that forcing me to write right-handed was horrible, and it had to stop. People were always charmed by my father, and when he talked in his firm manner, people particularly listened, and obeyed. That was the end of it. I was a lefty for life.

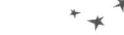

The Diet Doctor

In 1955, when I was in the second grade and seven years old, my mother announced at breakfast one morning that Dr. Veith had recommended that I go see a *special* doctor who would give me a *special* physical examination. Well, that got my attention. I knew enough about doctors even at this early age to know that when adults referred to them as special, it meant they really didn't want to tell you what was going on.

"Why can't I go to Dr. Veith?" That word "physical" set off all kinds of alarms. I knew I was overweight, and you have to understand that if you're a fat kid, you don't want someone looking at your body—no way. And when you go to see a doctor, you most definitely want to leave all your clothes on. Period. Dr. Veith understood that. When he listened to my heart and lungs, he would never make me take my shirt off. Instead, he would slip his stethoscope up under the shirt because he knew it was upsetting for me. I adored him for that. That's why I always tried to amuse him. When he came into the examining room, sometimes I would pretend I was the doctor: "Sit down. You don't look very good." I would take his temperature and listen to his heart. But now, I was being sent off to a "special" doctor who would probably make me take off my clothes. Oh, no.

When I came home from school that afternoon and saw a date circled on the calendar, I could barely eat my afternoon snack. In the circle was written, "Milton's physical—4:00 P.M." So there it was. I feared that date. I spent the next few days hoping the doctor would be called away on an emergency—to China. Or maybe he would get sick—that would be a twist. My mother reassured me that he was just going to check my eyes, my ears, my heartbeat—things like that. There was nothing to worry about. It wouldn't hurt a bit.

She couldn't have been more wrong. While my mother thumbed through *Life* magazine in the waiting room, a nurse escorted me into a small room with sickly green walls and a cold metal table. She told me to take off all my clothes except for my underwear, and then she'd be right back with the doctor. I undressed quickly, folded my khaki uniform, and placed it neatly on a nearby chair.

There I was in my underwear, with my body uncovered, when I first met Dr. Hallman. I'll never forget the first thing he said to me: "Whoa, you're a big fella." Well, maybe I was a little bigger than the other kids. But this was worse than being teased in school. There, I could expect to hear lines like that—I didn't expect it here in the doctor's office, where all I wanted was a sympathetic ear and a little snack. The nurse took my blood pressure and put me on the scale. She wrote my weight on a form and then, with a meaningful glance, showed it to the doctor. The room was so silent I could hear myself breathe.

They checked my ears and eyes. He listened to my heart and then made me cough while he listened to my lungs. He said, "I'd like to talk with you and your mother. Come to my office after you've dressed." He left the room without another word. Well, this was worse than having to go to the principal's office. As I dressed, I decided I must have some terrible disease. Dr. Hallman had barely been able to look me in the eye.

I joined my mother in the office and sat down next to her. I stared up at the many diplomas that covered the walls. The doctor didn't look up, but continued to write furiously in a file folder, adding to my worry. Only something serious could take so much time to write out. Finally, he took off his glasses and looked at me.

"We've got to get some of that weight off of you," he said in a very flat voice. He opened the drawer in the middle of his desk and pulled out two thin sheets of paper. This paper was the beginning of a journey I would take that would last nearly twenty years. Before he slammed the drawer shut, I caught a glimpse of a whole stack of these identical sheets.

"I want you to start tonight."

"Start what?" I asked, afraid of what his answer might be.

"I'm putting you on a diet." He handed one sheet of paper to me and the other to my mother. I thought maybe this was a chain letter and that I would wind up with something nice. I was wrong. This was a diet. The paper was hard to read because it had been copied so many times. There was no title, and nothing remotely personal about this diet. This is what was printed on that little sheet of paper:

BREAKFAST:

½ grapefruit		1 slice of dry wheat toast
hard-boiled egg	or	poached egg
beverage		beverage

LUNCH:

lettuce and tomato		3 oz. tuna fish—no oil
cottage cheese		salad with lemon
2 slices Melba Toast	or	2 slices Rye Krisp
lemon wedges		

SNACK:

carrot sticks		1 apple
celery sticks	or	

DINNER:

3 oz. lean meat		4 oz. fish
1 c. dark green vegetables	or	1 c. dark green vegetables
beverage		beverage

He told me in a stern voice to stick to this diet, and he'd see me again in six months. That was it. My time was up and he was on to bigger and better patients—well, maybe not bigger. He hadn't asked me what I'd been eating or bothered to explain anything more about this diet. He'd also forgotten to ask me or my mom if we had any questions. And I had a big one, which I asked my mother: "Why was I being punished?" I didn't understand. Shirley had always told me that a little baby fat was okay, and now this doctor was telling me I had to go on a diet.

That night at dinner, nobody mentioned my diet and no one said a word when I took a second helping of mashed potatoes. In fact, everyone, including my brother, seemed to be especially nice to me. Lenny didn't even complain when I swiped the last roll from his plate. If they were feeling sorry for me, that was okay. I figured I could put the whole, unhappy incident behind me and things would get back to normal. It was just another of our family's disappearing acts—the diet had vanished.

But I found out the next morning at breakfast that things were far from normal. The diet had not disappeared, but the food I loved had. No hash browns sizzling in a skillet on the stove for me. No omelets, no bacon or sausage, no pancakes. My bowl of sweetened cereal and my glass of juice were gone, and in their place was half of a cold, sour, lonely grapefruit—not even a cherry on top. I was supposed to eat that?! Please!

The day after my physical, I went from eating fried chicken, potato salad, and apple pie to a hard-boiled egg and a slice of dry toast the size of a postage stamp. I carried around a hard-boiled egg every day. I began to feel like a hen. My mother would cut it in half and put it in a piece of waxed paper. She'd sprinkle some salt and pepper on it. To say that I felt unloved and punished would be an understatement. But I decided that if eating this way would make me lose weight, then once I got down to a "normal" size, I could go back to eating the things I loved. I would give it my best shot.

* * *

The Cheating Begins

As it turned out, my best shot lasted three days. How I even made it through day three was a miracle. It was on the fourth day, the day my mother made me a tuna-salad sandwich to take to school for lunch, that

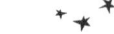

I realized life wasn't worth living without the food I loved. One of my very favorite things in the whole world was my mother's tuna-fish sandwich. She made it with big chunks of onion and celery and flaky tuna, all smothered in real mayonnaise. To tell the truth, I was looking forward to a real lunch—I was hungry all the time.

That morning, as I sat at the breakfast table, my half a grapefruit in front of me, I watched as Shirley opened the can. Back then, tuna was only packed in oil. She took out a strainer and she washed the tuna. She literally scrubbed it with a brush, pushing all the excess oil through the strainer. And then she put the sanitized tuna on the two pieces of rye bread—no butter, no mayo, not even a measly piece of celery or a sliver of onion. She squeezed a little lemon juice on it. Then she slapped the bread together, sliced it neatly, and wrapped it in waxed paper.

In the cafeteria at lunch, I pulled that sandwich out of the bag. It looked bad and smelled worse. I was depressed. I looked at the bottom of my lunch bag, and all that was there were some celery and carrot sticks. Frankly, they reminded me of some of my skinny-looking classmates.

That's when I decided I couldn't exist like this. What did I do wrong? I only did as I was told. I ate everything on my plate, and because of that I was being punished. I had thought I was loved. Wasn't giving food to someone suppose to mean you loved them? Well, if no one was willing to reward me for all the work I was doing on this diet, then I would just have to reward myself.

On the way home from school that day I stopped at one of my favorite places, the lunch counter at Woolworth's on Canal Street, and I treated myself to a real meal. I sat right down at that long curved counter and I ordered their special turkey dinner—which they still serve to this day—paying for it with money saved from my allowance. There were juicy slices of turkey with dressing, mashed potatoes, and homemade gravy, thick with the fat drippings of the turkey. There was a hot roll with real butter, cranberry sauce, and, for dessert, a thick slice of pumpkin pie with real whipped cream on top. I thought I'd died and gone to heaven. It wasn't Thanksgiving, but I was giving thanks. Finally, after three and a half days, I was no longer hungry. It was a good feeling.

But the good feeling didn't last when my mother asked me that night why I wasn't eating my dinner. I could barely finish the small slices of roast

t. But I decided that if eating this way would make me lose

beef and broccoli she'd given me. I lied and told her I didn't feel all that well. I felt bad lying to my mother, but I was still stuffed from my turkey dinner. I shouldn't have eaten that second roll. And this was just the beginning of more lies I would continue to tell over the years about my dieting and my weight.

From that day on, I learned how to fake a diet. At school I was Mr. Goody Two Shoes, eating my hard-boiled egg and cottage cheese. But after school, I'd make a stop at one of the three grocery stores on my way home. My favorite was the St. Louis Street Grocery. Or I'd go to McCrory's for a banana split or a hot fudge sundae.

In the evening, my mother or my father would ask, "How did you do today? Were you good today?" I was "good" if I didn't include the fried pigskins and the two candy bars I ate on the way home. I wanted to cry when my father told me what a wonderful boy I was. More lies.

That night, lying in bed, I was consumed by guilt. I vowed I wouldn't do this anymore. I'd get back on my diet and stick to it. And then a few days later, I'd find myself back at the St. Louis Street grocery store, buying a Hershey bar or a cookie. I realized I'd have to balance these food lies. I began to throw away my lunch sometimes—not throw up, which comes later, but throw away. I'd skip a meal here and there so I could treat myself to the sweets I craved.

Once a week, I would get weighed on my mother's pink-and-white scale she kept in the pink-and-white bathroom. She'd say excitedly, "Oh, look. You've lost two pounds!" She wouldn't realize I'd skipped lunch for the last two days and fed my breakfast to Mickey, our family dog, in order to lose the pounds. Poor Mickey. He didn't seem to care much for the dry toast I ate at breakfast. And as for the grapefruit—well, Mickey learned pretty quickly not to beg for my table scraps. Who wants to be best friends with someone who's eating sour grapefruit?

I yo-yoed back and forth, gaining a pound or two, losing a pound or two, and before I knew it, six months had passed. It was time for another visit to Dr. Hallman. I tried really hard for almost a week, and my efforts were rewarded. When I got on the scale, I'd lost four pounds! Nobody was more surprised than I was. And while these weren't the spectacular results Dr. Hallman may have expected, he told me to keep dieting.

And that's exactly what I did for the next several years. I'd gain and lose,

I'd gain and lose. I'd stop at Lucky's Hot Dog Cart and have three or four hot dogs, and I'd throw away my lunch the next day. And when I'd see another physical coming up on the calendar, I'd cut way back so I'd lose a few pounds when it was time to get weighed. And if I didn't lose, I'd make excuses. I had a cold or I had a terrible headache. The lying became a habit, just like overeating. I began to wear baggy clothes. I'd wear my shirt out, or tuck it in and billow it out a bit. I was becoming expert at how to wear clothing to camouflage my weight.

* * *

Mr. Perfect

During this time, my brother Len and I continued to share a room. Me on my side with my asthma umbrella, and him on his side with his books. We had little beds, and about once every year my father would change the look. One year it was stars-and-planets wallpaper. (I think my father was hoping I'd move to Jupiter.) Another year we returned from summer camp and the whole room looked like the woods we had just left, all painted in hunter green.

Lenny, in my eyes, was really a child prodigy. He began to talk before other children talked. He began to read before other children read. He loved to learn. While I collected food, he collected books. At an early age, while I was sucking on crawfish heads, he was busy reading about where crawfish came from and what *they* snacked on. Lenny had a natural curiosity about things and asked questions that would never have crossed my mind. Once, I remember, he went down to the Vieux Carré Commission Building to find out about our house. He wanted to know who built it, when it was built, what it cost originally, and who lived there before us. He wanted to know more about the crown molding, the style of the house, and the architecture. I was wondering whether there'd be seconds on the mashed potatoes, and my brother was wondering whether or not this was the original door of the house.

Lenny was always an adult—I don't think he was ever a child. And long before I did, he picked up my father's habit of doing things for other people, for neighbors, for projects at school. If a volunteer was needed for anything, Lenny was first in line.

Lenny was many things, but he was not neat. From the very beginning I was neat. I even changed my own diapers because I didn't like the way my parents did it. My room had to be neat. This was not my brother.

So, Lenny would be sitting at the breakfast table and I'd be running late. I'd walk in and say, "Whew, sorry I'm so late for breakfast. I just had to clean up the mess in our room because of Lenny." No one said a thing. It was hard to rile Lenny—he let everything roll off his back.

But there was this one little thing that would drive Lenny crazy. It was his special phobia. You couldn't touch his plate or the food on it. I don't know why. That's just the way he was. You can guess what I did at the dinner table. If things got too quiet, I'd say, "Oh Lenny, look over there." Then I'd reach across the table and take a forkful of mashed potatoes from his plate, or a roll. He'd catch the movement out of the corner of his eye, and quickly turn and look down at his plate.

"Why did you do that?" Lenny would calmly pick up his plate, walk over to the trash can, and silently scrape off all the food.

And my father would say, "Again! You did it again. You know your brother doesn't like his plate touched. Why did you do that?" Poor Lenny—I gave him such a hard time.

The major problem I had with my brother—and it really wasn't that big—was that he could sometimes be a snitch. I had very little patience when it came to waiting for presents—whether it was my birthday, Christmas, Easter, or whatever. My parents would hide the gifts around the house, and I'd go searching for them. Sometimes I'd find Lenny's presents. Then I would say to Len, "Lenny, you're going to be so excited this Christmas. You got a basketball and net!"

He'd walk right into the living room and announce, "Mom. Dad. Milton's been looking through all the closets and he found the basketball and the net." Then I would be punished, and my father would dribble me back to my room.

* *
*

Restaurant Row

*M*y life wasn't diets all the time. Once in a while when my parents could see that this was getting a little difficult for me to handle,

The French quarter was full of restaurants, and Len and Shirl

they realized there had to be a treat here and there. Or very often a holiday or a birthday would become an excuse for me to eat what everyone else was eating. Thank goodness!

The French quarter was full of restaurants, and Len and Shirl loved to go out and my brother and I went with them. Sometimes it would be too late to cook, and other times, especially during the summer, it was just too hot and muggy. Ugh. We were just a walk or a cab ride away from a great dinner. And there was no order-in—this was pre-take-out days.

My parents were also friends with many of the restaurant owners, and they along with the waiters and bartenders became part of that whole group my parents referred to as aunts and uncles. It was like visiting family when we'd stop in at the Blue Room, The Court of Two Sisters, Brennan's, Antoine's, or Tujaque's, to say hello to friends or to celebrate a special occasion. Then my parents were a little more forgiving if I strayed from my current diet and helped myself to the little potato puffs that were served when you sat down at Arnaud's, or if I had an extra crab cake at Commander's Palace. But the special occasion and the rich food were always marred by the reminder, "Don't forget that tomorrow you have to go back on your diet." That was always in the background.

My father and I frequently got into it when we went to restaurants. Are you surprised? And I was punished. Punishment by now was part of my relationship with my father.

When you're a little kid and you go to restaurants with your family, this is usually what happens: Mommy takes a little bit of her food and scrapes it off her plate onto the little butter plate. Daddy scrapes a little off his plate onto yours and mushes it together with Mommy's.

When my father attempted this with me, I'd look at him and say, "What?! Is our dog, Mickey, here? What is this?"

Other times, Leonard and Shirl would get menus, but the waiter would pass right by my brother and me.

And I'd say, "What did you bring me here for? Everybody's got a menu. Mom—can I see your menu?"

"Your mother's looking at her menu," my father would say. I couldn't understand why my father was so possessive over a piece of paper. What movies did he watch about raising kids?

The waiter would start to turn away and I'd say, "Excuse me."

"Yes?"

"May I see a menu, please?"

"Yes, I'll bring you one. Would you like another Roy Rogers?"

Lenny and I would almost be finished with the drinks my father had ordered for us: cherry juice and soda—for the boys it was a Roy Rogers, for the girls it was a Shirley Temple.

I'd answer, "No. No more drinks. I'd like the lobster thermidor. And the stuffed potatoes, please."

"What?" Leonard would ask.

"And oh, and don't forget the hollandaise with the asparagus. Thank you."

"Don't bring him anything. Thank you." Then Leonard would look at me, and say, "Lobster thermidor? Just a minute." He'd get up and almost run to the front of the restaurant, call a cab, and come back to the table.

"The cab will be here in five minutes," my father said.

"The cab's bringing the lobster thermidor?"

"No. You're going home."

"Oh, they're going to deliver the lobster to our house?"

"No. There's no lobster. You're going home, by yourself. Now."

And that was that. It was Leonard's show. But you know, I was never too upset, because there was always a refrigerator waiting for me at home. Was he sending me home to a closet? No, he was sending me to the house where I lived, with its refrigerator with no chains around it. He may have been punishing me again for the way I had acted in public, but the refrigerator would open its door to welcome me.

Part of the conflict with my father, I think, was that he was watching me grow into someone who was sort of like him, and he didn't want me to go through all the hurt that he had experienced in trying to get his show-business career off the ground. His life had not turned out exactly the way he wanted it to, so he was going to do his best to make sure the same thing didn't happen to me. The more I antagonized him with my theatrics, the harder it was becoming for me not to follow in his footsteps. I was cute and adorable, with lots of flair and pizzazz. (Giving yourself compliments is very healthy, you know!) I could go anywhere and was very comfortable being the center of attention, just like he had been when he was growing up. But you know, he was proud of me. He would tell his friends that I got good grades in school and that I was creative and funny, but he would never tell me that stuff directly. He just couldn't. That was just not his way. I would get all his compliments secondhand.

My parents would often take us to the Blue Room at the Roosevelt Hotel to see live entertainment. Back then we didn't get many road-company Broadway shows in New Orleans, but we did get performers like Peggy Lee, Patti Page, and even Liberace. Although I don't really remember it, my brother Lenny tells the story that I actually got up on the stage and performed with Liberace as if I were his brother George. Even though my parents had gone to great lengths to protect me from the world of theater and stage and to erase their own show-business past, I think I was just genetically programmed to perform, and nothing they could do was going to change that.

I loved the Blue Room. It was on two levels and very elegant. I would watch the waiters carry their big trays, delivering dishes to various tables, and if I saw a tray of something I particularly liked, I would excuse myself to go to the bathroom. But instead, I would follow that tray to the table. I'd introduce myself to the diners, hoping they would invite me to sit down and have a taste of what they were eating. I was in a little suit and so cute, just oozing charm, that everyone would act as if I were part of the group. Back at our table, my father would be like an ostrich watching me. I'd talk for a while, sometimes getting a sample of the food, and then I'd say good-bye and walk back to my family.

I'd sigh, "Well, I feel much better now."

"Why did you do that?" Leonard asked.

"I'm friendly. I love to make friends."

"That's all the friends you'll be making tonight. I just called a cab." My father knew the phone number of the Checker Cab by heart and could dial it with his eyes closed—and this was before touch-tone.

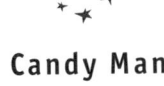

Candy Man

Besides the temptations I faced when we ate out, I had another food demon. I couldn't resist a New Orleans tradition, the delicious candy called pralines. I began to stop at a candy store called Leah's Southern

Confections, which was about two blocks from my house on St. Louis Street. They had the creamiest, dreamiest pralines in the French quarter.

For those of you who don't know, a praline is a round confection made from white sugar, brown sugar, butter, heavy cream, and lots and lots of pecans. You make a huge batch of the mixture in a large brass kettle and then spoon-drop them into little patties onto waxed paper to cool.

Unlike the other praline stores, Leah never used pecans that were broken. Instead, her pecans were perfect—they wouldn't dare be otherwise. I got into the habit of buying a praline on my way home from school every day. There were two sisters who worked in Leah's, Marie and Marguerite Garrison—not related to Leah. Miss Leah lived in Atlanta, and her niece, Elna Ruth, who lived above the shop with her mother, Edna Mae, helped run things for Leah. Marie, Marguerite, and Elna got to know me, since I was such a faithful customer. I started to stop in at Leah's as much to visit the three of them as I did for the pralines. And the visits got longer and longer, until one day I told Marie and Marguerite that since they were getting very busy, I wanted to work for them. So I gave them the whole *Citizen Kane* story, and they fell for it, lock, stock, and pecan. I was eight years old—certainly old enough to work. I saw this as a way to get free pralines. And part of what drove me was my desire for more independence. I was getting tired of spending so much time in my room for always saying the wrong thing in front of my father. I figured this way I would be out of the house more, and I would be my own breadwinner, making my own money. And like my father, I loved being around people.

Leah's was across the street from Antoine's, right around the corner from Brennan's, and two blocks away from Galatoire's, three famous, extremely popular restaurants. I would take some fresh pralines, break them up, and put them on a fancy tray. Then I'd walk with the tray to the front of these restaurants and say to the people lined up, "My, oh my, it's going to be an hour or longer before you get in there. How about a little taste of a praline?"

I'd give them a sample, and directions to the store, and then suggest they come by after dinner to purchase a praline for dessert. I loved doing this. Because I had a tray of candy, people were nice to me and they were always willing to talk. No one made fun of me, since I had something they wanted. Sometimes I'd even make friends with the people I gave samples

But better than the taste of a Leah's praline, of which I had

to. My father always told me there are no strangers in this world—we're all related in some way, so be nice. I talked to everybody. This was one of the many wonderful things Leonard taught me. He may not have been a regular father in a suit and tie, going off to work in the morning with his briefcase, but his understanding of people and his feelings of charity toward them were right on. Through my job at Leah's, I was becoming street-smart, and I learned how to start a conversation with anybody.

Very often I would invite strangers home for dinner. One time, I started chatting with a couple from Cleveland, Ohio, whom I handed some pralines to. They asked me for the name of a great place to eat.

"Well, we're eating at six. Why don't you come over to our house for dinner."

"No, we couldn't do that."

"Sure you could. My father loves to cook, and we always have people dropping by."

At six o'clock our doorbell would ring. My father would open the door and holler out, "Milton, are you expecting someone?"

I'd jump up from the couch and run to the door. "Oh, hi. I'm so glad you could come for dinner." I'd hug them. "This is my father Leonard and my mother Shirley . . . " My parents never seemed to mind this instant party, and they would easily pick up on the flow, my father offering them a glasses of iced tea. And that's how we would have guests for dinner.

But better than the taste of a Leah's praline, of which I had many, was my first taste of cash. I would go home at the end of the night with my pockets stuffed with tips people had given me on the street. I'd throw it all on the bed and count it. I loved earning money and working. I began to feel closer to my mother, who worked every day, and I started to resent my father even more, whom I saw as not earning his keep. I couldn't have been more wrong. My father did so much for us, but at the time, through the eyes of an eight-year-old child, all I knew was that my family had strange mixed-up roles, and I didn't like it.

One afternoon I was sorting out my pennies, nickels, dimes, and quarters, and my dollar bills—just like Leonard did—on my mother's gorgeous two-poster bed with the Victorian side drapes. Shirley walked in and sat down next to me. I looked at her and said, "I'm going to fill this bed with money, and mom, you're not going to have to work anymore." I thought to myself, Dad may not do things for you, but you can be doggone sure I am. And with that, Shirley leaned over and hugged and kissed me. "Oh, honey. You already give me everything I need." My mother never, never put down my father.

At Leah's, I worked hard and found ways to expand my duties. Through the years, I sold pralines over the phone, and during the holidays I made postcards urging people to buy their sweethearts pralines on Valentine's day, or reminding them that pralines would make a nice Christmas present. I may have been the first eight-year-old marketing executive in New Orleans.

Now, when I visit New Orleans and I stay in the French quarter, I stop by Leah's sometimes. Elna Ruth is still there. The women assure me that if I ever need it, my old job is still waiting there for me. I'm thinking about it. I still love pralines.

* ✶

Two Adults, Two Children

I don't want you to think that my life was only about food when I was growing up, because it was also about movies. Movies were a big deal. Most Sundays Lenny and I would go with our mother and father. Shirley adored heartthrob movies, with lots of passion, romance, and murder—real tearjerkers. We saw Joan Crawford movies, films by Alfred Hitchcock, and lots of movies like that. I don't remember seeing many other kids at these movies. I think they were in other theaters probably watching Jerry Lewis–Dean Martin movies or The Three Stooges or even Westerns. Ahhhhh! Please, please, never take me to a Western. I'll sing a Roy Rogers song—"Happy trails . . . to you . . . "—but never take me to a Western. I hated them. I hated cowboys and Indians. Once my parents gave me a Roy Rogers lunchbox. I refused to use it.

As I've said before, I don't remember much touchy-feely affection between my mother and father—no magic Kodak moments. So I think Shirley got her passion from the big screen. She just soaked it up, and it made her feel connected to the world.

The other good part about the movies were the snacks: Milk Duds, a large Coke, and popcorn with butter. I would say, "Could I have some extra butter, please? My mouth gets so dry during the movie." I'd put the popcorn on one side of my mouth and the Milk Duds on the other and just let them mix. Sometimes, if the popcorn was really fresh and hot, I'd put the Milk Duds on top of the popcorn and they would melt. The food was almost as exciting as the movie. I was always the first to finish my popcorn or empty the box of Milk Duds. I'd shake the box and wonder, "What happened to them?"

Then I'd whisper to my brother, "Lenny. . . "

"Shh, I'm watching the movie."

"Lenny, can I have some of your popcorn?"

"You ate yours." He was in his own little Bette Davis world. So I'd touch his popcorn and he'd put it down on the floor and wouldn't eat it.

And I'd whisper, "Well, if you're not going to eat it . . . "

And he'd hiss, "Shut up!"

"If you're not going to eat it, it's a waste!" But he wouldn't let me have it, because I had touched it.

I'd give up and wait for Lenny's conscience to kick in.

Finally, he'd pick it up and hand it to me. "Okay, you can have it."

I can honestly say my brother never did anything to hurt me—even though I drove him crazy—and he never caused an argument in my family. Never. It was hard living with someone so perfect.

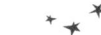

Mr. Milton Dick Simmons, My Uncle

During the summer when I was eight, in 1956, my brother Lenny and I went to Sarasota, Florida, to meet my Uncle Milton, the man I was named after. I was about to meet a "real" relative for the first time. I could hardly wait.

Remember, my parents very rarely talked about the relatives. But from what I could gather from the little bits and pieces of conversation that Leonard let slip over the years, Milton was the "rich relative." Thank God for rich relations. He had designed engines for airplanes during World War I, and it was rumored that he owned a country club in Ohio.

My father and Uncle Milton never really saw eye-to-eye on a lot of things. There was even a point in their lives when they didn't speak to each other. I never knew the reasons for their differences. It probably had something to do with the fact that Milton had been very successful, and Leonard less so. My father could be very stubborn, and I'm sure that my uncle, cut from the same Simmons cloth, was the same way. Milton had no children of his own. After his wife passed away, his sister—my Aunt Eva—moved to Sarasota to live with him. I didn't know what to expect, because father talked very little about either of them. These were the surprise relatives. There were no pictures, so I didn't even know what they looked like.

Finally! Lenny and I were going to Florida to meet a real live relative. Well, the real reason for our trip was a little more personal than that. Actually, it was a little embarrassing. We were going because . . . I had a rash. Really! It broke out on my right leg, going from my right kneecap on my inner leg all the way down to my anklebone. First, my father tried his own remedies, the Famous Four, including Tabasco sauce. When those didn't work, my parents took me to doctor after doctor, all of them experts. Each one would say they'd never seen anything like it. They tried salves, shots, and pills. They took tiny pieces of skin and looked at them under a microscope. Nothing. Meanwhile, they had my parents wrap and medicate the rash three times a day. It just got worse. It was itchy and painful. My parents, who by this time had been through quite a bit with me, were starting to panic. I was their little Frankenstein creature. There I was—under the vaporizer, in the Stride-Rites, with the salve and the gauze wrapped around my leg, eating a sandwich. What else could possibly go wrong with me?

My father, who knew that his brother Milton was smart about a lot of things, would occasionally turn to him for advice. He finally called Uncle Milton in Florida.

My uncle immediately said, "Send Lenny and Milton down."

Uncle Milton picked us up at the airport. He wore the typical retired man's Florida outfit: a safari shirt with the big pockets in the front, shorts, and sandals. He was probably in his mid-seventies. He was a very manicured man, like my father—a Simmons male characteristic. He had snow-white hair that glistened with silver threads in the Florida sun. He was a tall man and built like my father, though a bit on the brawnier side. And while my father had fair skin, Uncle Milton was extremely tan, probably because he played a lot of golf. He had a gruff look on his face. He may have looked strict, but he wasn't at all. I loved that man right away, the minute I met

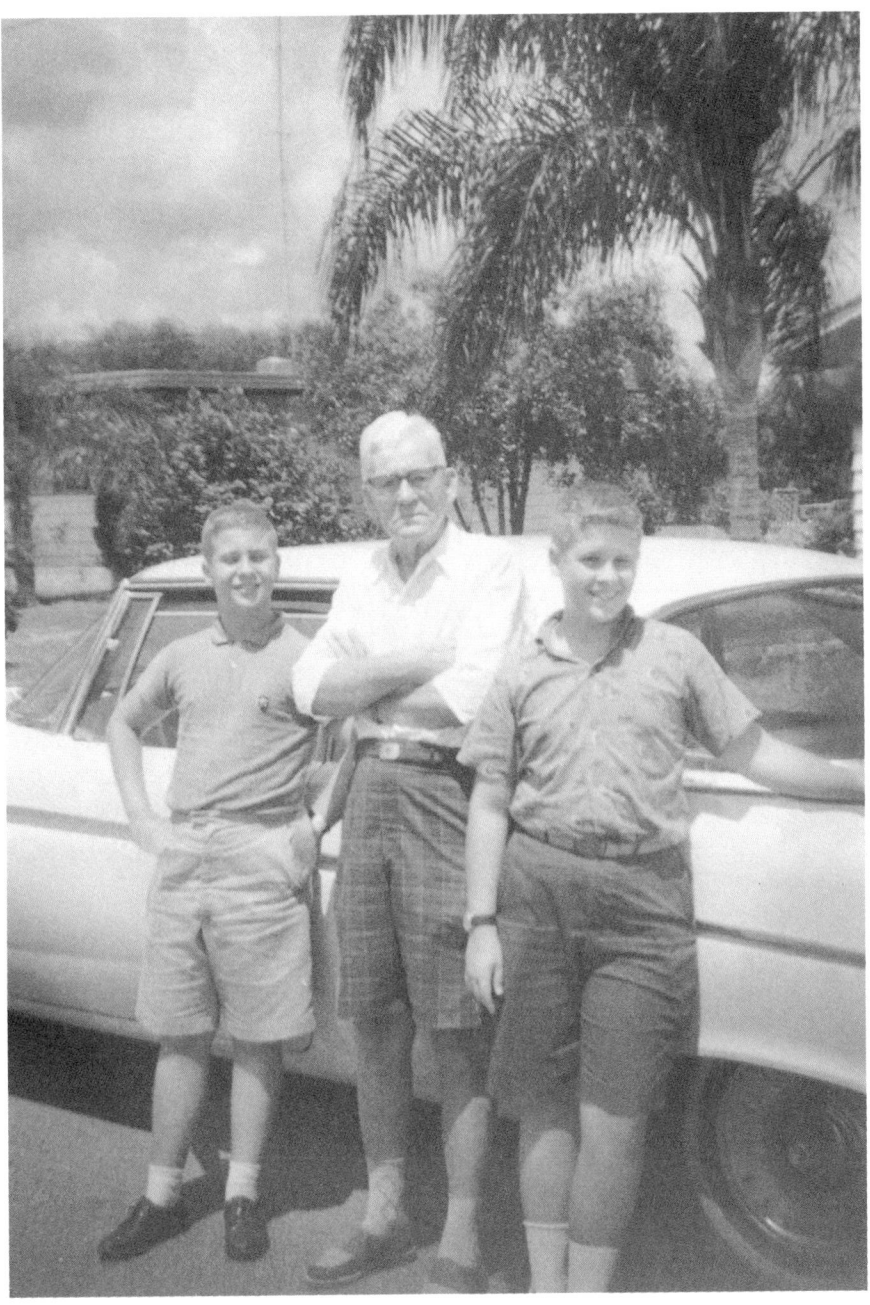

Uncle Milton—he looked tough, but oh! how I loved him.
That's me on the right, and Lenny on the left.

. *Well, the real reason for our trip was a little more personal*

him. So did Lenny. There was something about him that just seemed so honest and straightforward.

Uncle Milton owned a big Lincoln Continental; he bought a new one every year. He drove it about six miles an hour—it seemed like the plane ride was shorter than the ride to his house. Lenny and I didn't care, though, because we loved the leather seats and all the buttons and knobs in his car. He patiently explained over and over what each one was for. About three hours later, we arrived at my Uncle's beautiful house in South Gate.

The very next day, he took us to the beach. Although it was the middle of summer, I was really embarrassed about my rash, and I didn't want to go in the water.

But he packed us up in the car and took us to a secluded part of the beach. He laid a blanket down on the sand, and told me to take off the gauze and walk into the salt water.

I hesitated. "Go ahead, do it now," he said in his gruff manner.

Lenny was in the water already, in his bathing suit, swimming and laughing as he jumped in the waves. I was so mortified. The beach is one of the hardest places for someone who's overweight to go. When a young boy gains weight, he tends to gain it all over, but especially in his breasts. I felt like I had the biggest breasts at the beach, not something you feel proud of if you're an eight-year-old boy. I had figured out that if I wore a tight T-shirt under my regular shirt, it would sort of hold things in.

I looked at my Uncle and said, "Okay." I didn't want to disappoint him. I left both my undershirt and my shirt on and rolled up my pant legs until they were Bermuda-short length. I slowly unwrapped the gauze, and my uncle inspected my leg. I hardly knew this man, and here he was looking at my horrible rash. I was embarrassed all over again. I finally dragged myself down to the water and got in. As I put my leg into the salty water, the sore started to sting. The pain built until it really hurt! It was almost unbearable.

I'd start to come out of the water and my uncle said, "No—get back in. You have to get rid of that rash."

And the next day, he'd make me do it again. We went to the beach every day, and by the time we packed up after our two-week vacation, my rash was gone. The salt water had healed it. And I had a golden suntan that matched my Uncle Milton's. I still have the faint marks from that rash, and to this day I never really figured out what it was.

But he packed us up in the car and took us to a secluded part

During our vacation there, I noticed that everyone called my Uncle Milton "Dick." When I asked him about this, he explained that Dick was his nickname—and that was short for his middle name, which was Richard. He had changed his name all by himself. What a great idea, I thought.

Soon—too soon—it was time to say good-bye to Uncle Milton, and I didn't want to go. I'd gotten really close to my uncle. I wrote to him often, and this was the first of several summer vacations that Lenny and I would spend with Uncle Milton in Florida. Who would have thought a rash could bring a family together!

* * *

The Name Change

Once Lenny and I were back in New Orleans, I decided it was time to have a little heart-to-heart talk with my parents. I was so unhappy with my weight that summer that I looked for a way to make some changes. But rather than changing my eating habits, which was always a toughie for me to do, I came up with an easier way to transform myself.

One afternoon, I sat my parents down at the kitchen table to talk about this name thing. That had been inspired by my Uncle Milton.

"Leonard," I asked, "do you like your name?"

"Well, sure," he said cautiously, not knowing where I was going with this line of questioning.

"And Shirley," I continued. "Do you like your name?"

"Yes, honey," Shirley replied.

"Now, ask *me*," I dared them. "Because I don't like my name. I'm not a 'Milton.' I don't want to be a 'Milton' anymore." If you looked at my initials, it was M.T. Simmons. Empty Simmons. And that's how I felt a lot of the time, very empty. The "T" stood for Teagle, which was my mother's mother's—my grandmother's—maiden name (her name was Lola Solina Teagle).

After that, my parents started calling me Dick, like my Uncle. But that was too rough-sounding to me. My mother quickly cutened that to "Dicky." She figured she had added a "Y" to my brother's name, Leonard, to make him Lenny, so she would add a "Y" to mine, too. But to make matters worse, there was a famous brand of potato chips called Dicky's Chips

each. He laid a blanket down on the sand, and told me to take

that had a factory in New Orleans. When you're overweight as I was, you don't necessarily want your name to be synonymous with a potato-chip factory. It opens all sorts of possibilities for jokes. I thought about it awhile and finally decided that I would take the name Richard, which was my Uncle Milton's formal middle name. From that day on, if anyone called me Milton or Dick or Dicky or even Moby Dick, I simply wouldn't answer. I wouldn't turn around or say anything until they called me Richard. My mother would affectionately call me Dicky, and yes, I did answer her. She could call me anything she wanted (as long as it wasn't late for dinner). Now a lot of people call me Dicky, and I don't mind it because it's kind of endearing and it reminds me of my mother. Jay Leno calls me Dicky. What's funny is that if someone calls me Mr. Simmons, I look around, wondering who they're talking to. I forget that I'm not twelve anymore. I've raced through my twenties, thirties, and forties, and now I'm fifty, but I still don't feel grown up.

So, I entered the third grade with a new name, and felt at least a little changed, although many people still called me Milton. It's very hard to change overnight.

* * *

The Name Game

By the sixth grade, everybody in my class knew that I was Mr. Diet. When you resort to eating chalk, kids tend to realize that you're on a *very* restricted food program. And restricted was all I knew—Dr. Hallman's anonymous diet.

Being overweight—being different—made those early years very rough. With every new school year, the kids got meaner. By sixth grade, I had begun to avoid every situation where I might be taunted, or worse. After the bell rang for period change, I knew I'd have to leave the safety of my classroom and walk through the schoolyard, where the guys would be waiting for me. I really didn't understand why the boys picked on me, but because I loved food, because I was fat, it meant that I was a target for ridicule and name calling. I hadn't heard the word "discrimination" before, but that's what it was.

I'd hear, "Hey, pig," and "Hey, slob," as someone tripped me, pushing me down the stairs. I knew I couldn't go home with a bruise or a cut and not have a story ready for Shirley. If I told her the truth, she would have right away gotten on the phone to the other boy's mother—a fate worse than my bruises. I wasn't a snitch.

So I lied to Shirley: "You won't believe this, mom. We were all dissecting a frog in biology class today. Sister Rose handed me the knife, and she accidentally stabbed me. See? It's my own stigmata!"

Words like "tubby" and "fat" and "porker" were tossed my way—all those nice terms used to describe overweight kids. There was another word I heard quite a bit, and that was "sissy." (Not "*si, si*"—"yes, yes"—but sissy.) The first time I ever heard that word, or what I thought was that word, was in church when the priest talked about St. Francis of Assisi. So when one of my classmates said, "Hey, Sissy!" I just answered, "Hi!" I thought he meant I was a Franciscan monk. But I knew I wasn't a monk—not yet, anyway.

And then a classmate said to me, "Do you know what that means, what they're calling you?"

"Sure, St. Francis of Assisi. You see him, and he's got all those birds and the little animals and . . . "

"No, no. That's not what it means. It's a boy who acts like a baby, who acts kind of like a girl."

Well, I guess it was just all of my energy. I wrote it off as that. But looking back, I realize I was being attacked not only because I was overweight, but also because I was not Mr. Rough-Tough. I was different and stood apart from the crowd. Once I left the relatively safe world that my parents had created for us, I was always being made fun of. But all that never really stopped me from doing anything I wanted to do, or achieving any of the goals I set for myself. It made me all the more determined. I sharpened my self-defenses, especially my crazy sense of humor.

One afternoon I had a run-in with Moose in the school hallway—remember him from the bathroom? He walked by and said, "Hey, porkhead." By this time, I was getting pretty good at deflecting the insults. I turned around and joked, "Have you ever marinated pork? You can cut little slivers of garlic and stick it into the meat. It's very tasty." He didn't know what to say then, so he'd just give me that Jack Nicholson look from *The Shining*.

I endured all and laughed it off. I used my sense of humor when I could. And this helped me make friends with some of the girls. From the very beginning, the girls never judged me. They never laughed; they never pointed a finger. Joanne, Jeanette, Gloria, and Patricia became my confidantes, my friends. They stuck up for me when they could. But I remember once when no one could help me. Then I truly understood the meaning of the word "cruelty."

It was Moose again. He caught me just outside the gates of the schoolyard. "Hey, porker." Before I could turn around, I felt this crack. He hit me in the back of the head with a baseball bat. "Maybe I can put a hole in your head and some of that fat will come out," he sneered.

I lay on the ground with my head throbbing. I couldn't get up for quite a while. A group of girls came to my aid. Fortunately there was no blood— I was just a little stunned. There was one girl, Anna, who felt the worst about it. I knew her mother was overweight, and maybe that's why she was so sympathetic. She helped me get up, and then she walked alongside me for a bit to make sure I was all right.

She whispered to me, "Tomorrow I'm going to bring you something that's going to make you feel better." Well, maybe I will be all right, I thought. Maybe she'll bake me a cake. Anna was attractive, not overweight at all. She was Italian, with dark hair and those Ali MacGraw eyebrows that grew straight across her forehead. She was the kind of girl boys looked at.

* * *

One Pill Makes You Smaller

Anna told me to meet her before class the next day in the small alleyway on the side of the school. I was there the next morning. She reached into her schoolbag, pulled out a folded Kleenex, opened it up, and there, all by itself, lay a pill—a capsule. It was half red and half yellow.

"My mom takes these. She's overweight, too. It's helping her, so maybe it'll help you."

That was all I needed to hear. If Anna's mom could lose weight with a pill, so could I. My troubles were over. She told me that if the pill worked, she thought she could get more.

I took that pill right away, before class. All of a sudden, I was bursting with energy! Earlier that morning, just walking to school had been exhausting. When you're overweight, getting anywhere can be difficult and fatiguing. One small red-and-yellow pill later, and I had energy I'd never known before. I breezed through school, rushed home, did my homework, and cleaned my room. The best part was that I really didn't have an appetite. Food suddenly didn't mean that much to me. This is what it must be like to be normal.

I rushed back to school the next day to find Anna, still inspired by the energy I had the day before. I found her in the library.

"I've *got* to have more," I begged her. "They really work."

"Oh, I knew they would," she said. "I brought you these." She pulled a small butterscotch-colored prescription bottle from her pocket. I was so relieved, I hugged her. She told me the story: Her mother kept all her medication on a tray on the vanity, next to the toilet. Anna explained to her mother that she had knocked everything over and the pills fell into the toilet and were flushed away. I thanked Anna, telling her how clever her story was and how much she was helping me.

It wasn't until I was in class, already having taken another pill, that I had time to think about Anna and her mother. Not only was I lying to myself, to the doctor, and to my parents, but now other people were lying for me. Lying to get me diet pills.

Between classes, I found a quiet corner in the hallway, making sure there was no one else around. I looked at my pills. The little bottle still had a label with Anna's mother's name neatly typed on it. I counted them: twenty-five pills. I forgot about the lies and thought instead about how much thinner I'd be in twenty-five days. One day, with the help of these little pills, I was going to be just like everybody else. I would finally fit in.

After school, I went home and hid the bottle in my record case. I knew no one would look there.

I began to take a pill every morning before school. And the pounds began to drop off. It was magic—I wasn't hungry! I could walk by McCrory's or Woolworth's and I wasn't interested in food. Every night, I'd go home and have my dinner, and after dinner when my homework was done, I'd still have enough energy for ten people. During my weekly weigh-in, my mother was so impressed with my weight loss, she'd call the rest of the family in to congratulate me. Ten pounds gone! I'd never lost

at's going to make you feel better." Well, maybe I will be all

that much before by just dieting. I couldn't tell my family the truth. They were so proud I was on my diet and "sticking to it." The lie got bigger while I got smaller.

Three short weeks later, I went to my record case, retrieved the bottle, and noticed four lonely pills rattling around in the bottom. My "prescription" was running out. I'd have to do something. I'd have to talk to Anna.

I found her in the cafeteria with a couple of other girls. I told her I needed more pills. I'd lost ten pounds and those pills were the best thing that ever happened to me. Could she get me more?

Anna told me that her mother hadn't believed her story—the pill bottle couldn't have fit down the toilet. Anna had gotten punished. And to be on the safe side, Anna's mother moved all her medication to a locked cabinet. Anna's days as a pharmacist were over. I had a sinking feeling. What was I going to do? These pills were the first thing that ever worked. I needed them. How was I going to get more? I soon found that Anna's mom wasn't the only one taking diet pills.

Three of the four girls sitting at the table told me that their mothers had a little brown bottle, too. They all volunteered to help me. The next day, I had enough diet pills to fill my bottle back up. I got pills that were black on top and had little time-release capsules in the other half. I had red ones, pink-and-white ones. I didn't know what any of them were called. All I knew is that my weight loss could continue.

Each morning, I happily popped a new colored pill and waited for the rush of adrenaline that would come a few minutes later. But every day was a new adventure because all the pills were different. One day, I'd take a pill and nothing would happen. I'd get no rush and by lunchtime I'd be ravenous. It seemed that pill had no effect on me. Another day, I'd try a red one and my heart would pound, my mind would race, and my mouth would be so dry that I'd have to keep licking my lips. The worst part was, I couldn't take a deep breath and I couldn't concentrate. The red ones were strong. I'd save those for days when I was really tired.

Then I started that philosophy—the "if" philosophy. I was losing weight, but "if" I took a couple of pills at a time, I'd lose twice as much weight. Made sense to me.

One morning, I popped a couple of those black pills in my mouth before I left the house. Ten minutes later as I headed down the street on my way to

B u t   e v e r y   d a y   w a s   a   n e w   a d v e n t u r e   b e c a u s e   a l l   t h e   p i l l s   w e r e

school, I started to sweat—a lot. I began to feel very tingly all over, and a wave of anxiety hit me that constricted my breathing. An hour into school, I was almost fainting. I felt like my heart was going to explode. I asked permission to go to the infirmary, worried I was going to have a heart attack.

The nurse, a sweet motherly woman who had no idea I'd be desperate enough to take diet pills, thought that maybe I was having an allergic reaction. She was puzzled.

"It's probably just something you ate," she said.

I couldn't tell her it was something I *hadn't* eaten. She had me rest there. Rest was the last thing I was going to get. My mind kept racing, along with my heart. It was one of the most unpleasant feelings I had ever felt. Getting cracked in the head with a bat had hurt, but this feeling was something I had done to myself. Somehow, that made it worse. I was miserable.

Lying there in the infirmary on a low couch, waiting for my heart to slow down, I made my first serious decision—the first of many I would make about my weight. I decided that this was not the way for me to go. If I were going to lose weight, I'd have to find some other way to do it.

I went home that day and got the little brown bottle from my record case. I locked myself in the bathroom, dumped the pills down the toilet, flushed, and watched as they swirled around and around in the water before they vanished. The circle was complete. In a way, Anna hadn't lied to her mother after all. The pills were flushed down the toilet. I felt better already. I would just get back on my diet and continue to lose weight. Who was I kidding?

The minute I stopped taking those diet pills was the same minute the weight started coming back. I gained a pound, two pounds, three pounds. My appetite returned, bigger and better than ever. Those pills had done nothing to either change my eating habits or permanently change my desire for food.

Before I knew it, I'd regained all the weight I'd lost, and then some. I told my mother I'd been under a lot of pressure at school while I was taking exams. I lied when it was time for another checkup and told her I had too much homework—I had to study. She must have known there was something else wrong, because she didn't push me. She canceled my doctor's appointment. It was just another example of how my family never talked about the important stuff. All those issues just slid by.

nt. One day, I'd take a pill and nothing would happen. I'd get

* *
 *

Good and Bad Habits

*D*uring this time, I was still sharing the bedroom with Lenny, and I was always being compared to him, especially when report-card time came. We'd get our cards on a Friday. Lenny would walk home with his friends, and me with mine or by myself. We never mixed our friends together. We'd get home and have dinner, and then it would start.

"Okay, let's look at report cards. Lenny?" And then they'd say, "A in English, A in Math, A in Social Studies, A+ ... " I mean, how could a child get an A+?

And then they'd ask me, "Milton, where's your report card?"

"Mother Mary Porter died."

"Oh, my God," my mother would gasp.

"Shirley, Mother Mary Porter is not dead," my father would say. "Where's your report card, Milton?"

"You know, I had a really tough, emotional semester."

"Where is it?" I'd get my report card, and he would go down the list. I was not a school person. School to me was just another performance: Curtain going up! But I really didn't do that badly when it came to my studies. I got A's and B's. I was lucky. Conduct was the problem—I always seemed to get a C.

Leonard would say to me, "Getting C in conduct is almost failing." What could I say to that?

* *
 *

But despite my behavior, all the nuns did love my family. There were the strict nuns, the Mother Agnes nuns—you couldn't get anything past them. Well, sometimes I could, at least a little bit. And then there were the young nuns who were the real vulnerable ones for me. Them, I could charm. There was one named Mother Elvira, and she was from San Antonio, Texas. She was my sixth-grade teacher and I just adored her—something between us clicked right away.

One day I came home, and my father said, "You know your sixth-grade teacher Mother Elvira?"

And I said, "Yeah?"

"Well, she quit."

"Quit? She quit what?"

"She jumped the fence."

"Jumped what fence? She jumped a fence while wearing her habit? Did she hurt herself?"

"She doesn't want to be a nun anymore. That's why she quit."

"She's not a nun anymore?"

"No. She'll be here in about an hour. She's staying a couple of days until she goes back to Texas."

An hour later the bell rang, and there was this woman. It was Mother Elvira's face, but with clothes and hair attached! The habit and wimple were gone. She came in and sat down next to me on the couch in our living room. I had just seen her in class that day, and she never said a word to me. Now, she was sitting next to me, watching television. That's how much the nuns liked my father. They trusted him so much, they would confide in him. It was amazing. Even though Leonard wasn't Catholic, not even faux Catholic, his personality attracted even the most religious people—and occasionally the ones who were in a religious funk.

★ ★ ★

Even though my father did respect the nuns and was friends with them, he would always stick up for me if he thought they were getting out of line with me.

One day in class in the seventh grade, I was acting up, as I often did. The nun, Mother Catherine, turned to me, her nerves frazzled.

"You must be retarded!" she said. "Now sit down and be quiet."

I didn't know anybody who was "retarded," but I knew what it meant. Was Mother Catherine saying that I was a little slow? Was I? Was that why I didn't fit in?

During dinner that evening, I was still thinking about what Mother Catherine had said, and I wasn't talking much.

"What's bothering you?" my father asked. "You're not doing all the talking, the way you usually do. Something must be wrong."

"Oh, it's nothing really . . . " I was terrible at hiding my true feelings. My father knew I wasn't myself.

school person. School to me was just another performance:

"Richard. Don't tell me nothing is wrong. Why are you being so quiet?"

"Well, one of the nuns said something to me today that was very upsetting."

"Oh, and I'm sure you did nothing wrong. I'm sure it just came out of thin air and you did nothing to antagonize her the way you antagonize everyone in this family. What did she say to you?"

"She called me retarded," I told him. "Do you think I am?"

My father straightened up. "Who called you that?"

"Mother Catherine."

Well, he was ablaze. "Listen to me very carefully. You're not retarded. You're special. Crazy special, but special. There's nothing wrong with your mind. Always consider yourself a special person."

I think my mother was rather shocked to hear all this, because my father was not the type to talk about such personal things, especially out loud. That word "retarded" really upset him, I think because he didn't want me to get hurt. He had spent his life trying to protect me—something I didn't realize until I was much older. But he always recognized that there was a uniqueness in me, and from the very beginning, in his own way, he tried to encourage that uniqueness.

Even though I had my difficulties in grammar school, which went up through the eighth grade, I did have a few friends. They loved to eat as much as I did and were just as mischievous, too. We were quite a group.

I would go with them every week to a magic shop on Royal Street. (It's not there anymore.) I had been selling pralines for a while, so I had some extra cash. I'd always come away with something I could try on my family.

One week it was a special pen. I brought it home and said to Leonard, "Look at the new pen I got in school." As I handed it to him, I went, "Whoops!" and ink sprayed all over his white shirt and the dining room table. Everybody just froze. Then my father went off the deep end. He started screaming at the top of his voice, yelling at me. And then the spots just vanished—it was disappearing ink. He looked down, and I started laughing. I still got sent to my room.

Well, my pranks with the magic-shop tricks didn't stop there. I bought one of those hand buzzers and took it with me when I visited my mother at Maison Blanche one day after school. I went around shaking hands with the women who worked with my mother, and with some of her customers, too. You never heard so much laughing and screaming in your entire life! They almost called a floor walker to escort me out of the store.

My favorite trick was the plastic dog doo-doo. Ready for this? I would place three little piles of doo-doo in a row at the top of the escalator on the second floor, and then I would hide with my friends behind the Ship 'n Shore blouse rack nearby and watch. People getting on the escalator would open their eyes wide and do a little dance around the piles, while my friends and I would go into hysterics. Once we were discovered, I'd grab the piles and we would run out of the store.

Plastic vomit was even better, because you could use that anywhere. A bunch of us would be at a lunch counter, and after we finished, I'd throw the plastic vomit on the counter.

"Ohhhhhh, I'm so sick from this food." *Burp.* "I'm not going to pay for this—it's so awful." And all of us would get up and stagger out of the restaurant. Once we were on the street, we'd hold our sides from laughing so much.

Well, the pranks went on for a while, but eventually I graduated to more serious things. I guess it was all those cop shows I was watching. Yes, I got into stealing. One of my friends, Jack, taught me all about shoplifting. I had never done it before. I was curious to see if I could get away with it. Could I walk into a grocery store, take a candy bar, stuff it into my pocket, and walk out—without paying? I discovered I could. I was pretty nervy.

A lot of kids go through a stealing stage when they're young, but I went way beyond that, inventing my own playful twists. To me, it was all a game. I would steal things from the religious store in my school to give to the nuns. Now that's just recycling, not stealing.

Once, I took a really beautiful Aurora Borealis rosary from the store to give to one of the nuns. I had no idea the nuns made the rosaries to sell in the shop. So I took a box I found in one of my mother's drawers at home, put some cotton in it, arranged the rosary on top, and wrapped the whole thing up very prettily. You know where this is going, right? When I gave it to the nun, I told her this was special for her because she was my favorite. When she opened it, a puzzled look came over her face.

e until I was much older. But he always recognized that there

"You know, Milton, this is very strange. I made a rosary just like this to sell in our shop." A close call. I never got caught. And I don't shoplift anymore. I don't, I really don't. Well—maybe one Kit Kat candy bar.

Off with Their Heads . . .

Even though I had stopped the shoplifting, I wasn't able to totally walk away from my life of crime—not yet. Next was my Barbie doll phase. This is almost too bizarre for words.

One afternoon I was playing with Joy Lynn at her house just down the street from mine. She brought out her Barbie doll to show me. It was the cutest thing. While we were playing, her mother called to her and told her to get ready to go to her dance lesson. Joy Lynn said I could stay and play with Barbie if I wanted. Yes, I'd stay.

When I was alone with Barbie, I took a closer look and decided she needed a haircut. I saw a pair of scissors on the desk, so I started. I snipped and snipped, and snipped a little too much. Barbie looked like she just had a hair transplant. Oh no! What had I done? I quickly thought, If I run to Woolworth's, maybe I can get another doll and no one will ever know.

Off I went. I found the Barbies at Woolworth's, and as I was looking at one, the head snapped right off in my hand. What a terrific discovery! The bodies and the faces were always the same—it was the hair that was different. I found one head with the perfect hair, the perfect bubble style. I grabbed the head and replaced it with a Ken head. That would startle an unsuspecting shopper. I made the switch with my friend's doll, and no one was the wiser about my attempts to be a hairdresser.

But this started an obsession with the heads. You've heard of the headless horseman? Well now there was a Woolworth's in New Orleans that was full of headless Barbies. And I had a drawer in my room full of them, just the heads—you know, blond bubble, brunette bubble, redhead bubble, Barbie ponytail, Barbie evening . . . I would shampoo all that hair, cut it, highlight it, tease it, iron it.

My father had a voice I called the "Stern Voice." When I heard it, I always knew I was in serious trouble. Oh, no. There it was—the "Stern Voice": "Come here! I have to show you something!"

I   w a s n ' t   a b l e   t o   t o t a l l y   w a l k   a w a y   f r o m   m y   l i f e   o f   c r i m e — n o

And I answered, "Where? Where are you?"

"I'm in your bedroom!"

I went in, and the drawer was open and all the Barbie-doll heads were spread out on my bed. There were about fifty of them.

He said, "What are those?"

"Those are Barbie-doll heads."

"Where did they come from? No, don't tell me." He gave me one of his looks, and I knew my days of stealing Barbie heads were over. That look said, "You and your Barbie-doll heads have a good time in your room tonight." He turned and slammed the door. What could I do? I certainly wasn't going to take them back to Woolworth's and say, "Oh, I just happened to find these in a drawer in my bedroom." But my father's look put an end to it. Sitting on my bed with the fifty heads, I did a little soul-searching. I said to myself, "You know, one day I'm going to push too far, and he's just going to kill me." So I stopped stealing the Barbie heads. Actually, I was running out of places to hide things. But here's an interesting side note: Did you know that they now make Barbie dolls with heads that won't pop off? I like to think that I'm responsible for that.

* * *

Where's Baby Jesus?

One year at Christmas, my friends and I came dangerously close to getting into very serious trouble. (You can guess who the instigator was.) This was the grand finale of our "borrowing" adventures.

In the beginning of December, all the Catholic churches in the quarter would begin to set up their Nativity scenes, complete with the crèche: Mary, Joseph, and all the wise men and the angels—but no Jesus. On Christmas eve at midnight mass, parishioners would march down the aisle, carrying the little Italian- or Portuguese-made ceramic baby Jesus to put in the manger. It was a big thing—everyone would wait in the pews with anticipation. Is he coming? Is he coming? Are they bringing him out?

One day in Jackson Square, over a muffuletta—a New Orleans version of a club sandwich—I said to my friends, "Oh my, wouldn't it be funny if we just went to a couple of churches and borrowed Jesus?"

And that's what we did. Early on Christmas Eve, we sneaked into the

ext was my Barbie doll phase. This is almost too bizarre for

vestibules of several of the churches in the quarter, including the huge St. Louis Cathedral, where the baby Jesuses were kept for midnight mass. There was no one around, so we grabbed the babies and ran—we must have gotten about a half dozen of them. We took them back to my house and hid them under my bed.

At six o'clock, my father always watched Mr. Huntley and Mr. Brinkley, but before that he would tune into the local news.

"Hi, this is WWLTV. There has been a terrible scandal. Someone has stolen the baby Jesuses from several churches in the French quarter." Even though my father was not a religious man, as you know, he thought this was absolutely the most horrifying thing. I was at the table pretending I was doing my homework, but I heard the television.

My father called out, "Richard, come in here and listen to this!" I walked into the living room.

Then he said, "Look at this. What kind of a sick human being, what kind of perverted person would be going around stealing the baby Jesus before midnight mass? What kind of parents do they have? What kind of morals do these people have?"

From the T.V., I looked back into my room and, much to my horror, I saw one little baby Jesus hand sticking out from under my bed.

I said quietly, "I don't know. Excuse me, dad. I'm going back to my homework."

I got on the phone and called my friends. And there we were, sneaking around at night, with Maison Blanche shopping bags full of baby Jesuses. We had a big problem: Taking them had been easier than returning them. They all looked similar, but yet they didn't. They all had the hands up with the thumb and the fourth finger touching, and both feet were kind of up. But their eyes were different—some had glass eyes, and some had painted eyes, and some heads were bigger than others. We had to match each Jesus with the other statues in each Nativity. So two of us would talk to the priest while one would sneak up to the crèche to try and match the Jesus. Sometimes it was the wrong size or the wrong eyes. Then we'd have to try another one. It was like a religious scavenger hunt. But by the time all the midnight masses started, every baby Jesus was back in His proper church.

And my father never, ever knew. But I think my brother, "Judge Judy," suspected that I had been involved.

* ✦ ✶

Tasty Little Caramels

*D*uring my last year of grammar school, the eighth grade, there was a lot of pressure. I was taking tests and I was working hard to graduate. I'd gained back all the weight I had lost taking diet pills.

One night, while I was watching television with my mother, I sat right up when I saw a commercial for a new diet product. It was candy! What could be better? I loved candy! It had the unlikely name of AYDS. I still remember that commercial. A thin, attractive woman cheerfully told me, "These tasty little caramels will melt the pounds off you." She had such an honest face. She must be telling the truth.

I asked my mom if she would let me try them. She brought a box home the very next evening. I took it immediately to my bedroom and closed the door. Carefully, I took off the cellophane wrapper and opened the lid. There, individually wrapped, were rows and rows of little caramel squares. My mother knocked on the door and peeked in to check on me.

I turned to her. "Will you try one first?" I begged.

My sweet little mother, not even five feet tall and weighing practically nothing, unwrapped a caramel, a weight-loss product, and popped it into her mouth.

"They're good," she declared. She made me read the directions—"Take one or two before mealtime to control hunger." Finally, I tried one. It was luscious.

"If this is the way to lose weight, I'm in heaven!" I had struck gold in the form of a little caramel. I could eat candy *and* lose weight doing it.

So I started out with one. But after all, it was candy. I'd have another later . . . and another . . . and another. Then one afternoon, while my mother was at work, I couldn't stop eating. I'd tried to slow down by eating a few AYDS, but I was still hungry.

And then a brainstorm hit me. I could make candied apples. I went in the kitchen with my box of caramels and I unwrapped what was left of the sixty-four little squares. I put them in the double boiler, and while they were melting, I got a few apples and some sticks. Before you knew it, I had caramel apples. They were delicious! I could treat myself to a sweet *and* lose weight. No need to feel deprived.

ld be going around stealing the baby Jesus before midnight

A week later, I had gained two pounds. I couldn't understand why I wasn't losing any weight. Could it be that my liberation from a life of diets—my delicious caramel squares—could it be that they were a false hope? I considered the possibility as I finished off one last caramel apple. I'd have to try something else.

Culinary Puberty

I was now approaching the major event in a teenager's life: puberty. But you have to realize that I was raised in a very sexless way. I never saw my parents kissing each other, except the occasional peck on the cheek. Remember when I took you on a tour of the house and I pointed out the separate bedrooms?

And this whole issue of puberty was complicated by the fact that I was fat, and fat kids don't like their bodies or think of themselves as sexy. Certainly I didn't. It didn't occur to me that anybody else would find me attractive. That's why I was always the joker, the clown, trying to amuse people so they would like me.

The only time that love was thought of in our house was in connection with food. While other kids my age began exploring their sexuality, I spent time exploring food. Food became sex for me—it became my pleasure. And my taste was maturing. Puberty for me was graduating from Thousand Island salad dressing to Caesar salads. It was like going from hot dogs and hamburgers to beef stroganoff, or from ice cream in a cone to crème brûlée. So what if my pleasure came from a grocery store, and not from another person? I never really thought to look beyond the end of my fork.

I always got along well with girls. As I've said before, they were my protectors throughout grammar school. They wanted to go shopping or to the record store, or more often than not, they wanted to go out and eat. Over a plate of french fries with ketchup, they would tell me about their boyfriends. From the very beginning of my life, it was me playing the role of brother confessor, listening to people's stories, either to lend a sympathetic ear or, sometimes, to give advice.

While other kids my age began exploring their sexuality, I

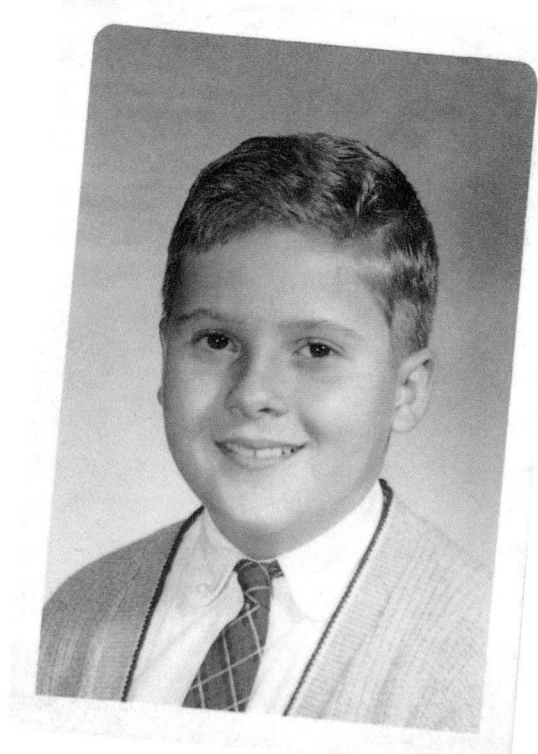

On my way to 200 pounds plus . . .

* *

Hello Motha', Hello Fatha'

igh school—the fall of 1962. By this time I had been dieting almost half of my very young life. I had started and stopped, and started and stopped. Truthfully, my parents had never made all that much of an issue over it. They'd spent a long time believing it was baby fat, saying I'd outgrow it. Well, I was still growing, but the baby fat became high-school fat, and instead of outgrowing it, I was growing out.

Sometimes, I'd get little stares at dinner when I reached for second or third helpings. My brother was notorious for the subtle throat-clearing warning. I'd reach for more twice-baked potatoes and he'd go *ah-ha-hem*. And that was supposed to make me stop. That worked about as well as if he'd kicked me under the table. He'd have to kick the fork out of my hand to get me to stop eating.

* * *

I went through a big transition going from St. Louis Cathedral—a parochial coeducational elementary school attended by a large number of students from the French quarter—to a strict, athletic-oriented all-boys high school. It was a modern, sophisticated high school with many kids from well-to-do neighborhoods. The stress was enough to make anybody want to eat. However, there was one good thing about it that sure did appeal to me—CorJesu (now called Brother Martin's) had a fabulous cafeteria. I mean, the food was great.

I had gotten used to the nuns in grammar school, and it was easy to get them on my side. Now I was going to be taught by the strict Brothers of the Sacred Heart. I was devastated that there were no girls. I just couldn't believe it. One summer I'm in the eighth grade and I've got my friends and protectors, and then all of a sudden I'm thrown into a room and it's thirty or forty guys, most of whom I've never met. But my parents wanted us to go to the best schools, so there we were. And I couldn't walk to school anymore. I had to take a public bus. It was only a twenty-minute ride away, but it was a world away from where I had grown up.

* * *

The Garbage Clown

The bus let me off right in front of CorJesu, my high school. Now I was in for four years of an all-boy high school. Just like in grammar school, the feeling of not fitting in followed me, as it had from my first day of kindergarten. I saw that the jocks were the most popular, and the rest of the student body was somewhere below them. And there I was—the token fat kid. So high school became a search for me, a search for a way to get rid of the fat and somehow fit in.

CorJesu was an expensive school. My brother had a partial scholarship, but for me, the Brothers worked out a special deal. I was to pick up garbage to help pay for my tuition. I had this pole with a nail in the end of it, and I was supposed to walk around the school yard, spearing trash. Picture me: a fat, asthmatic, flat-footed, unjockish trash picker. The first day I did this, I prayed: "Please, lightning, come my way and strike the nail and electrocute me." I was mortified. All the kids were pointing at me.

After a week or two of this humiliation, I decided I had to do something. I couldn't stand it. One morning I got to school early and hid a package in my locker. I had a plan. When the bell rang at three o'clock, I got the package out of my locker and went and found an empty classroom. Presto, I was like superman coming out of a telephone booth in his cape—except I was in a clown costume. And that's how I paraded around the school yard picking up the trash, and everybody was laughing because it was funny. To me, picking up trash was embarrassing. But as usual, I was laughing at myself before anybody else could. Being dressed as a clown camouflaged my weak self-esteem.

After I had enacted this scene for a couple of days, the principal, Brother Roland, called me in, looked at me, and said kindly, "I've made a decision. You just focus on your school work—you don't need to pick up the trash anymore. We'll find someone else to do it." I think after watching me in my clown outfit in the school yard, he figured that I had enough other issues to deal with, and maybe I just didn't need this one more thing.

Class Clown

One of the first things I found out in high school was a way to get rid of the school-yard bullies. Since my humor didn't always work and since I'd had asthma all my life, I learned to use my "funny breathing" as a crutch. When people made fun of me, I stopped telling jokes and started staging asthma attacks. So, if somebody were picking on me, I'd start wheezing.

"Hey, you big slob!"

"You talking to me?" I'd turn around, and start breathing funny.

"What's wrong? You got some kind of problem?"

"Who, me? No." Then I'd start doing more funny breathing, and finally I'd drop down in a heap, right on the concrete in the school yard. I'd pretend to pass out. Very high drama. These jocks didn't know what to make of it. Startled, they'd hurry off. I'd get up and dust myself off, no worse for the wear.

I have to admit I was a pretty easy target because I waddled a little when I walked. I was still in Stride-Rite shoes, my feet still flat as a pancake. I was

One summer I'm in the eighth grade and I've got my friends

overweight, and I wheezed because of my asthma. On top of that, I had curly hair when everyone else was wearing their hair straight with a part in the middle. And when I wasn't cracking jokes to shield myself, I was faking asthma attacks. No wonder I wasn't the most popular kid in class, but I was *always* a source of entertainment.

The worst thing about not being popular and going to the cafeteria is that no one wants to sit with you. There were a few guys who would still eat lunch with me, but I really developed a terrible habit: I'd pick food off other people's plates, with or without their permission. I used to eat so quickly that I was always the first person at the table with an empty plate. And that usually meant that I was searching for more food. So, if I were sitting next to someone still eating, I'd say, "Are you going to finish those fries?" or "Are you going to eat your pickle?" And before they could reply, I'd help myself. And, I must admit, I still do this today. I think this habit drove away my lunch mates. And that's why I'm never asked out for dinner today—especially by Lenny.

I was still a bit of the class clown, and I played it for all it was worth. That attracted some people, so I did run into some other guys who had a sense of humor, and I began to chum around with them during school. They were not necessarily fat, but each one was unusual in his own way— we each had our own little quirk or idiosyncrasy. One may have laughed a certain way, or had braces, or dressed in an unusual style. We were like the Little Rascals. If we saw a television show that was hysterical or had a really dramatic scene, we'd call each other and talk about the show. But because we traveled to school from different parts of the city, we didn't have the chance to go to each other's houses. At thirteen, we still didn't drive. If somebody was living on the other side of town, I didn't socialize with them at all. Once that three o'clock bell rang, you got on the bus and went back to your own neighborhood. No one from CorJesu lived where I did in the French quarter. Plus, I was still selling pralines, and that kept me busy after school.

* * *

The last two years of high school in some ways got tougher, because my brother went off to college at Tulane. I was always chasing after my brother, and living in his shadow. I saw him as more popular than me, with

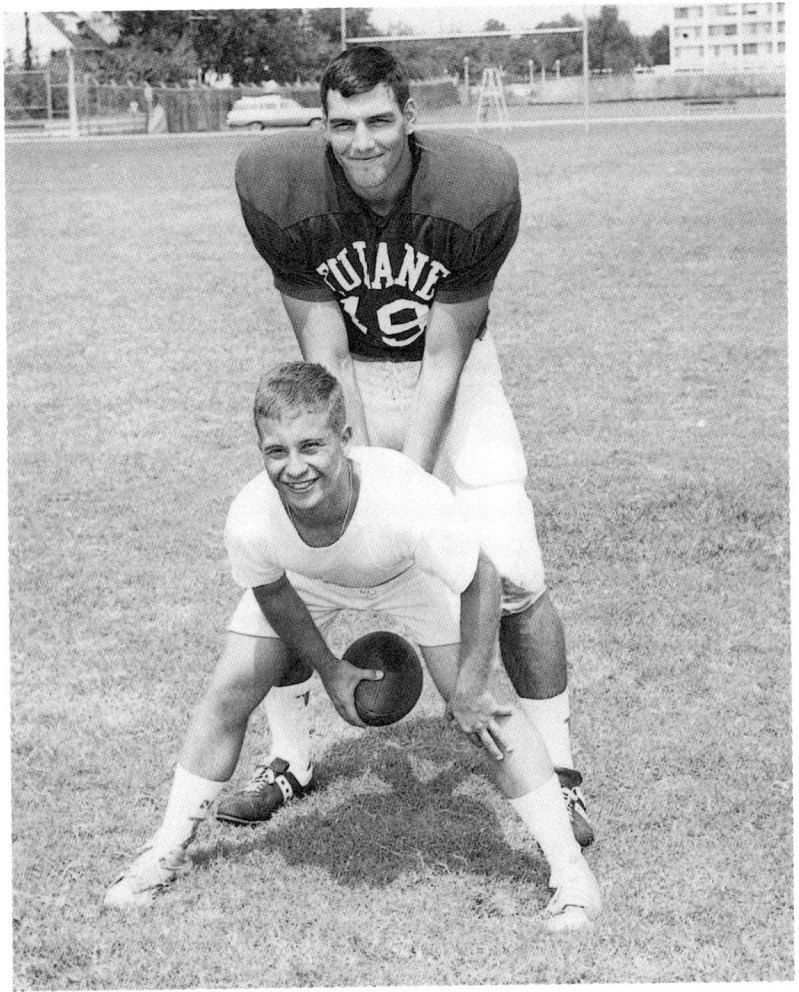

*My brother, an all-around guy, when he was manager of the
Tulane football team (he's in white)*

more friends. At Tulane, Lenny was the manager of the football team and
on the debate team and in ROTC—he was a take-charge kind of guy,
involved in everything, and busy, just like my father.

So after Lenny graduated from high school, all those years of wondering what was going to make me happy began to crowd in on me. What was
I going to do when I graduated from high school, and how was I going to
make a living? I couldn't always be the class clown. Certainly school didn't
interest me that much. But for the time being, one thing was for sure—
things were not getting any better at home between my dad and me.

* ⋆ ⋆

Button Pusher

I was still pulling off my usual stunts at home, and the antagonism between Leonard and me was getting worse.

For instance: One day, my father and I had another one of our arguments—which seemed to be happening more frequently. Who can remember what this one was about? Well, I had had it this time. I packed my suitcase and was ready to walk out the front door. My dad stopped me and told me in no uncertain terms that if I went through that door with the suitcase, I could never walk back in. When my father talked in that tone of voice, I knew he wasn't kidding.

I was really upset, and I decided I was going to have the last word. When no one was within earshot, I quietly called the Rent-All store and said we were having a surprise garden party the next day for my father, and we would need white folding lawn chairs, tables, and a white tent. I explained that I was Leonard Simmons's son—they knew who Leonard was—and could they deliver it the next afternoon, and then send the bill later to my father? They said they would take care of everything and keep it a secret. I knew that my mother would be at Maison Blanche and that my dad would be off somewhere, as he was every day.

As soon as the men arrived the next afternoon, I showed them where to set everything up, and then I went off to Leah's to sell pralines.

Later that afternoon, the phone rang at Leah's. Marie answered and then turned to me.

"It's for you. It's your father, and he sounds funny."

I walked over to Marie and took the phone.

"Hi, dad. I'm very busy here. What do you want?"

"What do I want? Guess."

"You want me to bring some pralines home?"

"No. Guess again."

"You want me to stop and get something for supper?"

"Stop. You just stop it, Richard. You get yourself home right now. Do you hear me?"

"Why?"

"Richard!"

"Okay, okay."

I could tell he was really mad. Maybe I had gone too far this time. He was waiting for me at the front gate.

"So, what are all the chairs and tables for in the backyard?"

"What?"

"The chair and tables—and the tent?"

"Someone having a party?"

"Richard!!"

Well, I had pushed him to his limit. No doubt about that. He made me fold up all the chairs and tables. Then I had to call the rental company and have them come and pick everything up. My father was getting tired of always sending me to my room. Obviously the old form of punishment wasn't working, and my behavior was really getting out of hand. So, this time he decided that I would have to pay for the rental, out of my allowance and praline money. And I still had to go to my room.

Another time as punishment, my father decided to leave me home with Victor and Hattie while he, mom, and Lenny went off for a short vacation. I can't remember what I did to get punished like that, but I'm sure it was something major.

Well, I knew how to maneuver around Victor and Hattie. I came up with a really good plan this time. I decided to put our house up for sale (remember, we didn't even own it!). If I sold the house, then I wouldn't have a room to be banished to! I made a "For Sale" sign and put it in the front yard. I straightened up all the rooms and covered everything with sheets to make it look as though we were ready to move. People saw the sign out front and actually stopped to look at the house. I explained that there had been a death in the family and that my parents were out of town making funeral arrangements, but I could show them the house. I conducted tours, pointing out the old front door, the moldings, the fancy fireplace mantel in the living room, and the French doors in the dining room.

Everything was going fine until my parents came home unexpectedly. My dad took one look at the "For Sale" sign, and he knew. Since I hadn't sold the house yet, you know where I was sent.

dad stopped me and told me in no uncertain terms that if I

*
* *

Pink Pigs

I still had a friend from St. Louis Cathedral whom I spent quite a bit of time with. Her name was Barbara, and she went to Holy Angels, an all-girl school. We'd meet at my house after school to watch T.V., usually *American Bandstand,* because her mother never let her turn that show on— too racy, I suppose. One day, Barbara invited me to her house to watch our favorite show, *Dance Party,* because her mother wasn't home. When I asked where her mom was, Barbara answered that she'd been going to weight meetings. My ears perked up.

"Where's she been going?"

"Weight meetings."

"What are the meetings called?"

"Weight Watchers."

"What kind of meeting is it?" I asked casually.

"I don't know." Barbara replied. "You should ask her."

And the next day, that's just what I did. There I was at her door, like Eddie Haskell from *Leave It to Beaver.* "Hi, Mrs. Cleaver. What a beautiful dress you're wearing." Only I had a million questions about Weight Watchers. How long had she been going? What did they do at the meetings? And most important, had she lost any weight? Barbara's mother told me the whole thing had been started by a woman named Jean Nidetch, who first held meetings in her own living room. In a short time, the organization started growing rapidly, spreading out across the country. Meetings were held in people's living rooms and in public halls. The main thing was that you weighed in at the beginning of every meeting. It was one big support group.

I was like a balloon ready to burst. I said, "Oh my God, this is great." And then I asked her—no, begged her—to take me to the next meeting.

I went home and told my parents that I was going to a Weight Watchers meeting. I was a little surprised by their reaction. They were so proud of me. Their son, on his own, had come to terms with the fact he needed to do something about his weight. In their eyes, this was such a grown-up sort of thing to do. From my perspective, it wasn't anything but going to a meeting and learning how to eat.

Barbara's mother drove us to a little building where the meetings were held. Inside, there were rows of folding chairs and a podium in the front. Over in the right-hand corner of the room, there were hospital partitions set up, and a woman sat on a stool, her legs crossed, smoking a cigarette. Next to her, she had a little file box. Since I was just observing for my first time, I took a seat as Barbara's mom went up front. As people lined up to weigh in—all women, so far—the lady on the stool thumbed through the files until she found the index card she was looking for. What I couldn't see was the scale behind the partition. The woman on the stool leaned over and took a peek at the scale as, one by one, the women weighed in. Then she'd write down the number on the index card. I watched as Barbara's mother waited her turn. She reached the front of the line and disappeared behind the partition. When she came out, she looked upset. Taking a seat beside me, she confessed she'd gained a little weight.

I felt so bad for her. All she was allowed to do was to remove her shoes. When I weighed myself at home, I had ten rules. They included: Make sure your ears are cleaned, nails clipped, hair absolutely dry, no gum, don't be holding anything, make sure the scale is firmly on zero, plus a few others I won't go into here. Barbara's mother never stood a chance.

After the weigh-in, the Weight Watchers leader stood up. This was a woman who had already lost weight on the program.

"Hi, I'm Sally, and I've been with Weight Watchers since 1961, and I'd like to welcome you all . . . " she chirped happily.

So far things were going pretty good, although I was the only guy there. I was also the only teenager. Then Sally became like a high-school principal. She pulled out a piece of paper with everyone's name on it. Suddenly, the mood in the room shifted, and you could feel the tension. Now it was report-card time.

One by one, she called each woman to the front. "Peggy has lost two pounds!" Sally would exclaim. The crowd would clap, and Peggy would receive a star that she pinned to her lapel. Barbara's mother, on the verge of tears, twisted in her seat beside me.

Sally continued to call out names and hand out stars. Then she fell silent for a moment. The room hushed along with her. Finally Sally said, "Now here are the people who have stayed the same. I want you to remember," she reminded us, "it's good to stay the same. For gosh sakes, it's not like you've gained weight. Maybe next week the scale will be your friend. Sadie, come on up here."

Sadie came to the front, and Sally pinned a turtle onto her. Turtle after turtle was pinned, until there was only one woman left. Wouldn't you know it, I had to be with the one lady who'd gained weight that week. Finally, Barbara's mother was called. Like a death march, she trudged to the front of the room, and Sally pinned a pink pig to her. Sally announced to everyone that Barbara's mother had gained 2½ pounds. She walked back to her seat with her head down. It was a sad Weight Watchers moment. I held her hand. She looked over at me for a moment, and then she said something that I'll never forget: "You better do something about your weight now, because it only gets worse later in life. Catch it now, before it's too late."

I'll never forget the look of shame on her face. Here was this happy lady, and one trip to the scale and twenty minutes later, she's crying, her mascara is running down her cheeks, and she has a pig on her shoulder. I knew from past experience that this system of reward and punishment probably wasn't going to work for me.

Barbara's mom drove me home. She was very quiet, and I could tell the meeting had really upset her. She had removed the pig from her shoulder before we'd even left the meeting. I asked her if she was going back. She told me that she was desperate and she had to do something. I felt so sorry for her. It's funny, because I was probably heavier than she was, and yet I felt the need to give her a pep talk, to try to make her feel better about herself again. Before I even realized what I was saying, I asked her if she wanted to be my partner, my Weight Watchers buddy.

Her face lit up. It was worth it to see the change in her. She gave me the list of foods and the instructions that went with them. We decided that next week she'd take me for my first weigh-in.

I'd call Barbara's mother every day, and we'd take turns listing what we'd eaten all day. We got to be very friendly. The next meeting, the same people, the same chairs, and the same scale were all there. But something was different. Barbara's mother had lost two pounds! She was thrilled and almost ran to the front to get her star when her name was called.

I weighed in for my first time, determined never to get a pink pig. The next week, Barbara's mother had lost another pound. I collected my first turtle, telling myself I was just off to a slow start, and I would get better. But what I did, in fact, was to return to my old habits I had formed with Dr. Hallman. I'd eat all week, and then two days before the meeting, I'd stop eating altogether. And then afterward, I knew I'd return to eating all the things that I'd given up.

I really liked going to the meetings. I liked Barbara's mom, and I liked the other women who stood up and told their stories. They'd talk about their obstacles and fears, what they ate or what was eating them. "My mother-in-law got sick and moved in with us," or "My husband used to love me. Now he's never home." It was a loving, supportive environment where these women could pour out their hearts, as if it were a Weight Watchers talk show. But while I listened to these women, I came to the realization that I wasn't really learning anything.

Two months later, I realized something else. I was now a pig collector. Every Monday, I had a date with Barbara's mom, and we'd go to a Weight Watchers meeting. I was helping her by being her buddy. For her, it was a team effort. But for weeks, it had been a one-person team, because I was lying again. I would eat what I wanted during the day, and then when I talked to her at night, I would read from the sheet and tell her I'd eaten a perfect Weight Watchers meal. The scale was the only one that wasn't lying. So each time I went to a meeting, I would gain. And gain. One day, as I was sitting in my room looking at my bulletin board filled with all the little pigs, I decided I couldn't bear to get another one. I had to continue the lie. I called Barbara's mother and told her I had a fever—my parents wanted me to stay home and I couldn't go to the meeting. When the next Monday rolled around, I told her I was studying for a final exam. I think by then she knew, because I'd barely spoken to her all week.

I wish I could have been honest and told her that I had been doing it for her, and that I wasn't doing it for me. But I felt like I was an embarrassment to her. But what was harder was the thought of facing Barbara. I ran into her at Walgreens in the nut aisle.

"Why haven't you called my mother? Why aren't you going to the meetings with her? You hurt her feelings, and you really let her down." That was the last time I spoke to Barbara. The fact of the matter was, everything she said to me was true.

+ *

A Catholic? Oy!

y father had always said that I could be baptized when I was a senior in high school. When I entered my last year of high school, I arranged for the big day—my baptism. I was eager to finally be like everyone else at CorJesu and end the faux part of Catholic life. Finally, I was going to be a legitimate Catholic! My brother Lenny didn't feel the calling as strongly as I did. He was baptized two years after I was, when he was eighteen and already in college.

For me, the baptism ceremony was my entry into a life with deeper meaning, and I continued to think about what I would do after graduation. Toward the end of my senior year in high school, I decided to explore a whole new calling: I was thinking of becoming a priest. Yes, a priest. Does that surprise you? Well, twelve years of Catholic school had been good training, and I did have this history of being faux Catholic.

But remember, religion was never discussed in our house, and there were conflicting messages. For instance, in the living room we had a menorah—the Jewish candle holder to celebrate Hanukkah. I had no idea what a menorah or Hanukkah was. To me, the menorah was just a candlestick holder—it was very ornate and very heavy.

Finally, an event happened—actually a trip—that revealed to me more clearly my religious roots. My mother came from a large family and I had heard her talking about her sister Marion, my aunt. But I knew we had all these fake Aunts and Uncles who came to visit us in New Orleans, so I didn't think Aunt Marion was for real.

Aunt Marion supposedly lived in New York, on Mosholu Parkway in the Bronx. I begged and begged to go see Aunt Marion. I'd play these scenes as if they were out of old black-and-white movies.

"I have no relatives. I know nothing about anybody. I'm feeling very alone."

My father shouted, "Stop. Stop. I've heard enough. Send him. Send him to Aunt Marion. Let Aunt Marion have him for a couple days."

So I went off to meet my relatives in the Bronx and visit the World's Fair—and see Barbra Streisand (but more about Streisand later). This was 1964, and I was sixteen.

I was Catholic. Bobby told me that wasn't so—that I was Jew

Aunt Marion was a very colorful, very upbeat woman, always smiling, very chatty. She was very different from my mother. She had a whole bunch of different jobs. One of them was working as a demonstrator for the Oster Blender Company. She'd go to Macy's department store at lunch time, make egg creams and malts in the blender, and then hand out little paper cups of free samples.

While I was staying at Aunt Marion's, I met three of my cousins: Bobby, Louis, and Janice. One afternoon I was talking with them, and Bobby began describing a bar mitzvah. Bar mitzvah? I had no idea what he was talking about. Bobby explained about this ceremony in the Jewish religion that takes place when a boy turns thirteen. I said I didn't know anything about the Jewish religion. I was Catholic. Bobby told me that wasn't so—that I was Jewish. His mother and my mother were sisters, and they were Russian Jews. I might have been going to a Catholic school, but my background was definitely Jewish.

Well, I didn't know any Jewish people in New Orleans. All I knew were Catholics. I was surrounded by Catholics. There were Catholics at the bake sale, Catholics at school, Catholics at church. No one had ever said "dreidel" to me. No one had said "kugel." There was no religion at our house except: Be nice to people, Don't steal, or I'll break both your hands next time.

So, it was a little bit of a shock finding out from my cousins that I was Jewish. But now I had everything: guilt, nuns, bagels, kugel—it was the best of both worlds.

When I returned to New Orleans and confronted Leonard and Shirley with a hundred questions about my Jewish relatives, they told me we couldn't talk about it because no one outside the family would understand. What was there to understand? I came from a family whose history I was just beginning to learn about at age sixteen. No problem!

For me, going to church, in addition to being sacred, was truly the first place I found out that God really didn't care if you were fat nor not. You know, there were just fat people, thin people, tall people, short people. You all went in and you took communion and lit candles. And you sang songs. It was teamwork. To me it seemed very nonjudgmental.

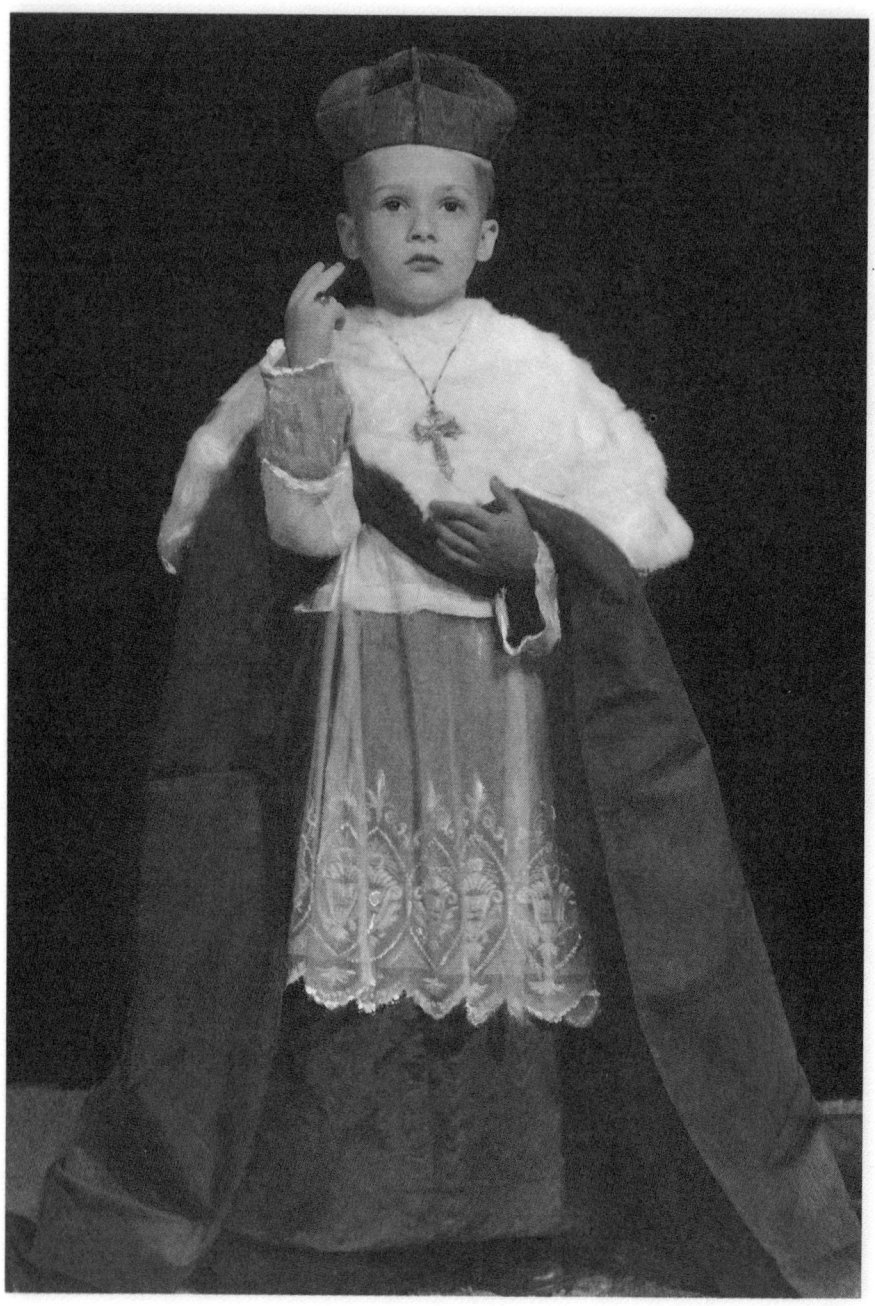

A blessing in disguise

I had all the moves down—waving my hand, looking solemn,

Leonard for some reason, however, had this fascination with the Catholic Church. My brother Lenny tells the story that when he was born, our father Leonard wanted him to be baptized Catholic. To this day we really don't know why, unless for some strange reason he thought that being a Catholic would make life easier for Lenny. Leonard called the parish priest and told him that he would like his newborn son baptized as a Catholic. He explained to the priest that neither he nor his wife were Catholic. The priest asked a few questions—and then hung up on him. This may be the reason why my father never went to church. But he still wanted the best education for his boys, so this experience with the priest didn't prevent him from sending us to Catholic school.

Probably one of the funniest events during grammar school that hinted at my later-to-blossom interest in becoming a priest involved my becoming a cardinal—no, I didn't dress up as a bird. I dressed up in red robes. Every year at St. Louis Cathedral, there was an elaborate coronation pageant, and one year I was in it. Students were picked to be a king and queen, and they were crowned by a cardinal during the beautiful pageant. In order for you to be either king or queen, it seemed that your parents needed to have done something special for the school. My friend Connie's parents were antiques dealers, and one year they donated a huge chandelier to be auctioned off at church for the school. So Connie became the queen for the pageant. Although my parents hadn't done anything extraordinary for the school, they often worked at the school bazaars and other functions, and as I told you, the nuns really adored my parents and me. As a reward for my parents' good works, I think the nuns just decided I would be the cardinal. So there I was, in the pageant, dressed in this adorable cardinal outfit. I had all the moves down—waving my hand, looking solemn, letting people kiss my ring, and making the sign of the cross. When queen Connie knelt down in front of me to kiss my cardinal ring, for some reason she bit my finger—I guess to be funny. But I really knew she was jealous, because my outfit was so much prettier than hers. Well, I wasn't going to let her get away with that, so I kicked her. She fell over, with a very big scream that drowned out the music. I hollered out, "It's okay. She just had a vision. But she's all right now." And I helped her up. It all happened so fast. So that was my short-lived elevation to the rank of cardinal. I was six then. But the event marked the beginning of my fascination with men of the cloth.

I really *did* look great in the cardinal's outfit. As a matter of fact, it took my parents three hours to convince me to take the robes off.

"Take those robes off. The pageant is over."

"No. No. I won't. I'm still the cardinal."

"Take it off."

"No. Don't touch me."

"Take that ring off. That whole outfit has to go back to the rental place."

"No, I want to keep it. Kiss my ring!"

Well, you can guess the ending. The cardinal was sent to his solemn chamber!

When I was in grammar school, I always wanted to try preaching. Often I would be in the St. Louis Cathedral all by myself. It would be early in the morning, when the church was being cleaned, and I would sit there, dreaming about preaching and becoming a priest. In the front of the church was a huge pulpit. It was so beautiful, like a huge, wooden bird cage. You had to climb a winding staircase to get to the top. When the priest was up there, he seemed very holy—he was so high off the ground.

One morning when I was there by myself, I just couldn't resist. I think it was the hand of you-know-who that nudged me. I walked quietly over to the pulpit, looking over my shoulder, making sure no one was watching. And then I climbed those stairs. When I got to the top, the view was just amazing. And there was a stand there with a little light, where the priest would put his sermon. There was a Bible and some pencils. Being up there was a little like being *Evita*—if I had stretched out my arms . . . It really was very powerful. I said to myself, I think I can do this. I can help change people's lives. I'm very good at talking and listening to others. In fact, next to eating, this is what I've had the most training for. I've been in Catholic school all this time. I mean, I knew the stations of the cross by heart. I knew the stories. I could take some Matthew, some Mark, a little Luke, and a sprinkling of John—I could take some subject and just go off on a tangent. I had seen *Elmer Gantry*. So when you put all this together, it made sense that I wanted to be a priest. But I didn't want to do the tent thing, a revival with the chairs and all that. And I wanted to be a little more flashy than the Brothers of the Sacred Heart at my high school. They wore brown—a very brown ensemble. And you already know how I feel about khaki. Next to khaki, brown was my least favorite color. One of the Brothers wore a sash around his waist with lots of keys. I had no idea what they were for—maybe one of them was the key to Heaven. But still, for me, I wanted something a little more exciting.

Once, I went with my brother Lenny to another church run by the Dominicans, and their robes were gorgeous. A Dominican I could be, I thought. The Dominicans wore black and white. And I was called Penguinette in school, so this was all beginning to fall into place. It was a sign.

During my senior year, my whole class went on a three-day religious retreat to a monastery outside of New Orleans. While there, we weren't allowed to talk. We were to "spiritually cleanse" ourselves and decide what we really wanted to do with our lives. Only once before in my life had I tried to be quiet. When I was in grammar school, I decided that I wanted to change and be like everyone else—because I really stood out, and sometimes I got tired of that. So, in school one day I tried to be quiet, and that lasted all of fifteen minutes. I fell asleep and I cracked my head on the desk. I just couldn't do it.

So for me to be quiet during this retreat was a real challenge. I had my own teeny little room with a teeny bed, a crucifix, and a little wooden cabinet. That was it. What this place needed was a little fluffing up by Martha Stewart. The class took walks together. We had seminars on religion and the Bible. We just listened, soaking up as much as we could, without saying a word. After all this, I could hardly wait to eat.

Well, we couldn't speak during dinner. After the meal, we had to say the rosary. This was one of the few times we could talk during the three days. It was hard, not being able to talk, but it did give me time to think.

I really had no idea what I was going to do with my life. But there was one thing that struck me about the retreat: No one told any "fat" jokes. It was really very intense, and you felt that you had some purpose. You felt that people respected you. So I began to think that if I chose a career that people would respect, maybe they would look right past my weight and not make fun of me.

Soon after the retreat, we had a vocational day. Actually it was a recruiting day. Representatives from the Army and the Navy came and set up their booths. There were businessmen there, too.

"Hi, I'm Barry. I'm from the Marines. And I want you." I don't think so, Barry.

The Dominican Brothers had a special booth, and I had already made an appointment. I was so excited to meet the Brothers that I arrived fifteen minutes early. Brother Joseph stepped out from the booth and introduced himself. He ushered me to a chair, and we began. As we talked, I kept looking at Brother Joseph and thinking about those loose robes. You could eat all day and no one would know. The robes were expandable, and this was long before Totie Fields muu-muu dresses. It was perfect for me.

Brother Joseph asked me, "Why do you want to be a Brother? What do you think you'll do, and how will you help people?"

I was off and running. And I was so enthusiastic about wanting to do all this, wanting to help people, because I thought it was my destiny. I got up and did little excerpts of what I had learned when I was in school. I recited little moral stories that I had practiced from the pulpit in St. Louis Cathedral. All this was probably my own version of Leonard's vaudeville routine. On and on I went. You can imagine how theatrical I was.

Brother Joseph was impressed. He said that he thought I would make a really good candidate for the brotherhood because my heart was in this and I loved people. He told me I could come to the monastery for a second interview. So we scheduled it, and I went to meet a whole crowd of the Brothers. I liked this. We talked for a while. All the Brothers got along with each other, and I had a very good feeling about the monastery.

Then one of the Brothers took out a box of robes.

"Do you take a small, medium, or large?"

"I don't know."

He pulled out an XL, and I tried it on. Not bad. Roomy.

Then he said, "How tall are you?"

"Why do you ask?"

He took out a tape measure.

"Wait a minute? What's that for? You going to measure my waist? I thought you weren't here to judge me!"

"Well, we still need to measure you."

"For what?"

"The coffin."

"A coffin? I beg your pardon. You want to know how tall I am for my coffin?"

"Well, we always like to know these things, just in case." I was a bit horrified. It was just a little too much Addams Family for me. The pulpit–bird cage thing in St. Louis Cathedral was a lot more fun than what this meeting was turning into. So I told the Brothers I needed to rethink this whole thing about the Brotherhood, and I would get back to them.

Over the next couple of days, the more I thought about my calling, I began to realize that it wasn't going to work for me. Sitting in a monastery without talking? Having my coffin already made and waiting for me? I called Brother Joseph and told him that my dedication was weakening, and I was going to put this decision on hold.

* * *

Taste of Camp

For high-school graduation, my classmates got cars, cameras, money. Not me. I got a trip to Camp Miniwonca on Stoney Lake, Michigan. My dear, saintly brother (who was a counselor there) thought it would be a great graduation present for my parents to send Dicky there for the summer. I pleaded with Lenny not to tell our parents how much he loved it. For him, camp was almost a religious experience.

But no. He wouldn't listen to me. He told them, "Oh, it would do him so much good. It's great. There's fourteen tribal teams, including the White Eagles and the Red Cherokees. There's a lot to do, and it's coeducational." My brother loved that camp. I had visions of him eventually buying the whole place and moving us all up there to live!

I lost. So before I knew it, I was at camp.

The camp was coeducational, so we did have a lot of activities together, and as usual, I made friends with many of the girls. There was archery— please! Me and archery? Maybe if they had painted pictures of pies or pieces of cake on the target instead of stripes—or used edible arrows—I would have been more interested.

We had scavenger hunts. Just as Lenny had described, we broke up into our tribes, dressed in our special Indian outfits with feathers, and we had to find things like a dried snake skin, a bluebird feather, a maple leaf, and rabbit droppings—well, maybe not the droppings, but it was almost that bad. If I were organizing the scavenger hunt, you'd have to bring back things like a prime rib, a rack of lamb, and a honey-baked ham. After a while, I just couldn't take it, so I stopped going to a lot of the activities. It was as simple as that. What were they going to do to me? Send me home? I wish!

During my second week there, I encountered the ritual of the s'mores. One night, I went to visit some of the girls in their house on the lake, and it was empty. I looked out the back windows, and there they were—all the girls huddled around a campfire. It was a cult! My family had sent me to a cult camp! I hid in the bushes, watching. The girls were laughing and waving sticks with marshmallows stuck onto the ends. On the ground were open boxes of graham crackers. Wait! Were those chocolate bars? I might like this cult. My friend Cindy heard me stepping on a branch. She turned around, and when she spotted me, she said, "Come over here." I did.

"Have you ever had a s'more?"

"A snore?"

"No. A s'more."

"A s'more? What's that?"

"Here. Let me show you. Get a little closer." Once again, I felt like I belonged. She put two marshmallows on sticks near the flames, not so close that they would burn, but close enough so they started to turn golden and get all puffy. One of the other girls had already placed a chocolate bar on one of the graham crackers. When the marshmallows were just perfect, Cindy slid them onto the chocolate bar, placed another graham cracker on top, and gently squeezed them together, squishing the hot marshmallows and melting the chocolate. I took a bite—the chocolate ran down the sides of my mouth and the marshmallow was warm and creamy, and the graham crackers held it all together.

I sighed, "Life is beautiful. This is God's sandwich."

When it came time to leave the camp, to tell you the truth, I cried. Even as horrible as the place was, I really did make some nice friends.

But now I had to get serious about school, and what I was going to do about the rest of my life.

College Years, Act I

The summer following my senior year in high school was fast coming to an end, and it would soon be time for me to go off to school.

Decisions about college had been made. The first hurdle was the money—there were not a lot of extra dollars in our family.

During high school, in addition to visiting my Uncle Milton in Florida, I wrote him from time to time, telling him how excited I was about going to college, even though I still hadn't figured out what I wanted to study. And I didn't know how we were going to pay for it. In the middle of all this worry, the phone rang one Sunday, and it was Uncle Milton. He talked to my father for a while, and then Leonard handed the phone to me.

Uncle Milton and I talked about my education and what I was going to do. Finally he said that I shouldn't worry about anything. He was going to pay for the whole thing. A week later, a check came in the mail. Uncle Milton was the first of many angels who would magically appear throughout my life, just at the right moment when I needed them the most.

The question now was, What was I going to study in college? I knew I liked art. Over the years, my father had taken me to all the museums in New Orleans, and he had taught me about different artists. I had taken a few art classes in grammar school and high school, and I enjoyed them. So I had this idea that maybe art was something I could do. There certainly wasn't anything else that held my attention. Math? Physics? I don't think so.

I had heard that the Rhode Island School of Design was a great place, and I decided that's where I wanted to go. Absolutely not, said my parents. I guess it was too far away and probably cost too much. My parents wanted me to go to Tulane—that's where my brother was. I suppose they thought that he could keep an eye on his brother, and as a result, things might be a little easier for me. Well, Tulane was a jock school, and I'd be following in my brother's footsteps again. So I said no to that. Back to the drawing board.

And speaking of drawing boards, my parents had heard that the University of Southern Louisiana in Lafayette had a great Fine Arts department: painting, sculpture, drawing, all that—and it was only a two-hour drive from New Orleans. Classmates had told me that the food there was good—plus there were a lot of restaurants in Lafayette. Suddenly, it was sounding better to me.

We all agreed that's where I would enroll. My major would be art, and I chose two minors: art history and English. I figured if I was going to paint, I'd better be able to talk about it.

belonged. She put two marshmallows on sticks near the flames

⋆ ⋆ ⋆

So off to U.S.L. I went. I couldn't wait. It was the beginning of my new life. This was college, with beautiful ivy-covered buildings and rolling lawns and people carrying books, talking in hushed tones. Everyone would be mature and dressed in nice neat clothes. And I would finally find respect from peers. It would be like a scene from the movie *Paper Chase.*

Then I moved into the dormitory. This was not the movie I'd expected. I was in the middle of *Animal House.* The dorm was all male—a jock dorm. I was assigned a single room with no roommate—thank goodness. It was a cubicle—a small, square, cinder-block room, painted beige, and not too much different from what I imagined a prison cell to be like.

Here, I learned quickly about "dorm food." By the third week of college, every paper I did was covered with food stains. Homework and eating were my new double major. Peanut butter and jelly, sub sandwiches, and pizza were at the top of my list. With no kitchen or hot plate available, I had two choices. I could eat in the cafeteria, which was not to my liking. Or there were four pizza places, a sub shop, and a few hamburger stands nearby. This was my introduction to fast food, only it wasn't called fast food back then. It was called "to go," as in pizza-to-go, subs-to-go, and burgers-and-fries-to-go. And "to go" meant bringing the food back to my dorm room, where it kept me company. I also spent a lot of time with the Colonel—we became very good friends. I loved the batter on the K.F.C. chicken, and even though it was fried, I told myself that eating chicken was healthier than pizza. So my diet consisted of hamburgers, hot dogs, french fries, onion rings, pizza, and poor boys. I was always eating—either snacking on the run between classes, or creating mini-banquets in my little room.

I kept myself very busy, studying and going to classes. I tried to leave the dorm as early in the morning as I could and return very late in the evening, so I wouldn't have to deal with the jocks. But I still got into trouble. It was just like I was a piece of raw meat, and the lions were there to devour me. I'd be studying late at night, munching away on a hamburger, and they would fill trash cans with water and pour them under my door. One time they even sprayed lighter fluid on my metal door jamb and set it on fire. Nice, eh? Well, once again I was the fat kid who stood out. At least in high school, I hadn't had to live there. Here, I was in dorm-hell. My parents quickly figured out that something was not quite right, so they told me I could come home on weekends.

I had other problems. College was harder than I expected, not because of the work, but because of all the walking to get from class to class. This was the first time I'd had to walk more than three blocks to go anywhere. It seemed I was always out of breath. But luckily, there were always places to stop and rest, and even get a bite to eat while I sat.

Besides the weight, there was something else that made me stand out in a crowd: my hair. Back then, everybody had straight hair with a part on the side—except me, of course. It's very, very hard to part an Afro. So the first thing I did when I moved into the dorm was go to the drugstore and buy a bottle of hair straightener. That's right, I straightened my hair. A whole bottle of hair straightener and a few hours later, there I was with my new look. Only, I had to put this gel on it every night and then comb it all the opposite way. I'd sleep on it like that, wake up the next morning, and then comb it all back the other way. After all that work, it would be straight and with a part. That is, of course, unless it was humid, which it was almost every single day. Five minutes later, my hair would frizz up and the part would disappear.

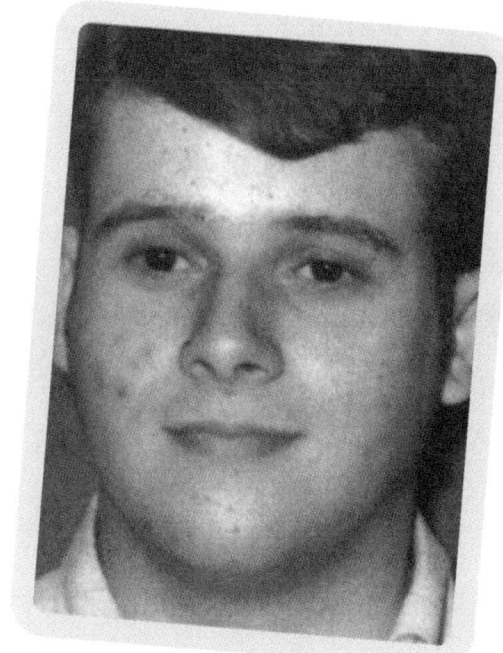

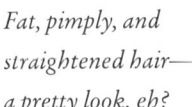

Fat, pimply, and straightened hair— a pretty look, eh?

And there was my skin: My fried-food-and-grease diet did not make for a beautiful complexion. Since I had never eaten like this before, I discovered pimples. I woke up one morning, after having snacked my way through an entire pepperoni pizza by myself the night before, and glanced in the mirror. Horrors! There were bumps all over my face! No, they were not bumps. They were mountains! I could almost hear Julie Andrews in *The Sound of Music* singing, "The hills are alive . . . " How much more could I take?

Now I was forced to use Clearasil, a flesh-toned cover-up for blemishes. Since I was compulsive about eating, I tended to be compulsive about everything. So, I'd begin with a dab here and there, and then decided I needed more to even it out. I ended up building layers of the putty-like cover-up. It looked great as long as I didn't smile or move a single muscle in my face. Otherwise, the Clearasil would crack and I'd end up looking like a "House of Wax" creature in an old Vincent Price movie.

But you know, other than my horrible jock-dorm life, breathlessly walking from class to class, and having funny hair and bad skin, I really liked the school. I loved my courses, and I loved the other art students. This was the first time I enjoyed what I was doing. I was good at painting and drawing, and at U.S.L. I learned a little about everything. It was like a buffet: a little papier-mâché-ing, a little acrylic painting, a little oil painting, a little sculpting. I loved it. And the art history—it was fascinating to me because all these famous artists started out as little kids who went to school and took courses, just like I was doing.

With my fellow art students, I discovered that they didn't care what I looked like. It reminded me of going to church when I was in high school—God didn't care if you were fat.

I was beginning to realize who I was and that I was good at certain things. I could paint and draw, and I was funny. This was who Richard Simmons was, and I wasn't going to change that. I was finally beginning to enjoy being me.

Until I went away to college, I didn't really have to shop much for clothes, since I always wore the same uniforms in grammar school and high school. But college was a different story. I had no uniforms to depend on. And now I had to shop for my clothes. I hated shopping for myself and trying on clothes. Even to this day, I hate it. Shopping for others—now that's a differ-ent story. I love buying clothes and gifts for friends.

While I was at U.S.L., I met a girl named Mindy, and we became good friends. She changed the way I dressed. Mindy was from the East, some-where in New York, and she had come to U.S.L. because the art program was good. Mindy and I were on the same eating tempo. She was short and in the same two-hundred-pound range that I was. But she flaunted it. She was very bohemian, designing and making her own clothes: long skirts and overalls. I loved her overalls. She smoked and said lots of words that girls were not supposed to say. And she was very funny. She was a brilliant artist: She could sketch, she could paint, she could sculpt. Her stuff was very different and progressive. We just seemed to hit it off.

Mindy lived with a bunch of other girls in a house only a block from my dorm, so I would spend a lot of time visiting there.

One day she said to me, "Here, try on a pair of my overalls."

I did, and they didn't look all that bad. She stuck a few pins here and there to make them fit better, and that was it.

A couple of days later she called. "Stop over. I've got a surprise." She had made me a pair of overalls out of some bright polyester material. I loved them because they were so comfortable. I had the silhouette of a farmer, and in those bright colors, I looked like a box of Crayola crayons. I had her make me a few more pairs, and they became my new uniform.

Mindy surfaced again briefly in my life, much later. When I was doing my own television show, *The Richard Simmons Show,* I got a letter with no return address. It was from Mindy. She said, "Look at you now! Remember me? I made you overalls when we were at U.S.L. And look, you're still wearing them. I'm very proud of you. I knew you were going to do some-thing really good with your life." The postmark was New York. I called information, but there was no telephone listing for her. The note was just her way of saying to me that once we had both been at the same place. Then one day she turned on the television and saw me wearing overalls, but now they were smaller. It was a very sweet letter.

I also became very friendly with another girl at U.S.L.—she was in one of my classes. Her name was Mary Lee Lecour, and she was beautiful. She had

things. I could paint and draw, and I was funny. This was who gorgeous Breck blond hair and was all smiley-faced. Her father was a prominent businessman from Louisiana, and everyone wanted to go out with her. Well, we just started to hang out together. She had this great car with a push-button automatic transmission, and she would let me drive it. It took me a while to figure out what the "R" and "D" meant. I thought how cute! R for Richard, and D for Dicky. We had a lot of close calls when I drove. Remember, I didn't know how to drive, and I didn't have a license.

Everyone was puzzled about why Mary Lee would want to hang out with me. People thought she could have anyone she wanted. Well, there were other things that were more important to her than looks. She told me one day, "You know, Richard, you're funny and very easy to be with. I like that a lot."

We finally got to a point, however, where she looked at me, and I knew she wanted to be romantic. I could tell it was heading in that *Love Story* direction, and I just couldn't figure it out. My whole life I was trying to understand why someone would be attracted to me. Why would anybody want to be intimate with me? I just couldn't figure it out. Well, *The Love Story* thing never happened, and we stayed friends.

A couple of months ago I was in Houston, Texas, where Mary Lee now lives. During a radio program I was doing, the interviewer asked me, "Who was the first girl you ever really liked?" I mentioned Mary Lee's name, saying she was the first girl I thought about marrying, and that she now lived right there in Texas. It was a very popular show, so of course everyone who was listening and who knew Mary Lee called her right away with the news that I was in town talking about her. At the next radio station I went to, there was a message from Mary Lee, with her phone number. I called her and we reminisced.

It's ironic how the two most important girls from U.S.L. resurfaced later in my life.

* ⋆ *

College Years, Act II

I spent two years at U.S.L., and I loved the art courses—I loved them as much as I loved eating. But I had other plans. I decided I wanted to go to Europe to study art, so I needed to find a school that had an exchange program, since U.S.L. didn't. After a little bit of hunting, I discovered that Florida State University in Tallahassee had a couple of programs, including one in Florence.

So, I convinced my parents that Florida State had a far superior art department than U.S.L., not mentioning anything about the exchange program, of course. My parents were already slightly bewildered by their baby boy with his straight hair and acne. I didn't want to worry them further by telling them that not only was I changing my look, I was also changing countries. I knew I had to take it one step at a time.

I made the switch, and all of a sudden I was in Florida, at Florida State University, living in Cash Hall. Thank you, Uncle Milton! It was the first coeducational dorm in the South. The school was expensive, and the dorm was gorgeous. The building had four wings, two assigned to male students and the other two to females. The wings formed a square with an interior courtyard sporting an Olympic-size swimming pool.

There were girls in my life again, and they were nearby. I was so relieved! I couldn't have been happier, all the while knowing that this was just a stopping place on my way to somewhere more exotic.

I had wonderful teachers. There was Gabrielle Dempsey, who taught me illustration and composition, and her husband Bruce was a teacher, too. I would often go to their house for dinner. They live in Florida now, and have children who look like works of art. I still keep in touch with them. Anne Kirn was another one of my illustration instructors, and I got to know her, too. This was part of my pattern again. I was always comfortable with people older than me, although at this point I felt I was starting to fit in more with my peers.

I was wearing more colorful overalls, and I was becoming identified as part of the art-student crowd. We were eccentric and strange, and we were accepted for it. We were Bohemians, pre-SoHo. I was still short, overweight, Catholic, and Jewish, but none of that mattered, because now I was an artist.

Another thing was happening. Although girls had always been my best friends and still were, I was starting to be more comfortable around guys my own age—the artistic ones, at least. I discovered that there were males who were created for other things besides beating up fat kids.

h me. People thought she could have anyone she wanted. Well,

I began to do more research on the foreign-exchange programs offered by the University. There were three.

The first was in England. I was tempted, mostly because I already knew the language, and it would be one less thing to struggle with. But on the downside, I also knew the food was horrible. My father had very few cookbooks with British recipes. The thought of kidney pie was enough to make me say no to England.

The second program was in Germany. Let's just say I'm not a schnitzel person, and leave it at that.

The third was in Florence, Italy. I knew right away—that was it for me! Every Italian dish I could think of made my mouth water. When it comes to food and love, the Italians really know what they're doing! The decision was cinched one day while I was talking to a girl in the cafeteria. She was very excited. She told me, "Oh! I just got back from studying abroad and it was so fabulous."

"Really?"

"Yeah. I was in the exchange program in Florence. It was the best, and the food was great."

That did it. I called my parents and announced, "I've just been accepted out of thousands and thousands of students to go to Florence, Italy, on an exchange program." I exaggerated, just a little bit.

They thought it was a huge honor, and they were very excited for me. What an opportunity it was for an art student to study in Italy! Visions of ravioli danced in my head.

* * *

College Years, Act III

On a crisp January afternoon in 1968, my plane touched down at the airport in Pisa, Italy. This was the closest airport to Florence, which was to be my new home for the next two years, along with about two dozen other American exchange students.

When I thought about how I had gotten to Italy, I was very pleased with myself. I felt I had accomplished what I had set out to do. By leaving the States, I had left behind everyone who knew me, and I had wiped the slate clean, just like my parents had. There was no burning of pictures for me—I just moved to a different country.

Although this may have been a new beginning for me, I was still carrying some old baggage—the weight. A quick look around the plane confirmed what I'd already guessed. I was the heaviest student. I was just over two hundred pounds at this point, and my life continued to center on what would be my next meal, my next snack, and, occasionally, what would be my next diet. And still with me were the overweight problems. I continued to get out of breath quickly when I walked, and walking itself was not easy because my feet were still pronated.

But despite all that, I was very excited. I loved Italy the minute I arrived. The architecture was breathtaking, the culture and history fascinating. Every other building seemed to be a restaurant—this place was created especially for me. But here's the best part: Many of the people were my size, and they seemed to be happy the way they were! They were like plum tomatoes and little provolone cheeses.

I said a silent prayer. "God, why wasn't I born here? Why did you make me suffer all those years in Louisiana and then Tallahassee (which, by the way, took me an entire week to learn how to spell)? You must have known that this was where I belonged."

And it was all beginning here in Pisa, which I assumed must have been the birthplace of my dear old friend, the pizza. And frankly, I was starving—so a pizza sounded great. There I was, dressed in my Mindy-made pumpkin-colored overalls, looking like a Jack-o'-lantern, with an hour to spare before our bus left for Florence. And I was ready to sample the food.

There were vendors everywhere. Around the base of the Leaning Tower of Pisa were little booths, serving all kinds of delicious Italian food. There was pizza, of course, but it was different from the pizza I was used to—this version was thick and square. There were also special Italian sandwiches, made with salty ham and hard cheeses and served on dense bread called focaccia. I'd eaten plenty of ham-and-cheese sandwiches in my life, but this was a sandwich like no other. I wasted no time. I bought a little of everything, creating my own Italian smorgasbord. It seemed the Italians loved food as much as the people in my hometown. This was like New Orleans, but with an Italian accent.

"Hey, I'm going to fit in here pretty well," I said to myself, as I finished my second sandwich and bit into a thick square of pizza.

Now it was time to try the tower. I began the climb, and after the third or fourth step, every remaining step was pure torture—I wheezed and gasped. I'd been in Italy less than an hour, and I had already learned a very valuable lesson: Never walk up a long flight of steps after you eat pizza.

We were loaded onto the bus, and off to Florence we drove. Next stop was the Villa Fabbricotti, the art school where I was going to live and study. However, this gorgeous villa had one drawback: To reach the front door, you had to climb two hundred steps—or it seemed like that many! Fortunately, I hadn't eaten anything on the bus.

All the classes were held in the villa. Some were taught in English, but most were taught in Italian, which was the whole point of the exchange program—to immerse each student in the language and culture. There were four adults in the villa who spoke English; but, of course, they encouraged us to speak Italian as well.

This was a bit of an obstacle that, in the midst of all my excitement, I hadn't anticipated. Not only was I in a foreign country whose language I really didn't speak, but I was also taking my classes in this same language. I had my work cut out for me.

In order to survive, I first learned the Italian phrases I thought were most important.

"*Ho fame,*" which means "I'm hungry." (Now say it again three times!)

"*Quanta costa?*" ("How much is that?")

But even given all this, I felt very much at home right away. Florence, the jewel of Italy, was very much like New Orleans. It was quite small, very compact, just like the French quarter. It was only five minutes from our villa to the hub of the city, and at its center was the famous Duomo, a beautiful cathedral with gorgeous carved doors. Everywhere you looked, there were elegant buildings, columns, statues of angels, fountains, and museums full of the most beautiful paintings. The whole city was like an art gallery. The streets were very narrow, and the Italians drove their small Fiats very, very fast. I loved all the craziness.

And just as I had done in Jackson Square in New Orleans, I soon discovered lots of places to eat, scattered around the open squares or piazzas.

There were pigeons everywhere, but trust me, I fed them nothing off my plate. Those pigeons had to fend for themselves.

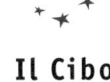

Il Cibo

The food was fantastic. There were cannoli stuffed with ricotta cheese, and hard Italian cookies similar to what my father had bought at the Four Seasons Bakery on Royal Street. There was pizza and a wide variety of sandwiches, including the ham-and-cheese I'd first tried in Pisa. I learned that this ham was called prosciutto and the cheese was fontina. I discovered another sandwich that was miraculous: a cross between a pizza and a turnover, called a calzone. I tried lots of different versions, but my favorite was at Vito's, probably because I liked Vito as much as I liked the calzones he made. Singing while he worked, Vito would take a round ball of dough, flatten it a little, dust it with flour, and then brush the inside with a little olive oil. He'd cut some ham and some cheese, place it on the dough, and fold the edges over to make a turnover. He'd sprinkle some chopped tomato on top and then slide the whole thing into an open brick oven. It was like watching Italian television. I'd stand in front of the oven and see my flat calzone begin to rise, the top getting all brown and the cheese oozing out the sides. Then Vito would fetch it hot from the oven. He drizzled a little olive oil over it, wrapped the bottom half in paper and handed it to me. I ordered a second one immediately. Every day I got into the habit of stopping for a calzone and having a conversation with Vito, much like I had stopped for pralines or a poor-boy sandwich on my way home from school in New Orleans.

The piazzas were always full of Italians smoking pungent-smelling ciga-rettes, drinking little cups of espresso—much stronger than ours—and of course, they were always eating. I was just so happy to be among them. Eating was finally acceptable. There was no doctor with a white piece of paper telling me what to eat. Whether I was speaking English or Italian, I never heard the word "diet." I ate what I wanted. I ignored the scale. And I learned certain Italian words that made people laugh. I was still using humor to get people to like me. This was how I lived my life during those early days in Florence.

There was another curious Italian custom that I came to love. Every day at noon, the church bells would chime, and shortly after, every business in town would close. The whole city came to a halt—the shops, the tours, everything. It became an Italian ghost town.

During this time, from twelve to three, people went to their homes for a big lunch: pasta, huge meatballs, homemade Italian sausages, breads, cheeses, and on and on. Then, after they were full and content, they took a nap. Two of my favorite activities: eating and sleeping. Around three o'clock, the city started coming back to life again. To me, it was almost like watching a play. Act I ended and then everyone ate and napped. Then it was time for Act II, and everyone went back to work.

Dinner, or Act III, didn't happen until late. At home in New Orleans, if it was six o'clock, you'd better be at that dinner table. In Italy, I was sitting down to eat dinner at nine, sometimes ten o'clock.

For dessert, or whenever I needed a little treat, which was often, I discovered gelato—a rich, creamy homemade ice cream. In Florence, there were many gelato stands catering to the tourists. But the locals had their special two or three out-of-the-way places where they went for their gelato. They were well-kept secrets—you had to have "connections" to find the *gelateria* in the Piazza S. Lorenzo.

One afternoon after I'd finished my third calzone at Vito's, I was feeling a little homesick. I told Vito he was like *familia* to me. I thought the man was going to break down and cry.

"You like-a family to me, too! I make you another calzone!"

While it baked, Vito filled me in on the best places to buy gelato. He told me to use his name. I was "connected."

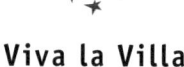

Viva la Villa

The Villa Fabbricotti was a very villa-looking villa, all done in marble. It had balconies and porches, and big half-circle entryways—wide staircases, high ceilings, and stained glass. The villa needed a little fixing up, and we did some while we were there. But still, it was really very nice. It was different from what I knew, but it did remind me of New Orleans, with all its antiques and old-world flavor.

I screamed and fell out of my chair. So there I was, lying on

My bedroom was on the second floor, and it was one of the biggest in the villa, with a pretty patio and two huge windows—you know, glass and then big shutters on the outside. I started out with a roommate, but that didn't last long.

I had brought very little to Italy. I did bring my bib overalls and some other clothing, and that was about it. With the money my Uncle Milton had given me, I went out and bought all my art equipment, my table, and all the materials I needed for art class. At this point in my art training, I was very much inspired by Aubrey Beardsley, a young artist from the turn of the century who illustrated the *Yellow Book* and worked with Oscar Wilde on many projects. His illustrations of people were very detailed black-and-white ink drawings, and in the very curvy Art Nouveau style. He died at the age of twenty-six. I read a lot about him and said to myself, "Well, I'm Aubrey Beardsley. Either that, or Edith Piaf."

So many of my early drawings were in Beardsley's style. I used a Rapidograph pen for the drawing. It had a very sharp point that stuck out about an eighth of an inch from the pen, almost like a hypodermic needle. They were a pain to work with. I was forever shaking the pen, since the ink got blocked in the tip.

One afternoon I was working very intently with this pen on a drawing. I had a roommate from Kenya, and he quietly came in. All of a sudden, he made a noise and startled me half to death, just as I was shaking the pen in front of me. Well, I was so surprised, I accidentally stabbed myself in the chest with the pen, point first. (When you see me now, ask to see my Rapidograph scar!) I screamed and fell out of my chair. So there I was, lying on the floor, with the pen sticking out of my chest! No one would remove the pen. They were afraid that blood would spurt out. Finally, I was rushed to a nearby hospital, where a nice doctor carefully extracted the pen. I was thoroughly examined, and the doctor announced that I would live, or at least that's what I thought he said. My Italian at this point was still pretty basic.

Well, word spread quickly about this student who had tried to commit suicide with his Rapidograph pen. My roommate was so unnerved by this that he found somewhere else to live and I had the whole room to myself. That was fine by me.

So now that I had this huge room to myself, I pushed the two beds up against one wall and turned the whole place into my studio. The room began to look like a little art store. There were cans everywhere—not A&P cans with lard, but cans full of brushes and paint thinner.

Over the weeks and months, my art style began to evolve. As I mentioned, I was very influenced by Aubrey Beardsley, as well as by Gustav Klimt—I had a very unusual style, and you could always identify it. It was me. And people liked it. I was beginning to think I would stay in Italy or Europe after I finished school. I would become an even better artist, make money, gain fame, and then I would triumphantly return home.

Even though I loved doing the art, the hard part for me was spending all that time alone while I created a piece. I just hated it, being alone. And the way I worked, I couldn't have any music, I couldn't have anybody around. It was all too distracting. But I did eat while I worked. It was just hours of eating—and this is when I really began to put on the weight. It was eating and drawing, eating and painting, eating and sculpting. People always knew that it was my work, because there was a food stain somewhere—a dried piece of pizza cheese, a mashed crumb from a calzone, a smudge of chocolate. But the good part was that I didn't have to share my food, because artwork doesn't eat.

The dining hall was the villa's original dining room. Instead of long tables, there were small, square tables, creating almost a bistro effect—you know, six at this table, four at this table, two at that table.

We had set times for each meal, and the food was pretty ordinary. There were no choices. No going in the kitchen allowed. As always, I was the exception. I got to know a few people in the kitchen. In fact, I got to know all of them! They lived in the villa. They loved me. I would do little favors for them and bring them gifts. If I wanted a snack or a little nibble, the kitchen was just a short walk away.

Since I was spending a lot of time in my room creating art, I began to stock food, just like I had in my bedroom at home in New Orleans. It was Dicky's own little grocery store.

There were these little candies called Baci's—hazelnut on the inside with a chocolate coating. No matter where you went, even in church, there would be a display of Baci's. You'd go to an art store—Baci's. Baci's were everywhere, and they were so quick to eat. That beautiful blue silver foil with silver stars on it—you couldn't wait to rip it off and pop the Baci into your mouth. So I had my Baci supply. Like my father, I began to shop for each meal or snack. I would buy a couple of calzones or several ham-and-cheese sandwiches and bring them back to my room. My little kitchen was once again open for business.

Since I was a loner, in my free time I enjoyed walking around Florence, just exploring. It reminded me of New Orleans, where everyone's door was open and the people were very friendly. I would talk with shopkeepers, who very often lived in back of the store, or above it. Occasionally one of the people I met would ask me to their home for dinner. It was quite an honor and somewhat unusual to be invited into someone's home for a meal. When this happened, I would have to get permission from Dr. Licht, who ran the school.

"I've been invited to dinner at the home of my friend who works at the *mercato*—the market," I told him.

"Impossible. With your broken Italian, you must have misunderstood," Dr. Licht replied.

"I don't think so. I mean, I know the words. *Mangiare* means eat and *pranzo* means dinner. That much I understand."

"Well, if you're sure . . . "

"I'm sure. I know all the food words," I told him. Dr. Licht certainly couldn't argue with me there. When it came to food, I was my very own person, no matter where I was.

I was settling easily into life in Florence. Since no one else seemed to notice my weight, I no longer paid any attention to it. My clothes may have been getting snug, but since everyone around me was eating, I figured when in Rome—or in this case, Florence—why not.

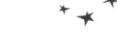

Two for the Road

For the weekends, we would pair up with someone from our exchange program and travel to a different city or country. Our mode of transportation? Hitchhiking. Back then, hitchhiking was considered safe. We'd leave around ten o'clock on Friday morning and usually be back by six in the evening on Sunday. Then we would write a report, in Italian, on where

g all that time alone while I created a piece. I just hated it, we had been and what we had eaten . . . oops, I mean, what we had seen. That was our homework assignment.

Well, I was paired with Katherine, who looked like she just came off the runway for the Miss America Pageant. She spoke four languages and was just one of those I'm-pretty-and-I-can-do-anything girls. She had gorgeous long, black hair, beautiful blue eyes, and long, long legs, higher than my head. Boy, was I happy. Dicky was with the beautiful girl again!

We were quite a pair: me in my Clarabelle overalls and her in a tiny skirt and a tank top. We never had a problem getting a ride. Even if a car passed us, it would screech to a halt and then back up at fifty miles an hour. It wasn't long before we started to get picky. Only a Mercedes for us—none of those cramped little cars. Katherine would explain where we were going, and we would just get in the car. They would treat us like they'd known us forever.

We'd tell them our destination, and they'd take us as far as they could. Then we'd hitch another ride, or maybe take a train from there. We traveled all over Europe that way. One weekend it was Rome or Venice, the next weekend, Berlin or Bern. That's how I learned about architecture.

Katherine was very good to me. Even though I was so slow and lagged behind the groups in the museums, Katherine slowed her pace to match mine. You know, when you have to take a hundred steps up a museum staircase to see a statue without toes or fingers or a head, and if you were my size, you didn't move too quickly. Walking was so painful. My feet hurt, and I had sores on the bottom of them. And because I'm so short and was so stocky, my knees and lower back just killed me. But Katherine was such a dear.

Each city during our weekend travels became a kitchen for me, a culinary adventure. Even though I had been exposed to many foreign foods through my father's cookbooks, this was now the real thing. I ate my way through all those different cities. On the one hand, it was a great experience because I was learning about so many cultures. On the other hand, my weight was steadily increasing. But I still wasn't concerned—yet.

I had lots of acquaintances at school, including faculty people. As in the past, though, I really didn't get close to anyone. There was one exception, which I've mentioned before: the kitchen workers in the villa. I especially liked Paolo, who had six kids. If I needed a car, he would lend me his Fiat. I was finally learning how to drive, but I still didn't have a license. His Fiat was the smallest and cheapest model—I think they made about two hundred of them a day!

* ⋆ ⋆

I'm Ready for My Close-up

One afternoon after class, I was in a café across from the Duomo, having a meal with some of my fellow students from the art school. I noticed a table of men across the way, staring at me. I just assumed they must be admiring my gorgeous curly hair or my new paisley, Gucci-knockoff overalls. By this time, I'd found a woman in Florence who made them for me in the most fabulous Italian fabrics. I did look pretty adorable, even if I was now quite overweight. One of the men came over and introduced himself, asking me if I knew Federico Fellini, the Italian director. I said I didn't know him, but I knew who he was. Well, the gentleman who introduced himself was the casting director for the movie *Satyricon,* and Fellini wanted *me* for a small role. And he wanted me because I was fat— but in Italian it sounded so much nicer.

Next question: Do I have an agent? I said no. I was told I must have an agent, and Primo was the main agency in Florence. No agent, no movie role. That was the story.

I walked into Primo, and there were the most breathtaking-looking people you've ever seen in your whole life. There were all these six-foot-tall girls with black hair, and the guys all looked like Michelangelo sculptures. And then there was me. I was the token heavy person. It was like the modeling agencies in the States that specialize in character people or people who have a certain look. So they signed me up for both the movie and commercials. If a client needed someone large, I was it.

A few weeks later, I found myself on the set of *Satyricon.* I was in a crowd scene—the "Tower of Babel" sequence—but there were a lot of people, so it's hard to pick me out. My best scene is where a man and woman had to leave their kids—I played one of the kids. The movie was exciting, and working on a set was everything I thought it would be. I had been bitten by the acting bug. This was show business—it was everything my parents had tried to shield me from, and I loved it.

Work just kept on coming. I started doing commercials. They were all in Italian, but I managed to get by because all my lines were short and simple and easily learned. There was a spaghetti-and-meatball commercial, and obviously I was not going to make it as the spaghetti. No, I was a dancing meatball, singing a little jingle. I played a bunch of grapes in a commercial for the Italian version of Fruit of the Loom underwear. In a peanut-butter commercial, I was a chubby Peter Pan who couldn't fly through a window. In a cheese commercial, I did a Lucy Ricardo thing, packing little round cheeses from a conveyor belt into boxes: The belt moved so fast, I'd pack one, then eat one, pack one, eat one. That was one of my more popular commercials. Once again I was the class clown, but now I was getting paid for it.

I had done a commercial for Big Boy jeans, and now there was a photo of my big butt in those jeans plastered on the sides of buses and buildings. People also recognized me because I seemed to be the only person in Florence who wore these wild-colored bib overalls. And I had that big head of hair. There really was no one in Florence who looked like me—I did not blend in.

From time to time I would telephone my parents to tell them how great things were going. (I love the telephone, and even today I spend half my life on the phone.) My father—Mr. Frugal—would answer.

"Hello? Who is this?"

"Hello, daddy. This is Richard, calling from Italy!"

"Who's paying for this call?"

"Daddy, I'm paying for it. Don't worry."

"Here's your mother."

From these telephone conversations, I could tell that my father was not happy with my acting career. Not at all. He and Shirley had spent a lot of time making sure that I would never get near show business. Well, all that effort didn't seem to have worked.

Most of the money I made, I sent home. And it wasn't until later that I learned my father put it all in an account for me. He called it my "lucky money," and he never touched it. He always thought this show-business stuff would never last and I would eventually fail, as he had. So he was going to protect me and plan for my future.

All this success with the commercials came with a weird side, involving a very mixed message for me. I was becoming a celebrity of sorts, making good money, but it was happening because I was fat. I was rewarded for being chunky and chubby and husky and cute. Underneath this success, I was finally becoming a little concerned about my weight. My overalls were really starting to become snug—I even had to move the buttons.

* ⋆ *

Good-Bye, Uncle Milton

While in Florence, I went through one of my first really tough emotional experiences—not that I hadn't had some difficult moments already in my life. After I had been in art school for a while—it was 1969 now—my brother Lenny was inducted into the army. There was a very good chance he would have to go to Vietnam. My parents were extremely upset, because they lived with all the grisly images of the war on television every day. I was constantly worried about Lenny. I called home on a regular basis to get any news my parents might have about him. While I could pick up a telephone any time, Lenny couldn't, since he was in boot camp. He would write to my parents or to me in Florence, but those letters took a while to get to me, so my news was never really current.

When I called home, the first thing we always talked about was who had gotten a letter from Lenny and where was he? Had he been sent overseas yet? Hearing my parents read their letter from Lenny was the next best thing to hearing from him directly. Then, one afternoon while I was studying in my room in the villa, I received my first telegram. I had only seen telegrams being delivered in the movies by a man in a crisp uniform with a peaked hat. I always thought, "How chic!" That's not what I felt now. I was filled with dread—afraid that something had happened to Lenny. What was I going to do?

As I ripped the telegram open, I thought, "Oh my God, please don't let this be a note asking me to come home."

It wasn't about Lenny, but it still stopped me short. My Uncle Milton had passed away—the man I'd been named after and the only relative I had ever really known. I was crushed. He was the one who helped me go to school. He had always been very supportive of anything I wanted to do, and I didn't even get to say good-bye to him. I'd never lost anyone whom I'd loved before. I called my parents, and when I heard my father's voice, I started crying. My father was not an outwardly emotional man, and it was very difficult for him to show grief or sadness.

"Uncle Milton is gone!" I sobbed.

"Richard, this crying is costing us thirty-five dollars," my father said calmly, keeping all of his emotions tightly in control—like my tears had a price on them. I was facing one of the big realities of life—death. My brother was about to be shipped off to the war, and my Uncle Milton was gone. And all my father could think about, at least on the surface, was the cost of the telephone call.

There was no one I could turn to with my grief. So I turned to food. My sadness triggered my eating, and I ate as if I would never fill myself up.

When I wasn't eating, I threw myself into school and my art projects. My career in commercials was really taking off, so that was a distraction. I just buried myself in everything so I wouldn't have to think about Uncle Milton or Lenny.

A few weeks later, I was called from my room to take an urgent call on the phone in the main lobby of the Villa Fabricotti. It was my father—and I knew my father would never spend money on a phone call unless something horrible had happened. My father was calling to tell me that Lenny had been shipped out to Vietnam. My parents' fears had come true. I could hear the sadness in my father's voice.

The Note

Not long after I had gotten the phone call about my brother, I was doing a personal appearance at a supermarket, autographing packages of gnocchi. It was time for me to leave for my next appointment, the filming of the peanut-butter commercial where I played Peter Pan, tights and all. Just before I left the supermarket, a huge rainstorm drenched everything. When I peeked out into the parking lot, the rain had slowed but it was still drizzling. As I rushed to the car—the little red Fiat I'd borrowed from my friend Paolo—I saw something under my windshield wiper. At first, I thought it was a parking ticket. As I got closer, I saw it was a handwritten note. The rain had made some of the words run. I pulled the damp sheet of paper from under the wiper and got in the car. I wiped my face and then read the note. It may have been slightly smeared but the meaning was very clear.

RICHARD—YOU'RE VERY FUNNY, BUT FAT PEOPLE DIE YOUNG. PLEASE DON'T DIE.

It wasn't signed. Someone who knew me had left this, and they were obviously very concerned about me. I had been gaining a lot of weight during the past couple of months. Even though I may have not noticed it, others had. Putting on weight is so easy. First you put on five pounds, then ten pounds. Then the weeks go by, and before you know it, you're in trouble— big trouble.

The more I thought about the note, I began to realize that despite the good intentions of whoever had left it, he or she really didn't know me. They hadn't been with me through all the years of grapefruit and hard-boiled eggs, of pills and Weight Watchers meetings. They didn't know that in all this time, in all the years I had struggled with my love for food and my desire to be "normal," I had never once thought of dying. Death had never been an issue. Instead, I had tried to lose weight so I could fit in. I was going to be successful, I was going to meet people, I was going to be popular—I was going to be all those things I'd heard you became when you lost weight.

I didn't have much experience with death. Because my parents were older, I had never known my grandparents. I had no aging relatives, no ailing friends. I'd been lucky and had never faced death. But now, a faceless person had noticed that my weight was slowing me down, and that maybe I was in trouble, in serious trouble. I drove the Fiat off to my filming of the Peter Pan commercial.

Three blocks away from the school, on a street in front of a grocery store, was an old scale, the kind where for a few *lire*, it would read your weight and tell your fortune at the same time. There, standing on that scale, I discovered something I'd been avoiding since I first got to Italy. The scale hit me right in the face with reality: I weighed two hundred and sixty-eight pounds, and I was short. I didn't need to read the fortune.

I panicked. I had to take immediate action. I had to find the enemy, the

My sadness triggered my eating, and I ate as if I would never

reason I was overweight—and turn the tide as soon as I possibly could. I knew I didn't want to die.

So who or what was the enemy? I knew the answer: food. In a single day, food went from being my friend, my comforter, my pain reliever, to being the thing that could kill me.

I had tried all those diets and even diet pills when I was younger, but I was still eating. I had tried the AYDS candies, but I was still eating. I sat through those Weight Watchers meetings, but I was still eating.

I knew what I had to do. I had to stop eating. That was it, plain and simple. And that's what I did. I stayed very busy, I drank water, I walked everywhere, and the weight began to come off, and I do mean the weight began to come off. Almost like a sugar rush, I began to feel a sort of heady euphoria. It became a game. Every day, I found new ways to avoid eating.

If I were going to a party or someone's house, I'd fill up with water, quickly drinking seven or eight glasses before I went. I had never drunk water before, unless it was in iced tea or Kool-Aid. Now it became one of the most important things in my life. At dinner with others, I'd play with my food, pushing it around the plate, or I'd hide the food in my napkin and throw it away when no one was looking.

Every day I'd roll the dice. How many days could I do this? I was interested in two things: the numbers on the scale and my waist measurement. That was what I lived for.

The first week, I lost seventeen pounds, and after that, I lost about ten pounds a week. It was amazing. Before my very eyes, I saw the weight falling off. I looked in the mirror every day and found body parts I didn't know I had. I saw ribs and collarbones emerge overnight. I watched my waist as it went from forty-eight inches to forty, and out of the forties to a thirty-eight. Then I reached the milestone of thirty-six, what most "average" people are. And I just kept on losing, until I finally reached an amazing twenty-eight-inch waist, which now meant that I could go into stores and they wouldn't have sizes small enough. It was exhilarating. This is what I'd worked so hard for.

Finally, I called the talent agency and told them I wouldn't be doing any more commercials. I said I was so busy at school that I just didn't have the time. I didn't tell them the real reason—I was quickly shrinking because I was concentrating on my new weight-loss plan.

After two and a half months, I had lost a hundred and twelve

Had I looked in that mirror a little closer, I would have also noticed that my skin was becoming dry and turning a grayish tint. I had always been barrel-chested and had carried a great deal of weight in my stomach. My skin began to get saggy, especially in my torso. In addition, my fingernails became brittle and unhealthy-looking. Worst of all, I was beginning to lose my hair. In the morning, I'd wake up and, literally, clumps of hair would be on my pillow. But I had an answer for everything. Over the years I had learned how to convincingly lie to myself as well as others about my weight. This was much easier than confronting the truth. The truth may set you free, but I wasn't ready yet for that. Instead, I told myself this was part of the process of losing weight, and that my hair would just grow back as soon as I started eating again. The mirror had two faces—I ignored one, and adored the other.

The Thin Man

After two and a half months, I had lost a hundred and twelve pounds. Now, for the first time in all my attempts to lose weight and fit in, I was finally "normal."

I began to take long walks around the city. I had so much more free time now that I wasn't eating. One afternoon, on one of my outings, I was on my way to a stationery store across from the Ufizzi Gallery to buy marbleized note paper. I started to feel nauseous—my head was spinning. I began to feel unbalanced, like I was losing control.

I woke up in a hospital. I had no recollection of how I got there. Like the note left on my car, my experience had been anonymous. People had helped, but I had no idea who they were.

There I was, staring up at the ceiling, hooked to an I.V. pole. I turned my head a little and saw that I wasn't even in a hospital room, but in a long corridor, lined up with a lot of other beds that were separated from each other by white curtains.

A very motherly, gentle-faced nun was leaning over me when I opened my eyes. I was at Santa Maria Nuova Hospital, not far from where I had collapsed. And in fact, a bystander had called an ambulance for me.

The sister spoke practically no English, but by now my Italian was pretty good. She told me that I was very dehydrated and that my kidneys and lungs were not working very well. That was quite a shock to me. They were trying to get fluids back into me, not only because I was dehydrated but because my electrolytes were way out of whack.

Then she asked me the $64,000 question: Why wasn't I eating? What was I doing to myself? Didn't I know how dangerous this was?

I gave her my simple answer. "I want to be skinny." I went on to tell her my whole story—I just had to tell someone. I was doing so well and it was all going so perfectly, until I fainted. She pointed out that my note almost came true. The method I chose for losing weight almost killed me. She told me I would have to stay in the hospital for at least a couple of days.

"We're going to have to get some color back in your cheeks and you're going to have to learn to start eating," she said.

So there I was. It had been quite a trip. I had been on both sides of the ruler. I had been on the overweight, obese side, and then I had quickly see-sawed to the very, very thin side—too thin. At this point in my life, I was no better off, no more intelligent, and had no more knowledge than I did when I took that first diet pill in the sixth grade. Now it was time for me to try to find some balance, some middle ground, for the first time in my life.

Well, actually . . . first, I had to go shopping. Now that I was skinny, I didn't mind buying clothes. It was a new experience for me. The Italian designers were so exciting, but I didn't just limit myself to Italy. I was still traveling on weekends with Katherine, so I had all of Europe at my disposal. I bought dress shirts in Paris, a hand-stitched vest in Madrid, and a sweater from Brussels. Something I picked up in Switzerland became one of my favorites. I bought lederhosen—suede shorts held up by suspenders. They showed off my slim waistline and my cute knees. This was the first pair of shorts I loved (and as you know, not the last!).

I Want You!

Then all of a sudden, my world came to a screeching halt, again. I got my second telegram. This one wasn't glamorous either. Uncle Sam was writing to say, "Hi, your number's up, and it's not for the lottery." I was to report to Whitehall Street in New York City, where I would take my physical for induction into the army. I had been drafted.

So long, Italy; hello, Broadway! I'm a Yankee-doodle dandy, and all that jazz. Although I was terrified of war, I was willing to do my part; and in the back of my mind, I also thought that maybe I could be with Lenny, who was in Vietnam. Now, you already know how I feel about physicals from my days with Dr. Veith. And just because I looked good in clothes didn't mean I was happy to take them off for some doctor with a very cold stethoscope.

Wearing my new lederhosen and a floor-length suede coat, I packed up and got ready to fly to New York to take my physical.

Classes were over, and I was finished with the program in Florence. I was still living like a traveling salesman—traveling light. All my art supplies and stuff that I had accumulated during the two years, I left behind. I had only my clothes and my portfolio, and that was it. I had been thinking about staying in Italy, since I'd been offered some apprenticeships. There was still a lot of restoration work going on in Florence after the floods, and there was some work at the Vatican. Can you imagine, me and the Pope? (In fact, we did meet years later.)

Arriving at the Army's testing office in downtown Manhattan, I guess I looked a little out of place in my leather shorts and long coat. Another draftee asked me what country I was from. But before I could answer, a blunt, rough, crew-cut man in a uniform told us we'd be taking a written test, because they didn't let stupid people into the army. That was a relief. I wouldn't want to be fighting beside someone who was a bad speller!

I must have passed with flying colors, because soon I was ushered into a locker room filled with a wall of wire baskets.

"Take off all your clothes, except for your underwear and your socks," Mr. Crewcut told us.

"Excuse me." I said politely. "Would you happen to have a hanger for my coat? It's suede and I really don't want to shove it into that little basket."

Well, there was so much yelling going on in the changing room, I couldn't get an answer right away. About twenty minutes later, I found out they didn't have hangers. I folded my clothes carefully, just like I did when I had my physical with Dr. Hallman, and I took my place in line among the other candidates, who were wearing only white and light-striped boxers and briefs. As you can imagine, my choice of underwear was a little more creative. I was always ahead of my time. In Rome, I'd bought underwear with a beautiful scene of the Colosseum on them.

A doctor came in to examine each of us. He looked at me and asked if I'd been sick. I explained that I'd lost weight. He pulled me out of line and had me meet with another doctor. The two of them took a look at my pronated feet, my swollen knees, my sagging skin, and the bald spots here and there on my head. They determined that I was certainly not Army material.

"It would cost us more to keep you than to just let you go home." They put me down as 4-F—"excused for medical reasons." Things hadn't changed much since my days at CorJesu—I was still getting medical excuses from P.E. But I wasn't happy with their decision. I wanted to go, I wanted to be with Lenny in Vietnam. I begged, I argued. That's when they suggested maybe I should see the shrink. I decided to go home instead.

* * *

Welcome Home?

I returned to New Orleans, both relieved and disappointed. My father and mother picked me up at the airport. They took one look at me, with my new body, my striking clothing, and my hair combed over like cotton candy to cover my bald spots, and I'm sure they wondered exactly what had happened to their baby boy. But, they were very kind. They told me I looked great. I guess they were too stunned to say anything else.

I was amused by the horrified look on my father's face as he inspected my floor-length suede coat. He refused to ride in the same cab with "it." So he got a separate cab for my coat, and my father, mother, and I rode home, with "it" following behind.

I felt all warm and safe being back with my family, but my father was determined that I shouldn't get too comfortable. He'd already bought me a one-way plane ticket to New York and told me I was leaving in six days. The underlying antagonism between my father and me had not gone away during my time at college—it was still there, unresolved. Since there had been no attempts to talk about any of the issues that kept us apart, what would you expect? But my father was right about one thing—it was time for me to start my life. It was 1970, and I was twenty-one years old.

*   *
 *

The Big Apple

I called Jeff, a friend from college in Lafayette who was living in New York, and asked if I could stay with him. He told me he had plenty of room as long as I didn't mind sleeping on an overstuffed chair that folded out into a bed.

Jeff was brilliant, the egghead type: tall and skinny with glasses, and the perfect student. He was one of the very few of my classmates whom I kept in contact with. He hadn't been an art student, but he was in some of my English and history classes, and because he stood out from the crowd, I guess that's why we got along. He had moved to New York City and was studying to become a dentist.

Carrying my Bachelor's Degree in art and my portfolio, I got on a plane and flew to New York City to seek my fortune as an illustrator and a graphic designer. And suddenly, I was on my own again.

Moving to the Big Apple was almost like the new beginning I'd hoped to make in Italy. No one knew what I used to weigh. No one knew the pain I'd been through. So this time, I had really wiped the slate clean. And, for the first time, I was skinny.

I had lived in a variety of unusual places during my first twenty-one years, starting with that shotgun house in New Orleans that I was raised in. Now I was standing in front an apartment building in Greenwich Village, New York City, a building that looked like it was ready to fall down. It was one of those dark, tenement-looking places. It had one elevator. Jeff's apartment was on the fifth floor, and since the elevator didn't usually work, I was forever climbing the stairs—no easy task for me, with my bad feet.

Jeff proudly took me on a tour of his apartment, like it was the Ponderosa. It was more like a shoebox. When you walked in, you entered a hallway, and to the left was a study, with the little convertible chair-bed that Jeff had told me about over the telephone. There was also a little kitchen, a little bathroom, and a bedroom that was Jeff's. My father had been kind enough to send me a box of my things, and that became my closet. I was in a box, living out of a box. I didn't really mind all that much, though. I was young, and New York was full of exciting possibilities. The Village reminded me of a movie set. It was quaint-looking, and teeming with

was determined that I shouldn't get too comfortable. He'd

people at all hours of the day or night, just like New Orleans and Florence. It was all very adult. I felt right at home. And I lived in that apartment until I left New York a couple of years later.

I decided that in New York City the big thing was to become a fashion illustrator at *Women's Wear Daily,* or to become an illustrator at a department store like Arnold Constable or B. Altman or Saks. If you looked at newspaper ads, all you saw were fashion sketches and illustrations. And it was very good money, because you got paid by each illustration you did. In those days there were very few, if any, fashion photographs like there are today—just illustrations.

I never got a job as a fashion illustrator, but I eventually got a free-lance job at an advertising agency named Cole, Fisher, and Rogo. They called when they needed me to do paste-ups and mechanicals, which is basically arranging other people's artwork on a page to create an ad. In those days, it involved a lot of gluing with rubber cement. I'd go home with pain in my shoulders from being hunched for hours over a drawing table, and a headache from smelling glue all day. Not a fun job.

A friend of mine, Karl, who worked at the agency, decided to leave New York and move back home. He had a job in the evenings working as a waiter in a restaurant. He knew I was always looking for ways to make extra money, so he suggested I apply for his old job.

Waiting on Tables—East Coast

Three days later, I was working at the AutoPub in the General Motors building on Fifth Avenue. It was the "in" place, right in the middle of everything, across from the Plaza Hotel. The interior of the restaurant itself was unique. In one section, there were antique cars. The inside of each car had been removed and replaced with a table, so customers ate right inside the car. There was another area with booths, and all around these booths—and, in fact, all around the entire restaurant—was a track on which miniature cars raced. Another room was set up like a drive-in movie theater. It was the Disneyland of restaurants. And I was in the middle of it. It was like the Fellini movie set or a set for one of my Italian commercials. Just one more performance.

Boy, was I a great waiter. The bread was always hot and the

The AutoPub waiters and waitresses all wore gas-station-attendant zip-up jumpsuits. It seemed to me that everybody who worked there was an aspiring actor or model. Everyone was gorgeous, except me. I looked like a poodle who worked at a gas station, with my little jumpsuit and my round curly hair. I was still teetering with my weight, and let me tell you, those coveralls were not the most flattering look. I was still afraid of food. At this point, I weighed about a hundred and thirty-five pounds. But then I would overeat and go up to one-sixty, and I'd find myself terrified of being over-weight again. And even though I'd almost killed myself by starving, and even though I'd read the books on nutrition and exercise, I'd still starve to lose weight. It was the only thing that worked for me. I didn't know any other way to do it.

Boy, was I a great waiter. The bread was always hot and the salad plates and forks were always cold. If a napkin was dropped on the floor, I'd be there to pick it up and hand my customer a new one. As much as I had loved meeting people when I was handing out praline samples in the French quarter, this was even better. I loved talking to my AutoPub customers while I was grinding fresh pepper on their Caesar salad. I was there to make sure people had a good time, and if they did, they would like me and not really care what I looked like. You know, things had not really changed since my praline-selling days.

* ★ *

The Ritual

I also loved the people I worked with. They were my new "family." There was one girl in particular, named Josie, whom I became friends with. Josie was from Brooklyn. She was thin, and her makeup and her hair were always perfect. She had a heavy Brooklyn accent—very exotic, I thought, and certainly different from anything I'd heard before. She had a quick sense of humor and was very blunt and to-the-point. I loved that about her, because she really helped me through my early training at the AutoPub, giving me advice on what the best sections were for tips and which days I'd make the most money.

There was something about Josie that always fascinated me. This woman ate like a thoroughbred, but she never put on weight. At the

AutoPub, we served a loaf of bread—a small loaf of fresh, whole-wheat bread. I'd get it straight out of the oven, put it on a bread board, stick a knife in it, and rush it out to my table. I'd even warm the butter, because nothing is worse than cold, hard butter on warm bread—the bread just rips and becomes a mess. I'd be in the kitchen warming up my butter, and I'd see Josie gobble down huge pieces of bread while she was waiting for her orders to come up. She could eat two or three loaves of this bread slathered with butter each night. Plus, she'd eat a full meal and then polish it off with a slice of blueberry pie.

One evening, we had begun our nightly cleanup, wiping ashtrays and refilling salt and pepper shakers as the customers lingered over the last of their meals and coffee and dessert. In the kitchen, I spotted Josie eating one of her feasts at nearly two o'clock in the morning. I hadn't eaten so much as a cracker all night, and I was starving, and more than a little envious.

"Josie, what is the secret here?" I asked. "I have trouble just keeping at the weight I am now. I feel guilty if I have even one french fry, and you're eating a plateful."

"It's so easy," she replied, smiling secretively. "Come with me."

She took me into the employee's bathroom, locking the door behind us. Josie chattered away about a customer who had kept her running back and forth all night, and then had given her a very small tip. As she talked, she washed her hands, dried them, and gestured for me to join her in the stall.

Now, I felt like I was in the *Twilight Zone*. I had no idea what she was up to. I'd also never spent time with a woman alone in a bathroom stall. I couldn't imagine how I'd gotten myself in this situation.

Standing next to the toilet bowl, Josie instructed me to watch her. She bent over and placed her index finger and her third finger in her mouth. Then she slowly started edging the two fingers to the back of her throat until her face became red—and she threw up.

Now, let me just say that I've always hated throwing up. Even as a child, I'd do anything to avoid it. When my mother would say, "If you throw up, you'll feel better," I always preferred to stay sick rather than throw up. Maybe it was because I was so attached to the food that I didn't want it to go anywhere. The idea of throwing up made me, well—nauseous.

Josie ignored my stunned look and gave me a few more pointers on the art of making yourself throw up.

"Hold your breath and pull your stomach muscles in when you do it," she said helpfully.

She flushed the toilet, washed her hands again, and touched up her makeup, all the while chatting about her weekend plans. I was speechless. Not too many things had ever shocked me in my young life, but I had never seen a pretty woman eat like Josie could, then just throw up and not think anything of it—and be so willing to teach me, besides.

All the way home on the subway, I said to myself, "That is just so disgusting. It is so horrible." And then, "Maybe I should try it. I'm going to try it." Yes, no, yes, no. My mind went back and forth. Sure, it looked horrible, but that's the reason Josie looked so great. If it worked for her, it could work for me. And maybe I wouldn't have to starve myself anymore.

By the time I got home, I decided I wanted to try the ritual. That's what Josie had called it—the ritual. I didn't want my roommate Jeff to hear me, so I washed my hands and then left the water running. I mentally psyched myself up. Standing over the toilet, I kept trying to picture what Josie had shown me. I put my two fingers down my throat. I felt blood rushing to my head, and I gagged. I threw up a little, and then I started choking. I just couldn't do it.

I washed my hands again under the running water. As I shut off the tap, I looked in the mirror. My eyes were bloodshot, there were tears rolling down my cheeks, and I was all hot and flushed. It wasn't pretty.

"So much for the ritual," I said to my red face. I was done with throwing up—at least, that's what I thought until my birthday a few nights later.

My friends from the AutoPub took me out for a birthday celebration— I was twenty-two. We went to a Chinese restaurant and were seated at a long table in a private room in the back. Before you knew it, the table was filled with appetizers and dishes that were passed around and refilled when they ran out—just like at home in New Orleans. There were egg rolls, potstickers, chicken chow mein, barbecue pork, and shrimp foo young—and that was just for starters. Everything we ordered was fried and sauced, or covered with peanuts or oil. I didn't care—it was my birthday. I ate and ate and ate. I ate to the point where I was ashamed. Sometimes, I felt like I still had my fat suit on, my shadow from the past that always followed me. You know, that's how fat people feel, even when they're skinny. They always see themselves as fat and unattractive. But this night, I had my obese suit on. I could have been back in Italy at two hundred and sixty-eight pounds, eating my fourth or fifth calzone. I felt awful.

So I excused myself from the table, and I went to the bathroom. I locked the door. I washed my hands and performed the ritual just like Josie had taught me. Everything I'd just eaten was gone, in a minute. My God, it was like I could take back my guilt! There I was, wiping the slate clean, once again.

I washed my hands, splashed cold water on my face, and returned to the table. My friends took one look at my red, tear-stained face, and asked what was wrong.

"Why are you crying?" they asked.

I thought fast. "Well, I just miss my family," I told them. Lying to cover up my efforts at weight loss was getting to be a habit with me—in fact, it was already a habit.

Still, it was worth it. This was the perfect formula. I knew that I could not only eat anything I wanted, but I could even lose weight, just by throwing up.

After a month or two of using the ritual as my weight-loss method, in my typical fashion I became obsessive. I began to weigh myself pre- and post-ritual. Sometimes I'd lose a pound, a pound and a half. Well, if 3,500 calories equal a pound, then like Josie, I could eat bread with butter, french fries, and pie for dessert and not even think twice about losing the calories I'd eaten.

One morning, I woke up and got ready to go to work. For some reason that day, after months of throwing up, I took a long, hard look at my reflection in the mirror. It was that double image in the mirror again: the thin me and then the other unhealthy one. My eyes were extremely bloodshot; I looked very fatigued and worn out. I thought I might be coming down with a virus, so I decided to get a checkup. It didn't dawn on me that I was headed down the same road I had taken in Florence.

Well, the days of Dr. Hallman were over. I did find a kind, patient doctor, like Dr. Veith, who took the time to explain things to me. He looked down my throat, felt my glands, listened to my heartbeat, and examined my fingernails.

"Are you throwing up?" he asked me.

"What do you mean?" I asked, shocked that he could read my mind about my secret ritual.

He asked, "Are you sticking your fingers down your throat and throwing up?"

"Of course not!" I replied.

"Let me tell you what will happen to your body if you are." He sat with me for a long time and patiently explained what I'd been doing to myself. I'd been shocked when Josie had first shown me how to throw up. And now I was shocked again. The doctor told me that over a period of time, I could break capillaries in my eyes and face that eventually would become so worn out that they would not repair themselves, ever. He also described how stomach acid could erode the enamel on my teeth, making them gray and discolored. He told me that people who threw up on a regular basis could eventually do it by just contracting their stomach muscles in a certain way. I had already reached that point where I no longer needed to use my fingers. He went on for about thirty minutes. I felt like throwing up.

Well, that did it. After my visit to the doctor, I went home and got ready to go to work at the AutoPub. I vowed to myself that I would never throw up again—never. And to this day, I haven't, even when I've been sick. When I finally make a major decision about something, I stick to it.

A couple of days later, I noticed that Josie had been out sick for a while. The week before, she hadn't looked that well. Her face was drawn and pale; her hair was limp-looking. When I asked the shift manager where she'd been, he told me that she was in the hospital.

The girl who had taught me the ritual had developed colitis. I bought some flowers and went to visit her. When I walked into her room, she started crying. She told me that she was so sorry that she'd ever taught me something so destructive. She hadn't known the consequences. I told her about my doctor's visit, and I assured her that my days of using the ritual were over. I think she felt a little better after that. She never returned to work, though, and later I heard she'd moved back to Brooklyn where her family could help her recover.

So, no longer using the ritual, I saw the numbers on the scale stop going down and slowly start to climb back upward. I'd lost and gained and had still learned nothing about what would make my body healthy and happy.

* ⋆ *
⋆

Put On a Happy Face

By now, in the restaurant, I had a lot of regular customers—people who lived in New York and people who came to the city for business. One of those people became my next angel, a stepping-stone to another change in my life.

There was an older man whom I noticed coming into the restaurant occasionally. After I had been there awhile, he began requesting a table in my section. He looked like he was from a royal family. He was always very well dressed: His handkerchief matched his tie, his cuff links were gold, and he had a gold collar pin. He was very manicured, just like my dad. His hair was silvery white, combed straight back—very Errol Flynn. He was always watching me, and he would leave generous fifty-dollar tips. But he never really spoke to me, except to order.

One day I just decided to ask him. "What gives here? I don't want to be too forward, but I'm curious. You've been very generous, but you never speak to me. And I was wondering why you always request my section."

"I come here because I love to watch the way you handle people," he said. "You're so much fun, and everybody enjoys themselves. I think there's a bigger and brighter future waiting for you. How about coming to work for me? Would you like to come in for an interview?"

Now I had no idea who this man was. When he said all this, I began to think he was some big producer, and I started having Busby Berkeley dreams of me becoming a fabulous star, with my name in lights on a Broadway marquee. When he handed me his card, I glanced down at it and discovered that he was not a producer. He said to me, "I'm a marketing executive at the Pfizer chemical company, and we make Coty cosmetics. And I know what to do with your talent." The cosmetics world!

I went for the interview. The dapper man explained that I would travel to major department stores to market new Coty cosmetic products, including a new line for Dina Merrill. I'd test the products on customers, at the same time showing them how to apply makeup and convincing them to try a new fragrance. I told him that my mother had sold Coty for years, and was still selling Coty products in New Orleans—the fragrances Emeraud, Lamont, Jacqueminot, Vertige. We were a Coty family!

"Like mother, like son," I said. All those years of sitting on the edge of my mother's bed and watching her putting makeup on were going to pay off—something I'd never really expected.

I said yes to the job. With me, these kinds of decisions were like taking the next train: You got on and never looked back. I was taking another chance, and I was ready for it. Studying art in college, going to school in Italy, dancing as a meatball, coming to New York—these were all risks for me. True, I was young, but I seemed to thrive on always turning a new corner. So now it was happening again.

I went back to the AutoPub, gave my notice, cleaned out my locker in five minutes, and off I went.

I started my job with a brief training period. I learned about colors, palettes, and strokes. I learned to put foundation on the lips before the lipstick, so you'd see the true color. When applying eye shadow, I learned how to put the light color on the lid and then the dark in the crease of the eyelid to make the eyes look bigger. And most important, I learned how to apply eyeliner and add a little flip to the corner of the eye. It was almost like my mother's hands were guiding me.

Now it was time to put all this knowledge into practice. I started working the Coty counter in Bloomingdale's department store, promoting new products. What I didn't know, I improvised as I went along. Again, this was just like the AutoPub: another performance, except with makeup.

The big push was at twelve noon, when all the women rushed in during their lunch hour. I always had some special products going for Coty, whether it was a fragrance or new makeup or the new palette of blushes and colors. The really big hit of the season was eyelashes. Twiggy, the model, had made a big splash with her lashes, so now everyone was wearing them. Coty must have had fifty different kind of lashes: There was flutter, and flutter 2, and evening flutter—I mean, there were so many boxes of eyelashes, they all looked like little butterflies.

So I had to put lashes on these women, who were all in a rush. Well, at first I was not too successful at it. Ever try putting lashes on someone if they're in a hurry and you're impatient, like I was? In the beginning, I'd make terrible mistakes: I was putting the upper lashes on the lowers, so there'd be these huge curly things covering half the cheek. Or I'd put too much glue on the lashes, and the woman couldn't open her eyes, and I'd say, "Okay. Let's see now. Open your eyes." Completely shut. And then I'd make a mistake with the liner. The hardest thing to do is to draw a thin line on a woman's eyelid when she's talking to you and she has a nervous twitch. It was a learning process.

And once again, my performance attracted the crowds. I went back to my roots as the class clown and used my humor to get people to try the new products. I made people laugh, and while they were in a good mood, they bought and bought. "Ma'am! Yes, you. I think you've been shopping too long. Come over here. Take a seat. Relax and rest those feet. I'm going to show you how you can look years younger, not that you don't look beautiful already. And it's so easy." Who could turn down an offer like that?

One day while I was doing a make-over, the man who hired me stood behind a pillar, watching me doing my shtick. He walked over and told me to come and see him when I was done at the end of the day.

"How do you like what you are doing?"

"Well, how could you not like this? This is so much fun. I mean, it's a party here. It's dress-up time."

"Richard, you've been doing such great things for the company, I've decided to give you a promotion. I would like you to move to Dallas and use that as your home base. Then, I want you to travel to other cities and stores, and report back to me on how the new product lines are doing, and whether the stores are displaying and selling our products properly."

In a flash, I packed my bags (Coty had given me new luggage) and moved to Dallas. No looking back. I traveled a lot, doing four or five cities a week, hitting two or three stores a day. Dicky was on the move again. And I was making ten times more money than I had made at the AutoPub. I loved the traveling. I'm sure my parents' early show-biz days on the road had something to do with it.

But after a while, I began to wonder how long I could take this pace— and more important, where was all this going to lead me? Was I just going to die with a mascara wand in my hand in some department store? Was I going to make a career out of being a makeup artist? I couldn't figure out how I was going to grow in this job. I knew that I was the youngest person in the company to have so much responsibility. I was twenty-four and everybody else was about twice my age, all very conservative and stuffy.

Los Angeles was going to be my new home. I had no idea what

But I couldn't see myself with this same company in twenty years. Then, one of my trips took me to Bullocks, a large department store in Pasadena, California. I was to conduct a seminar on some new products in addition to a new fragrance that Coty was introducing.

City of Angels

As our plane flew over the mountains and began to make its final approach into Los Angeles International Airport, I looked out the window and started to get very excited. I thought, "This is Eden." I got this strange feeling when I walked into the terminal from the jetway. I knew, without a doubt, that there was another angel waiting for me in this city. In fact, this was a city of angels. I've always been blessed by the angels in my life, so I thought, I might as well meet a few here and stay. Los Angeles was going to be my new home. I had no idea what was waiting here for me, but I was so full of hope and excitement.

I did the Coty seminars and they were very successful, but it was time for a change. After the last seminar, I returned to my hotel, where I immediately picked up a phone and called my boss in New York to tell him I was giving my two-week notice. This was the hard part.

"Hi, this is Richard Simmons."

"Oh, hello, Richard. How did the seminars go?"

"They were really great. Everybody loved them. But there's something I must tell you."

"Oh, what is that?"

"Well, I've loved working for Coty and I really appreciate everything you've done for me. But it's time for me to move on. It's not the money, it's not the job, it's not you. It's just that I feel I belong here in L.A., and that I should be doing something else."

"I'm very sorry to hear that, Richard. But wait a second. Think about this. If you like Los Angeles so much, we can arrange it so you can work for Coty there. Think about it. You could have quite a future with this company."

"I appreciate that, sir. But I've already given it some thought, and I feel that it's time for me to explore some other things."

"What can I say. I respect you, Richard. If you've decided this is not your life's work, then you should move on. Whatever you do, Richard, I know you'll do it well."

"Thank you. Like I said, it's not the job. It's just that I feel there's something else waiting for me here, and I need to find it." I was deeply touched by what he said to me. I thanked him. And that was it. One more time, I was making a fresh start and wiping the slate clean.

The timing seemed perfect for me. I had managed to save a lot of money during the last year, so I had a financial cushion. And I remembered that you could never truly start something unless you stopped something else.

No more traveling for me. L.A. was to be my new home, and after a little more than a year on the road, I was settling down. There I was again, making one of those monumental decisions, and doing it quickly, without a second thought. Call me impulsive, but it's always worked for me. One of my teachers in high school once told me, "If you're taking a test with multiple choice or fill in the blank, usually the first thing you think of is the correct answer." If you begin to think too much, you wander into strange territory. I had never forgotten that lesson, and now I live my life that way—or at least that's how I try.

I didn't know anybody in Los Angeles. I had no idea what I was going to do here. I only knew that my life had already been like a novel—or an autobiography—and now I was about to start a new chapter.

Because of the cosmetics seminar, I was already staying at the tall, tubular Holiday Inn in Brentwood, right in the middle of several major freeways (it's still there). It was like a tube of lipstick, and every window faced a freeway.

Every day, I searched through the Help Wanted section of the *Hollywood Reporter* and *Daily Variety,* two local trade papers geared to the entertainment industry. I still didn't know what I was looking for, but I figured I'd know it when I saw it. And I was willing to wait until the right job came along.

About this time, I moved out of the Holiday Inn into a small apartment in Brentwood, which put me more in the center of things. Living next door to me was an Italian dentist who made false teeth. Really! We became friends, and he offered me a part-time job, sorting imported plastic teeth. When a shipment of the teeth came in, I would go over to his apartment where I would separate them by color. Let me tell you, this was not easy. There are twenty-six teeth in the mouth, and the plastic ones come in nine shades of white. You've heard that Eskimos have a whole bunch of different words for snow? Now I understand why. There were all these little boxes, just full of loose teeth. I couldn't tell the difference between "real white" and "real, real white" and "sparkling white." So while I was looking for a job, this is how I made a little money. And to this day, I'll look at people and say, "I think you're a C-1. No. Make that a C-2."

Today's Special Is . . .

As I was eating lunch in a coffee shop one day, reading the classifieds in the *Hollywood Reporter*, I saw the ad I'd been waiting for: It said, "Looking for a waiter with a fun personality." Well, I had been a waiter and I certainly was fun. No question about it! This was the job for me.

Immediately, I went over to a little hotel called the Beverly Comstock on Wilshire Boulevard. I took the elevator to the second floor to a restaurant called Derek's. When I got off the elevator, there was a heavy wooden door. I thought, "There couldn't possibly be a restaurant here. It looks too private." But I opened it up and there it was, this little gem of a restaurant. I felt at home right away. There were twelve round tables. All the seats were deep maroon vinyl and each table was lit by candlelight. The walls were dark wood paneling, giving the place a very cozy feeling.

Derek, the owner, a Welshman who had been a chef for several famous Italian restaurants in L.A., such as Carmines, had just finished making an order of veal saltimbocca with prosciutto and spinach. And I knew about prosciutto from my first day in Italy, in Pisa. I spoke with him and his wife, Judy, as I ate the delicious meal. It was love at first bite. Derek told me that he and Judy had taken all their money and decided to open a restaurant— their dream. They'd been in business three days, and they were looking for a waiter with a sense of humor who could really keep things lively. They asked me when I could start.

I said, "How about now?" And that was it. Once again, impulsive Dicky had made his decision, just like that.

Judy was much younger than Derek, and she was all Irish, with dark hair and a happy, round face. She was rather plump and could talk anybody into anything. So Judy and I worked the front room—I waited on tables and she did the hosting. We were quite a pair.

Because the restaurant was new, business started off slowly, and at first, I did a little of everything. I washed dishes, I waited on tables, and I answered the phone if Judy wasn't at the front. Derek was always in the kitchen, and Judy was always mingling. There was also a bartender named Franz, and that was it—just the four of us.

For the first few months, things were slow, so they gave me a little extra salary to cover my expenses. They had no budget for advertising and were hoping to build business by word of mouth, slowly—and that's exactly what happened.

Word got around about this little Italian restaurant in the neighborhood where the food was excellent and the waiter was very funny and very outrageous. The area of Wilshire Boulevard where the hotel was located is called the Wilshire Corridor—it's a string of high-rise condominiums with extremely wealthy tenants. Within a couple of months, the restaurant became very busy. At times there was a two-hour wait for a table. People didn't mind. They waited. And just like the AutoPub, there were great tippers. But I was always thinking of ways to make extra money.

All of a sudden, it occurred to me: I'll make jewelry. I'd had a course in art school where we had to make parts of the body look like art. So that's what I did now. I designed jewelry pins and charms in the shape of a heart, liver, spleen, pancreas, kidney, lungs, and a special 24-carat-gold uterus with opal ovaries. Really, I did. It was anatomical jewelry. I found a factory downtown that could make them from my designs. Then, from a jewelry shop in the neighborhood, I got a velvet-lined traveling case so I could display all the pins, and I took the case to the restaurant.

After a table had finished dessert and was sipping coffee, I would bring the case over and sit down.

One of the diners would ask, "What's that?"

I'd take out a pin out and say, "That's a liver."

"A liver? Oh, what a lovely liver."

"And look, I also have a spleen!"

"A spleen?" She'd turn to another diner at the table and say, "Look, Doris. It's a spleen. Isn't it adorable?"

And then I would sell a liver and a spleen. After a while, practically everyone at Derek's was wearing one of my anatomical pins or charms.

I was also infatuated with the way circles looked, so I designed cloisonné rainbow circles, and they became very popular with the Derek's crowd.

One evening, the very famous designer Rudi Gernreich came in. He spotted my rainbow pins on some of the customers and instantly liked them. When he found out that I had designed them, he walked over to me and said, "I love that circle you designed. I'll need about forty-seven thousand of them. I want to put one on every dress that I'm doing in my new line."

I said to myself, "This is good. I may have stumbled onto something here." I got busy manufacturing those pins.

In the meantime, I took the extra money I'd made from the jewelry and I moved to an apartment in a building called Le Chateau on Rossmore Avenue, across the street from the Ravenswood, which Mae West owned and lived in, located in an area called Hancock Park. This is where a lot of old-time movie stars such as George Raft, James Cagney, and Edward G. Robinson built apartment buildings. My new home had more history and more character than the apartment in Brentwood.

And at Derek's, as business picked up, the tips just kept rolling in and I kept moving on up, just like the Jeffersons. A short time later, I moved into another apartment, on South Maple in Beverly Hills.

There was one area, however, where I wasn't making any progress. I'd put some weight back on because I'd been eating. At first, when the restaurant wasn't busy, I would "sample" the dishes. As we got busier, I found I was eating "on the run." But the biggest reason I was eating was because the food was free. I've always said that food is great. Well, free food is even better. (You know that I couldn't write a book without saying that somewhere.)

And the food at Derek's was like no other. When customers were seated, I'd greet them with a basket of french-fried zucchini, which had been tossed into a bowl of Parmesan cheese and shaken around. People would drool as they saw me approaching with that basket.

rhood where the food was excellent and the waiter was very

There were no menus at Derek's. Instead, I would sit on someone's lap, usually a man who could handle my weight—rather than a woman, whose legs I might break—which made everyone laugh. Then, I'd say, "Hi. Let me tell you about what we're serving tonight."

And I would paint a portrait with food. I'd describe the jumbo shrimp cocktail with fresh tangy dipping sauce or the mozzarella marinara—thick pieces of cheese rolled in bread crumbs and ground filberts, deep-fried until golden brown, and the cheese inside oozed out when you cut into it with your fork. I'd tell them about the veal piccata: veal sliced very thin and sautéed with capers and finished with a light lemon sauce. Or I'd describe cioppino, a steamy bouillabaisse-style dish with shellfish. They'd have been willing to eat their napkins if I had described an Alfredo cream sauce to spoon over them—the napkins, that is.

I became very meshugana—even more of a cutup. I felt like I had found another little stage, this time inside an Italian restaurant. And all these people came to eat—and to see me.

People would come in with fur coats and I'd say, "Oh, let me get your beautiful coat." Then I'd take their expensive mink and throw it in the corner like it was a towel. They would all howl with laughter. And if two people came in, and the restaurant was crowded, I would sit them at a table with people they didn't know. If I brought a customer the wrong dish, I'd say, "Look. It's hot, you're here, you're hungry. Let's just go for it, okay?" Or if someone would say, "I wonder what that mozzarella marinara tastes like?" I'd go over to a table that had the mozzarella, and say, "Excuse me. Can I have that fork? Give me a little bite of that," and I'd take it over to the other table. Sometimes I'd be on roller skates. It was like a party—a huge party, where I was the guest of honor. And I was never sick—I never missed a night. I was always there. (I had never missed a day in grammar school or high school, either. Write me, if you want to see my gold stars.)

All the celebrities and producers came in. People would bring in their friends and not tell them anything about what was going to happen, and then sit back and watch the reaction as I cut the necktie off a well-dressed man (no ties allowed at Derek's). If someone would loiter too long, I'd blow a whistle and tell them they didn't buy the table—get moving! I was so outrageous, and I made such unbelievable friends. I made up for every party I had missed going to as a child. I could do no wrong.

Derek's was becoming the hot place. All kinds of people came there, but mainly rich people from Westwood and the Wilshire Corridor. There would be entertainers like Johnny Carson, Ed McMahon, Mitzi Gaynor, Ray Stark, Dionne Warwick, and Tom Jones, and just plain rich people like the guy who created the Kerr canning jars and people who owned the big contracting companies. And sometimes there were politicians. Many times people would come in by themselves—like Robert Conrad from *The Wild, Wild West,* one of my favorite T.V. shows—and I would just sit down and talk with them.

I remember once I took a reservation for the Carpenters, and the whole family came in: mother, father, Richard, and Karen. Although there had been a lot of articles about Karen being heavy, by this time she was very thin. They ordered everything: the mozzarella marinara, the french-fried zucchini basket with Parmesan cheese, the baby shrimp whipped into a cream sauce and put into a light pastry shell, the Caesar salad, veal dishes, and pasta.

I noticed right away that Karen cut her food and sort of moved it around the plate, but she ate very little. She never touched her entree. I had been there. I knew the consequences of starving, and I was a little worried about her. When I cleared the table, there was still a lot of food on her plate.

I joked, "Come on, Karen. Finish this up." And then I started singing, "Close to you . . . " And they all laughed—all except her brother, Richard. He didn't think I was so funny.

Not too long after this dinner, Karen died. I read newspaper reports of her longtime battle to be thin. I felt a great sadness. How I wished there was something I could have said or done for her, something that would have helped her to understand that she was on a dead-end path. Would she have listened? I would never know. But I was deeply troubled by her death. She and I were closer than I thought.

I met someone at Derek's who would soon become another one of my angels, in a big way. His name was David Weisman. David came in quite frequently, and we bonded immediately. He was in his thirties and big and

ight—rather than a woman, whose legs I might break—which

burly, about six foot four, just like the Bounty paper towel man, and not the slimmest of people. He loved food. And I would see him around town, not only at Derek's. He was a very successful man, a self-made millionaire. He had a company that made these dresses that were on the seductive side, very tease-me—the hottest thing in juniors.

David did everything with gusto. When he came into Derek's, he would order a huge amount of food and stay late, and just laugh and laugh. You could see that he was a hard worker and burned the candle at both ends. And he was a gambler. He gambled at everything in his life—nothing had ever been handed to him.

After the restaurant had really started to become popular, I noticed a lady who began coming in. I later discovered that she was the restaurant critic for the *Los Angeles Times,* and she had a reputation as a terror. If she wrote bad things about a restaurant, that was it. It closed, because no one would eat there anymore, based on her review.

She came in one night with a man who I assumed was her husband. Remember, I didn't know who these people were. At Derek's I treated everyone like family. That's what my father had taught me—no strangers. I sat on her husband's lap. I did my whole menu thing, and they loved it.

Well, this couple kept coming back over the next two or three weeks, bringing all their friends with them. And I became especially friendly with her. One night as I was serving the basket of zucchini sticks, I said to her, jokingly, "You've been here so often, are you planning to move in? Oh, wait a second. I know. You're a restaurant critic. Are you writing a review?" And I just laughed.

The next Saturday night after work, I stopped as I always did to pick up the Sunday *L.A. Times.* When I got home around two or three in the morning, I took the phone off the hook and went to bed. When I finally got up late Sunday morning, I sat down and started flipping through the paper. All of a sudden, I saw this huge write-up on Derek's. I mean, it was a whole page of the "Calendar" section, and it was all about me! The food was mentioned: The veal saltimbocca was very delicious, the shrimp with the green fettuccine, the mozzarella marinara, the Caesar salad—all to-die-for. But it was just a paragraph about the food. The rest was about this outrageous

The article was like a movie review. It was another performanc

person who you had to see—you had to go to this restaurant to see the waiter. The article was like a movie review. It was another performance where I was four thumbs up (plus a chicken breast). After the review appeared, there was a three-hour wait to get in for dinner. The article was both good and bad. It was certainly good for me. It was about Richard, but it wasn't about Derek's. From that day, even though the restaurant became even more popular, things would never be the same. I was more of the star than Derek or Judy were, and I think they both began to resent me.

A couple of days after the restaurant review appeared, Derek had a heart attack. I was the one who discovered him in the kitchen, face down in a plate of linguini with clams. I immediately called an ambulance. I was pretty sure that the review had caused it. I was getting the star billing and taking over their dream. It was hard for me to come to terms with all this, because I was doing exactly what I was getting paid to do, and that was to bring in customers.

While Derek was in the hospital, Judy and I ran the restaurant by ourselves until he got better. And the craziness continued, even during the hospital visits. Because Judy and I worked late, we couldn't get to the hospital until after regular visiting hours. So, to walk past security, we would dress up as nuns. That's right, you heard me—nuns. Nuns can go anywhere. (Always keep a nun's outfit in your closet, because it's going to get you places. But don't make a habit out of it!)

Dieting in Beverly Hills

Since I had been living in Los Angeles, I noticed that there were many more diet fads on the West Coast than in New York. In L.A., it was the diet of the week—like the blue plate special. Every time I heard about a new, fast way to lose weight, I'd try it. You'd think by now I would have learned my lesson.

One evening at Derek's, I was waiting on a table of models. It was toward the end of the night and the restaurant was clearing out, so I sat down with them for a few minutes—you know how beautiful people are attracted to each other! The three women worked at a Saks department store in Beverly Hills as runway models. As we chatted, one of the women reached for her wallet in her purse, which was on the floor next to her feet. The strap was caught under her chair and when she lifted it, she spilled the contents of her purse onto the floor. As I bent to help her retrieve her things, I noticed a large family-size candy bar. I picked it up, and then realized it wasn't a candy bar—it was Ex-Lax, disguised as a candy bar. It was one of those embarrassing moments where we made eye contact, but no one said a thing. I discreetly shoved the Ex-Lax back into her purse before anyone else could notice, and continued to help her pick up pens and change and makeup from under her seat.

When she and her friends were leaving, she pulled me to one side.

"Oh my God, thanks for doing that," she said. "I just can't live without them."

"Live without . . . Ex-Ex-Ex-Lax?" I asked. I could easily make a list of the things I couldn't live without, such as my robe and fuzzy slippers or a plate of veal cordon bleu. But I don't think a laxative would be anywhere on my list.

"This is how I keep my weight down," she told me.

"What do you mean, this is how you keep your weight down? This is supposed to make you go to the bathroom."

"Exactly." She smiled at me. "I have a couple of squares before I eat, and then I just go to the bathroom. It's like I never ate." This woman was a size six. I immediately thought of my friend Josie from the AutoPub. But this woman looked great. She didn't look tired, she didn't look sick the way Josie had after a few months of the ritual. Besides, what could a few Ex-Lax hurt? What was the big deal?

So, the next day, I went to a nearby Rexall Drug Store and bought a bar of Ex-Lax, the family-size. When I got home, I removed the outside wrapper, too embarrassed to be seen with a laxative that big. To dispose of any trace of evidence, I flushed the wrapper down the toilet, something that would come back to haunt me as I clogged the plumbing in my apartment forever.

I was left with a gleaming silver bar. It was milk chocolate and delicious! If you didn't know any better, it could have been a large Hershey bar—not bad. I added another instrument to my tool chest of diets.

And that's how I began. I'd have two squares before breakfast, eat, and then go to the bathroom. I'd repeat the pattern at lunch and again at dinner.

And then I did what I always did. I followed the theory of "more is better." I began taking three squares of candy per meal, and then four. My giant bar was gone before I knew it.

I'd been shopping at the same Rexall Drug Store for a while, and everyone knew me—it was difficult not to. I didn't want to keep going back there for my Ex-Lax—people might begin to talk. So I began to shop as though I were buying an illicit drug, going from store to store in the neighborhood, trying to find different places where I could get my fix and people wouldn't recognize me.

Once again I was spending my life in the bathroom, just like I did when I was sticking my fingers down my throat. If only I had bought stock in Scott toilet paper, back when I was practicing those commercials in front of the mirror in New Orleans! The Ex-Lax was doing its job. I wasn't feeling any serious side effects, other than getting to know my bathroom very well. But I was always uncomfortable and sore. And, I never knew when I was going to have to go, so I'd always make sure there were rest rooms nearby. I was losing weight, but not as fast as when I starved myself. It began to dawn on me. Was I starting down that same road I had traveled in Italy? I began to worry. Maybe the laxatives were not such a great idea. I had to try something else.

* * *

Just as I was wondering what that something could be, a friend asked me if I would try a diet with him called Metrecal. Metrecal stood for "metered calories." It was a liquid shake that took the place of meals. You mixed a powder with water, milk, or juice.

It was 1973, and all of a sudden these diet shakes became all the rage in California. It was like the powder wars—everyone was sipping a drink instead of eating a meal. One night, one of my regular customers asked me what my astrological sign was. She told me she went to a place where they blended a powder that was matched to your astrological sign. Mine was Cancer, but not just plain old Cancer. I was Cancer with chocolate rising.

At the time, there were two things I liked about the shakes. First, most of them were given out by doctors. And second, the shakes took the place of "real" food. So since you weren't eating, you lost weight. This all made perfect sense to me: doctor-supervised, and no eating.

I tried all the powders and shakes. I developed a very close relationship with my blender. I'd have one drink for breakfast, another for lunch, and a third and final shake for dinner. There was no food involved, so no choices to make. No grocery shopping, none of that. It was so easy. And the other nice thing was that, unlike the laxatives or throwing up, I didn't have to hide. I could do this right out in the open. Everyone was doing it. In fact, drinking these shakes became quite popular in Los Angeles. People began bringing their powders into the restaurant to be blended, while the rest of their friends ate.

Just like when I was starving myself in Italy, I felt the same euphoric high. My body didn't have to go through the digestive process. Initially, I did begin to lose weight. Of course, every morning, I would want to eat my blender, I was so hungry. I had to find ways to make the shakes more palatable. I discovered that they did taste better if I added a scoop of vanilla ice cream. Or when I substituted half-and-half for the water, they were really quite tasty. If you put a scoop of peanut butter in the chocolate flavor, you had a Reese's Peanut Butter Cup—well, almost. And this was before Ben & Jerry's became popular.

One day, I was at home, getting ready to go to work at Derek's. I was fixing a shake for myself. I added the powder, the ice cubes, and the milk. I flipped the "on" switch on the blender, and instantly I was covered in a gooey mess. There was liquid dripping from the kitchen ceiling, my appliances, and my face. I'd remembered the correct ingredients, but because I was in a rush, I'd forgotten to put the cover on the blender. I was reaching my breaking point. I was beginning to feel punished.

I was sipping my shake at the bar in Derek's that night and complaining to the bartender. I needed to lose more weight, but I'd had my fill of these stupid shakes. He said, "Hey. See that lady over there in the corner? She has a place called the Willow Tree."

"Willow Tree? Sounds thin and wispy," I said. "What is it?"

"It's a place where you can get some special kind of shots," he told me. "H.C.G., or something like that." I had no idea what they were, but I was

Then, a woman in a lab coat took me to a private room and to

willing to find out. If it didn't involve starving, throwing up, taking laxatives, or sipping shakes, I was eager to try it.

The woman gave me her card, and the next day I called and made an appointment. The Willow Tree wasn't quite as private and serene as it sounded. It was just a little place in an office building on Wilshire Boulevard. I arrived for my appointment, and an assistant behind the desk weighed me. Then, a woman in a lab coat took me to a private room and told me to drop my pants. She slapped my butt and gave me a shot. In the lobby, I received a white sheet of paper. But unlike Dr. Hallman's diet, this piece of paper was pretty. There was a picture of a willow tree on it. The sheet had a 500-calorie diet I was to follow. And finally as a treat, I received one sucker from a West Coast gourmet candy store called See's Candy. After I paid them forty dollars for the visit, that was it. I was on my way. No questions about my medical history, no discussion about what H.C.G. was. And truthfully, I didn't think to ask. I was too excited because I thought this was the answer to my weight problems.

I got a shot three times a week. Each time I went in, the nurses would crowd around the scale and applaud. The numbers were going down rapidly. Unlike my Weight Watchers experience where I fibbed, this time I was really working the program. I had discipline. I was coming in, getting my shot, and paying forty dollars each time. I was religiously following a 500-calorie diet. And I left with a sucker. Wait a second. On a 500-calorie-a-day diet, anybody could lose weight. Even a parakeet. Who was the sucker? It was me!

Then one morning, I picked up a newspaper. My eyes widened. There was an exposé about my latest weight-loss program. H.C.G. was a hormone derived from the urine of pregnant women! Can you believe it! I'd done it again! I bet if the pretty paper with the diet on it had read Pee Tree, rather than Willow Tree, the office would have been empty. But because the treatments had a medical-sounding title, and were administered by people in lab coats, the whole thing seemed legitimate. I read on to discover that no studies had been done to determine that H.C.G. was either safe or effective. Fear set in. I wasn't any better off than when I had starved myself in Italy.

For almost the past two years, I'd spent a good part of my restaurant tip money on powders, shakes, laxatives, and shots. I was running out of diets. I had tried all these things, and I was still in no better shape mentally or physically than I was when I took that first diet pill in sixth grade. But never in my wildest dreams did I think I was going to become involved in something that I swore I would never, ever try.

Sweat—What's That?

When I was growing up, gym class, as far as I was concerned, was the worst thing in the world. As I told you before, I never participated. I always had doctors' excuses because of my asthma or my flat feet or anything else I could think of that would get me out of class. So I'd never done any physical activity my entire life, except, of course for that horrible experience of climbing the leaning tower of Pisa. To me, walking through a cafeteria line was exercise enough.

But California was about to be hit with the exercise craze. And because I was a person always looking for the newest thing to help me lose weight, I was about to be swept away.

At Derek's, there was a woman in her early sixties who was very slim and toned. She ate at the restaurant almost every night, since she lived directly across the street. One evening, when our conversation turned to weight loss, she told me she had a fabulous way to stay thin.

"Oh my goodness, you've got to go take a yoga class with me."

"Yogurt? You mean there are classes on how to eat yogurt?"

"No, my dear. Yoga. It involves breathing and stretching. I've been going to this yoga man, and he's very exciting. You must come with me, as my guest."

If yoga helped this woman stay thin, then maybe it would work for me. Breathing and stretching—how hard could that be?

She took me to a place called Bickram's in Beverly Hills. Bickram himself taught the class. He was a man in his early twenties who was short and thin, originally from India. He put on some slow, peaceful music, almost like a chant. We all sat down on mats and then he began, softly and soothingly, to give us directions.

"Bend your head to the left and your arm to the right like this," he said, contorting his body gracefully. Some positions or exercises had their own names. "Breath of Fire," he'd call out, and everyone would begin breathing rapidly through their noses. I was the only one doing "Breath of Fainting." All that breathing made me dizzy.

He'd call out "Cobra," and everyone would get on their belly and twist themselves up like a pretzel. It took me at least five minutes to get myself out of the cobra. I got a little stuck.

I thought Mr. Bickram was a wonderful teacher, but after class I knew that yoga was not for me. For one thing, everyone was so serious. No one cracked a single joke, even though they had their bodies in these really funny positions. I thanked Mr. Bickram and the woman who took me, but I knew I was never going to reach a Zen moment with yoga.

The next wave of gossip was about another kind of exercise called Pilates, now very popular again. Everyone was working out with a man named Ron Fletcher. So there I was, on my way up the stairs to Ron Fletcher's in Beverly Hills. The next thing you know, I'm exercising with Ali MacGraw and Cher.

Pilates is a form of exercise that uses resistance. It's done on a Pilates machine, which looks a bit like a long box with springs and a pad in the middle. You lie down on your stomach or your side, and then move your body slowly through a variety of different positions. The room was very quiet. There was no music. And all you could hear were people breathing. Everyone who worked there was very serious. Even the phone rang quietly, and the receptionist whispered when she answered it. This place made the Beverly Hills Public Library look like a fraternity party.

Ron himself was a wonderful and dedicated man and a very good teacher. And I couldn't wait to get out of there.

New places featuring techniques I had never heard of kept opening— and there was always something new to try. And I kept trying.

One afternoon, I found myself at Alex and Walter's. Alex and Walter were two men, originally from Russia, who had worked with Russian gymnasts, preparing them for the Olympics. I remember the first day I went. Alex

d me she had a fabulous way to stay thin. "Oh my goodness,

and Walter were dressed in the little white tank tops and long white pants and suspenders that gymnasts wore. One of the men (honestly, I couldn't tell them apart) went to the wall near a matted area and let down a rope. Magically, two silver rings appeared from the ceiling.

"Grab the rings," the other man said.

Okay. I could do that. I grabbed the rings, and then both of the men started pulling on the rope. Still holding the rings, but now hanging on for dear life, I rose up in the air like a balloon from Cirque de Soleil. I was three feet off the ground, then five feet, and then I was fifteen feet up. My hands were burning, but I couldn't let go. I was too high up.

Now both of them said together, "Try your best to keep your arms straight, and bring these rings to the side so your body forms a T." "T" obviously meant torture.

"Get me down." I said, trying not to scream. "Lower those ropes. I'm afraid of heights." This was not starting out too well. So down I came, but Alex and Walter were not ready to give up on me.

"Let's tumble," they said to me.

I was no gymnast, and I was willing to admit it. After one session with Alex and Walter, I swear my arms had stretched several inches. I was glad they'd helped all those people win medals. But there was no medal in my future.

Still, there were many more avenues to investigate. Driving on Ventura Boulevard in the Valley one day, I saw a sign that I just knew would be my salvation. It was made for me. It said, "Get in shape in thirty days—fifty dollars at Vince's Gym." I'd already spent a lot of money on exercise. Each place I'd go, I'd sign up for a series of visits, but I would barely make it through the first session. I figured Vince's Gym could even things out for me. I went around the block a few times, getting my courage up, and finally pulled into a small parking lot, next to a very unattractive, small, dark-wood building. Vince's gym would be my next step up.

I was already feeling like a failure. But I thought that as long as I kept trying to exercise, hopefully I wouldn't have to deprive myself, punishing my body with endless diets.

I paid my fifty dollars up front and walked into the gym. It was one big room with benches and free weights for circuit training. Some of the dumb-bells were twice the size of my head. I had never picked up a weight in my

I put on my muscle-man attitude so I'd fit in. The truth was,

life. The heaviest thing I'd ever picked up was a party platter at Nate and Al's Delicatessen.

At the front, a weathered-looking little man, who bore a remarkable resemblance to Burgess Meredith in the movie *Rocky,* came over to me. He slapped me on the back, which practically knocked the wind right out of me. He told me we were going to do some real work.

I took a look around the gym and realized that everyone in the place looked either like him or like Rocky. This was a man's gym. There were guys in this gym who were three times my size. They were mountain men, policemen, prizefighters, and construction workers. They could bench-pressed me without even breaking into a sweat.

I put on my muscle-man attitude so I'd fit in. The truth was, I felt like turning and running out the door—that would have been a good workout. But I'd already paid my money, so I decided to stay and at least try it.

Vince himself patiently showed me how to use each machine and walked me through each exercise. There were weights and pulleys and cables. I did biceps curls and lifted barbells next to a man who told me he was a retired policeman. He'd been shot three times and he was willing to show me the bullet holes to prove it. On the other side was a truck driver with a weight belt. They all made grunting noises and scrunched their faces each time they hoisted a weight. Everyone was in gray sweats that you could tell had never seen a washing machine or a box of Tide. I had selected an emerald-green jogging suit with narrow white piping on the side, which I'd purchased at the sporting-goods store the day before. I may not have been able to lift a Volkswagen like some of these guys, but at least I could coordinate a colorful outfit.

Vince had me do squats with a forty-five-pound barbell that I had balanced on my shoulders. After I'd lifted weights, Vince had more surprises in store for me.

"All right, now. Do you like push-ups?" Vince asked.

Did he mean the kind in the frozen-food section with the sherbet inside? Sure! I'll have a raspberry one! Was he going to give me a push-up? Apparently not, because when I looked at him he was on the mat doing twenty fast push-ups.

"Okay, your turn. Start with twenty."

I did two.

"Okay, we'll work on those next time." Vince was unfazed. "Let's do some situps. Give me fifty."

Fifty! He held my ankles. Maybe if he'd been holding a candy bar, I would have had a reason to sit up. I managed to do five . . . but not very well.

"Okay, those need work, too."

Then, he had me go up and down, up and down, on this little set of three steps, about a thousand times. I was going nowhere fast. Finally, Vince said I could rest. He should have added, "in peace." As I was lying on the mat, he told me to come back tomorrow. We had a lot more work to do, and he wasn't going to be as easy on me as he had this first day. Oh, really? Needless to say, I would not be back.

I got in my car and tried to lift my hands to the steering wheel—it took me a few minutes. Every muscle was cramped and everything hurt: my neck, my back, my legs, my arms—it even hurt when I blinked my eyes. I drove home and got into a hot bath. Lying there, unable to lift the soap out of the tray, I thought to myself, You know, maybe this is just the way I'm supposed to be—this is how the cards were dealt. I would always be a little overweight, and I would always struggle to do something about it. Is that such a bad thing?

The Turning Point

I really felt like a failure at all the exercise places I'd been to. I just couldn't seem to fit in. One night at the restaurant, I was telling all this to Darolyn, a friend of mine. I explained that I had tried a whole bunch of different exercise places, but none of the shoes fit. I had come to the conclusion that exercise was not fun. What was I going to do now?

She said, "I know a place for you. It's where I go, and believe me, it's fun. I love it. As a matter of fact, the lady who teaches the class is a customer of yours here at Derek's. Her name is Gilda Marx. She teaches a class on Pico Boulevard."

I had nothing to lose. I met Darolyn one afternoon, and she took me to the class in a dance studio. A very striking, very powerful-looking woman stood at the front of the room. She was like Xena, but blond. She had red nails and red lips and was wearing a red leotard. It was Gilda Marx.

During class, a man named Steve played the piano. I loved it. Maybe I was finally getting somewhere. The workout was a combination of many of the other exercises I'd tried. But this was to music, and we danced! This was fun! Gilda was very high-energy, she was exciting, and she had the most beautiful smile. As I looked around the dance studio, I noticed I was the only guy. But almost everyone else in the room was someone I knew from Derek's—models, actresses, and other show-biz types. And they knew me. We cracked jokes together as we danced, and maybe I did sing a number or two. Exercise could be *fun*, for me, anyway! I finished the class, right to the very end, and then I paid for the entire series.

I was finally on my way to finding true fitness. I was so excited and invigorated that I just wasn't ready for the next rejection. I didn't see it coming. And maybe that's why it hurt so much.

That evening, Gilda and her husband came into the restaurant. After they had been seated, Gilda got up and walked over to me and handed me an envelope.

"I'm sorry, Richard."

"Sorry about what?"

"Here's all your money back for the classes."

"Why? Is the money counterfeit? Should I print some new bills?"

"No. I don't think you can come back to class. The truth of the matter is, the women are not comfortable with a man in the class."

"They're not comfortable with me? But they all know me. They're my friends. And we had such a good time this afternoon. Gilda, I just don't understand."

"I'm sorry, Richard."

I was very upset and almost in tears. I didn't really believe that the women in class didn't want me there. I think it was Gilda's decision—I was just too much of a cutup, too much of a disruption for her to handle. But for me, I couldn't remember a happier day than when I'd taken that class. It was the first time I felt that my body was really alive.

The music in Gilda's class had taken me back to my childhood, when I used to listen to my 45 r.p.m. records in my room. Her class had opened a new door for me, and then it got slammed shut, right in my face. My heart was broken, and I was so furious with Gilda.

Years later, my path crossed with Gilda's again. I was on a television show in L.A., and someone was saying that Jane Fonda had started the whole exercise movement, and I said, "Hold it! Wait a minute. Jane Fonda did not start it. Jane Fonda went to the same studio I did, and it was Gilda Marx's—she was married to a son of one of the Marx brothers. And no one teaches a better class than Gilda."

After the program was over I went back to my exercise studio, and there was a telephone message from Gilda. I thought to myself, What do I do now? Do I call her back, do I ignore the message? I hadn't seen or talked to her since that night at Derek's, when she handed me my money back. I wasn't sure I wanted to revisit this whole rejection issue with Gilda. I swallowed hard, and decided I should at least find out what she had to say. I dialed her number.

"Hi, Gilda. This is Richard. Simmons."

"Richard! Oh, my God! How are you?" She acted as though we had just seen each other the day before. "All my friends have been calling. People who I haven't talked to in years. They all saw you on T.V., talking about me and how I started the exercise movement. That was so sweet of you, Richard."

She had no idea of what she had done to me years before. I was very quiet while she talked, and then I just started crying.

"Richard. What's wrong?"

"Gilda, it was so hard to call you. It was easy to talk about you on T.V., looking into a camera. But I've never really faced you with this."

"What are you talking about?"

"For all those years I had been looking for something that would help me lose weight and a place where I could feel alive. And then I found you and your exercise class. It meant so much to me to finally feel part of something so positive. But then you rejected me—you threw me out. The whole thing just made me feel real low and upset."

Now it was Gilda's turn to be upset.

"Richard! I had absolutely no idea that this happened, and that you've been carrying this around for all these years. I'm so sorry. What can I do to make it up to you? Can we have dinner?" That's what the whole world does: Patch things up over dinner.

"Gilda, despite what happened, I still respect you. I meant every word of what I said on television."

"Richard, I'm so glad we had this talk. Do you forgive me?"

"Absolutely. You know, in a way, you did me a big, big favor. When you wouldn't let me come back to the class, I didn't just sit in a corner and wallow. I got busy teaching myself the principles of exercise, then I opened my own little place, and I've been here ever since."

And Gilda had moved on to the exercise-clothing world, creating her own multimillion-dollar flexitard empire. With this phone call, I resolved my feelings with Gilda, and I put my anger to rest. Now finally, after all these years, I had made my peace with the lady.

At about this same time, something else happened that added to my unhappiness. There was a man, an actor, named Jim Stacey who used to come into Derek's often. Jim was everything that I knew I wasn't. He had been a football player and was currently an actor on a T.V. Western. He was a very good-looking, classic masculine type, who always brought gorgeous girls into the restaurant. He'd come in with a new model or an actress in a tight dress, with great curves, big hair, and major lips, and he'd give me a big hug. He just thought there was nobody like me—and of course, there wasn't. We were always kidding around.

One afternoon while getting ready for work, I was watching the news. My heart stopped. The newscaster was talking about Jim Stacey. There had been a terrible accident on Coldwater Canyon. Jim had been on his motorcycle with a girlfriend, and a truck had come around a bend and sideswiped them. It was horrible—in the accident, Jim had lost one of his legs and an arm.

I was in shock. I couldn't believe it. I found out which hospital he was in, and I tried to visit him a couple of times, but they wouldn't let anybody in except for the immediate family. I did finally manage to sneak into his room. He was unconscious, and there were machines and tubes everywhere. I turned and walked out of that room, devastated. I couldn't believe that one minute we were in a restaurant laughing and cutting up, and the next moment he was like this. Life is so precious.

The experience with Gilda, and now Jim, was a wake-up call for me. I realized that you could never know what's around the corner, waiting for you. Every minute, every second of life counts, and time shouldn't be

wasted. What was I doing with my life? Judy and Derek and all the customers at Derek's were like my family. I had made them all laugh, but now,
nothing seemed funny. And I was caught in a paradox. During the days, I
was trying to exercise to control my own weight, trying to eat less; and in
the evenings, I was serving fattening food to people in the restaurant. It just
didn't make sense.

I knew I was ready for a change, again. But what that change was going
to be, I couldn't figure out.

On one of my nights off from Derek's, I went into Chuck's Steakhouse in
Westwood, by myself. I was doing a lot thinking these days, and some ideas
were starting to take shape, vaguely. I sat down at a table and ordered a
steak, which included a trip to the salad bar. Well, the salad bar was puny
and hidden in a dark corner, like it was being punished. Some of the greens
looked as though they had been picked the season before. I made a salad
with tons of croutons and nuts. Sitting there eating, I said to myself, "So
here I am. And just look at my life so far. I'm still working in restaurants,
struggling with my weight, and I was kicked out of the only exercise class I
ever liked. I need to make some sense of my life and figure out how to get
more connected with people in a way that helps me. You know, what I
think I really want to do is open my own exercise studio. I think I'm onto
something here. I could learn the exercise steps, and I know some exercise
teachers. I love music, and I know a lot about it. And maybe I could add a
salad bar somehow." The ideas were starting, but they weren't gelling yet.

A few nights later, I was at a Chinese restaurant on Rodeo Drive. And
who should I bump into but my Derek's customer David Weisman. I
joined him at his table. He sat there smoking as I ate plates of steamed fresh
fish, moo goo gai pan, and chow fun noodles. He was in his usual jovial
mood, and we just talked and talked. I told him about Gilda's classes, my
salad bar idea, and everything else.

He said, "What do you really want to do?"

"Well, I really think if I built a little place and had a little salad bar and
exercise studio—I think it could be successful. I've got some teachers in
mind. And I know a lot of people in this town, and they would come."

He looked at me and said, "Well, stop by my office in the morning. I'll

Now I had the Willy Wonka golden ticket. I had David's chec

give you some money, and then you'll go find a place. Could you pass the egg foo young?" It was just as easy as that. He believed in me.

The next day, I drove downtown to the merchandise mart where I met him in his office. As I sat down, he reached into his desk, took out his checkbook, and wrote me a check. "Go find a place and get started. You're wasting time."

My next stop was to talk with Derek and Judy. I told them that this was it—I wasn't happy there anymore, and it was time for me to move on. I told them my idea about the studio, and they wished me luck.

Now I had the Willy Wonka golden ticket. I had David's check, and I had saved enough money from all the great tips that I had made. Now it was time to start the next journey, finding a place for my exercise studio.

Home Sweat Home

A few days later, I was driving around the shopping district in Beverly Hills. I turned a corner, and there it was—this little private street. It was like something out of the French quarter in New Orleans. There were bushes along one side, and parallel to them was an unused set of train tracks. And in the middle of the block was the old Wilson House of Suede warehouse, with a "For Lease" sign on the door. I peeked in the windows, and I could see that the space was long and narrow, just like a dance studio. And it wasn't that big, so it couldn't be expensive.

I immediately drove over to see my accountant and told him all about a terrific place I had found on Little Santa Monica in Beverly Hills. Well, this confused him, since there were two streets named Santa Monica: Santa Monica Boulevard, the one everyone knew, and then this little one that was about a block long that I had discovered, and that nobody could ever find—and still can't. When I took my accountant back there to show him, we got lost and drove around for about an hour, searching. He said to me, "You know, this isn't funny."

I said, "It's here! I know it is. I was just here a couple of hours ago." It was like the *Twilight Zone.* Someone had removed the street. For two weeks I searched, trying to remember that tricky turn. Then one day I finally found it. But the "For Lease" sign was gone. This *couldn't* be happening to me.

Next to the door was a small sign with the name of the owner of the building and a telephone number. I called right away, and to make a long story short, I talked him into letting me have the space, which had already been leased. And for twenty-five years now, I've been renting on a month-to-month basis. Four years ago, the name of the street was changed to Civic Center Drive, which made the studio a little easier to find. The people in the nearby Beverly Hills library are much happier now. There are fewer people who stumble in, shouting, "This doesn't look like Slimmons!"

So my plan was to have the exercise studio and a salad bar. I still thought that was a great combination. You could eat healthy and exercise—all under one roof. We went to work on it, and two months later, I opened Ruffage and Anatomy Asylum. Ruffage, the salad-bar part, actually had a bar that was twenty-five feet long. Attached in the back was the Anatomy Asylum, an exercise studio. Anatomy Asylum?! What kind of name is that? Well, if you're a little crazy in the head, you go to the insane asylum. If you're a little crazy in the body, you go to the anatomy asylum. It took me four weeks to come up with that name. (Later, I expanded the studio into one large space, just for exercise, and I changed the name to Slimmons. And Slimmons it remains today.)

Ruffage and the Anatomy Asylum became instant hits. This was my life, divided between salads and sweat. There had been a few salad bars in town, but they were part of larger restaurants, such as steak houses. Mine was the first salad bar where salad was the primary item served. Everyone flocked to it, including all my old friends from Derek's. Every person who thought a salad was a wedge of iceberg; every vegetarian who had never seen a real salad bar—this was their Field of Dreams . . . oops, I mean greens.

I had gotten Charles Burke to design the interior of Ruffage. He was a hot designer who had such a flair for designing clean, happy, whimsical rooms. The walls were textured cement, painted white, so when you walked in, it was like walking into a room of frosting. The floor was white tile, the tables were Plexiglas bases with glass tops, and there were director's chairs with white backs. To give it that enchanted feeling, Charles took the white umbrellas you see in photography studios and hung them upside

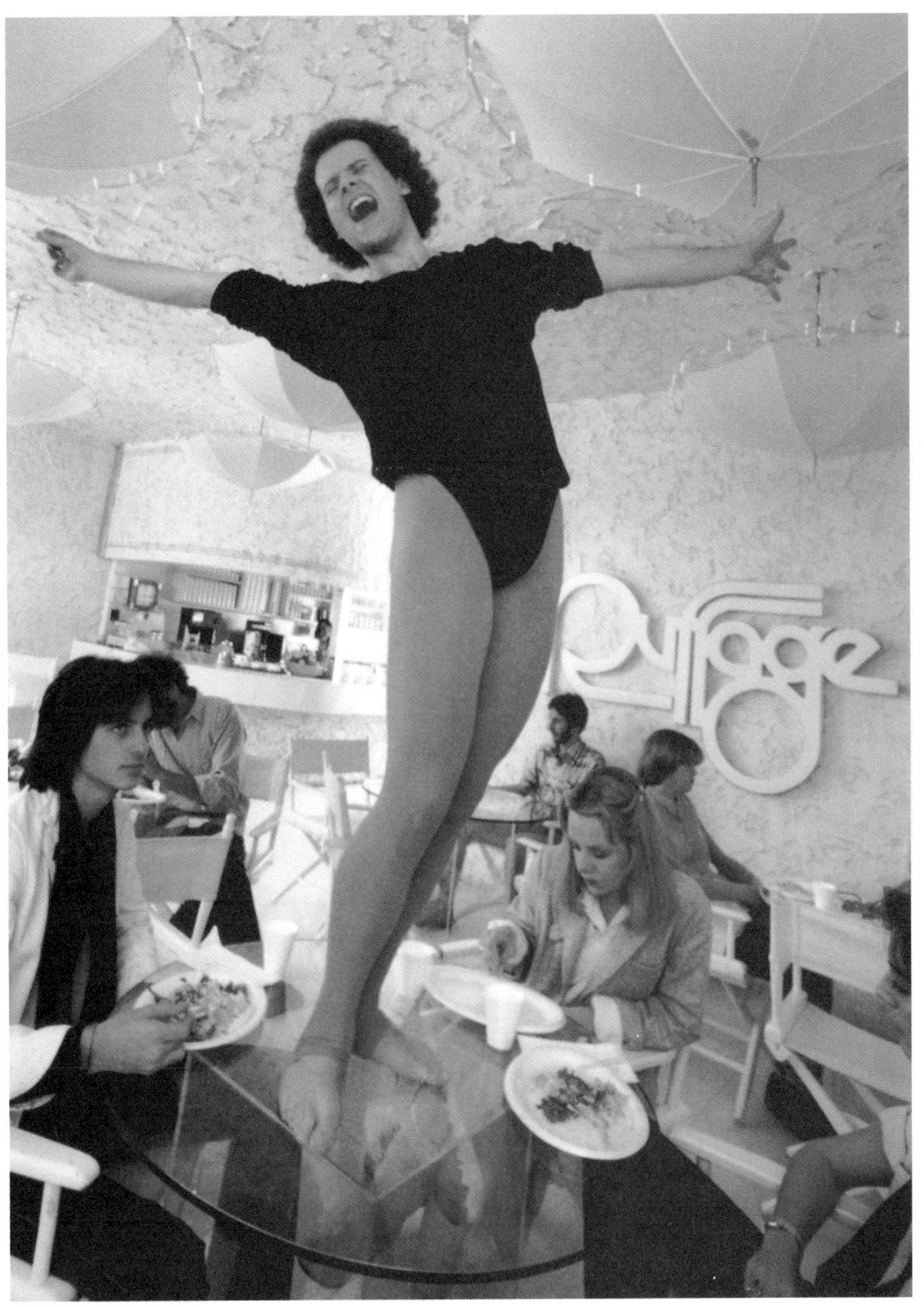

"Food, glorious food . . ."

n. If you're a little crazy in the body, you go to the anatomy

down from the ceiling. He took tubes of twinkle lights and arranged them all around the room. The tiny white lights gave the room a soft glow. The only colors were in the salad bar: the chopped fruits, vegetables, salad dressings, and juices—the carrot, watermelon, spinach, orange, and grapefruit juices that the Beverly Hills Juice Company delivered fresh every morning. California is produce heaven. The color of the food is what made the restaurant so appealing. And every day, I made a fresh vegetable soup.

The work at Ruffage was easy and came naturally to me because of all my experience at the AutoPub and Derek's. And remember, there was that kitchen on St. Louis Street, right next to my bedroom when I was growing up. I knew restaurants and I knew food. As I searched through recipe books and experimented with healthy low-calorie soups, breads, and side dishes, I heard my father's voice. As I talked to vendors about the fresh vegetables and fruits and spices that I'd need for the salad bar, I saw Leonard shopping at Solari's, the A&P, and the French Market.

But the other half of my business—the exercise—is where the real excitement was for me. I loved teaching classes. I loved the fact that I was exercising. It made me feel great, and I was truly having fun.

I had met a wonderful woman named Nina. She had been an aerobics teacher in other studios, so she taught me all the moves. I learned a lot from Nina, and the two of us took turns teaching classes.

I had hoped to have a piano player, but I couldn't afford one, so I brought in all my own favorite records from my collection. The first song I exercised to was on a Chuck Mangione record that Nina had given me, and I still use it even now. All that music I listened to while growing up, when I was overeating, was now the music I was exercising to.

I'll never forget the woman whom I regarded as truly my first student. She'd just been fired from a job at a hospital and felt it had something to do with her weight. Her knees and feet were constantly aching, and she was having trouble breathing. When she came in, she was both self-conscious and curious about the studio, and I saw a look on her face that tugged at my heart. I had been in her Stride-Rites and I knew exactly how she felt. I asked her if she was ready to take the first step, and I told her that I would be there with her.

I taught classes that were more like dancing, and they made you sweat. I included situps and push-ups, a little leg and arm work, and I did them all

I found out I was right about my studio. There were so man

with energy and humor. I always began every session with a warm-up. Then we began dancing, and finally we ended with a cool-down of stretching. I'd go to the nearby Beverly Hills library and I'd read everything I could about exercise and the body.

I found out I was right about my studio. There were so many people out there who were in my situation. There were people who hadn't thought that exercise could be fun. There were more people who'd never set foot in a gym or a dance studio because they were embarrassed by their size. There were people who had harmed themselves trying to fit in and lose weight. I welcomed all of them into my studio.

So, David Weisman had made a wise move when he decided to back me. As the years went on, David would call from time to time to see how things were going, or he would stop in and see me. I really think he liked the veal piccata and the fettuccine Alfredo at Derek's a whole lot better than grazing at my salad bar.

Besides Nina, who taught classes, there were two other women who helped me out at Ruffage. First, there was Roberta Kent, a woman I'd met at Derek's. She was a writer who later became a stand-up comedian. She soon became a close friend (and still is to this very day). She did a little of everything, and she fit right in when it came to telling jokes.

I had also hired a Filipino woman named Edna to help me in the kitchen. I'd met Edna at a place called Lindbergh's, an all-pink store that sold vitamins and beauty aids. Lindbergh's also had a counter with pink stools where they served healthy dishes. I used to love to go there for a half a sandwich and a cup of vegetable soup. Edna was like a human Veg-O-Matic. She could chop, dice, and slice like no one I knew, and she did it all with a smile.

This was a typical day for me: I'd get up early, about 4 A.M., and I'd go to a wholesale produce company called Mushrooms, Incorporated, to buy all the fresh produce. I'd bring the produce back, and Roberta and Edna would begin their work while I went in to teach the first exercise class at 6:30. After class, I'd join Edna and Roberta in the kitchen to help them prepare the food for the salad bar. Then, there'd be another exercise class at 9:00. After that, we'd set up the salad bar and prepare for the lunch crowd. Then there'd be an exercise class at noon. That's when the salad bar would really start getting busy. Just after one o'clock, the noon class would come

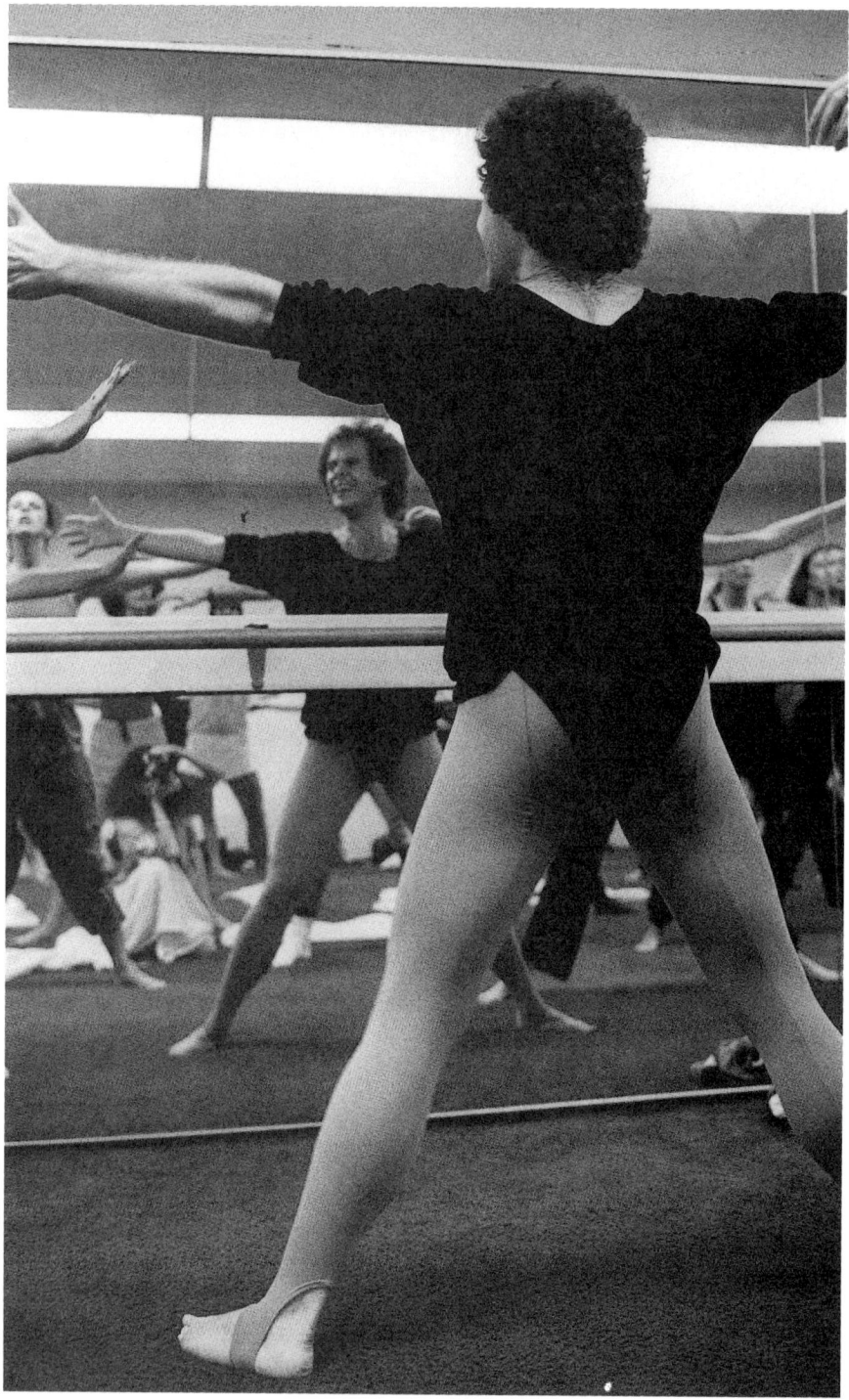

My early classes at Slimmons

The days may have been long, but I was very happy. I foun

out and have lunch. I'd spend my time restocking, cleaning, and going from table to table. There were more classes at 4:00, 6:00, and finally 8:00. Nina and I would take turns teaching these classes.

The days may have been long, but I was very happy. I found that when I kept busy, my desire for food did not speak to me so loudly and clearly. And busy I was, since I oversaw all the aspects of both businesses. Somehow, it all just seemed to work, and things kept moving along smoothly. Could one person be doing all this? I was so energized.

In class, my first student brought a friend, and her friends brought their friends. People who'd come to get a salad could hear the music. They'd watch us, and sometimes they'd come back the next day to take class. Little by little, we built up a big reputation.

In the exercise classes, I quickly developed a loyal group of students who all became friends. They were healthy, they were exercising, and they were feeling good. They began to call themselves the Richard Simmons Angels. There was such camaraderie and motivation that seemed to build every day. To my knowledge, there'd never been a place—an exercise studio—where out-of-shape and overweight people were both welcome and made to feel comfortable. In the Anatomy Asylum, there were overweight people next to overweight people. But then Cheryl Tiegs would be third from the left and René Russo would be in the back row. I think it was the combination of the music, the unique atmosphere, and the fun that made it a hit.

In my classes, everyone was wearing leotards and tights, a look influenced by the ballet. I decided that since I was at my thinnest, I should give it a try. Remember, I was into uniforms. Now I was entering my Rudolf Nureyev stage. I went to a place on Fairfax called Carabelle's, where I tried on a black leotard (size small) and flesh-toned tights, and they all fit! There wasn't a lot of material there. But like my fat clothes, this would become the uniform I put on every day. And I knew that uniform would not allow me to slip back into my old habits. I went everywhere barefoot, in my leotard and tights. As I dressed every morning, I'd think to myself, "I'm going to eat healthy, I'm going to exercise, and I'm going to fit into this tiny little leotard." By building my career around this philosophy, I hoped I was guaranteeing that I would stay that way.

In the early days, when I was still struggling to establish myself, I would look for extra ways to use the studio to make money. I hadn't changed much from the days of sorting teeth and making organ jewelry for extra cash. Because I was so close to Beverly Hills, I offered the studio for private parties. I began to have "healthy" birthday parties and showers. But I especially held a lot of Bat Mitzvah parties—religious coming-of-age parties for young Jewish girls. The girls would bring me their favorite records and we'd exercise, and then they'd have a salad. We'd finish with carrot cake, and then they would open their presents. It was certainly different—an aerobic Bat Mitzvah. The kids just loved it, and as the word spread, I found I was booked for an event every weekend. I wasn't the Wedding Singer—I was the Bat Mitzvah Sweat-er.

Each day seemed to bring in a new face. And each day brought in a person with a new problem—a problem to be solved. For many, my studio was a very healing place. I was there to listen. And while I wasn't a doctor or a psychiatrist, sometimes people talked to me about what was bothering them; sometimes they didn't. They came to Ruffage or the Anatomy Asylum to get away from their problems, to watch me cut up and to laugh. They felt good being there. And I felt good by being there for them. And it let me get beyond my own problems by helping others.

I was very open with everybody about my history—all the years I'd been facing this food war. I didn't hold anything back. If they wanted to hear it, I told them my whole story. I found that people trusted me because I was so honest about my own trials and tribulations. And in return, I heard stories that would affect me and stay with me for life. Sometimes, those stories weren't told to me—sometimes they happened right before my eyes.

"Bearly" There

I remember a sweet, young girl named Ellen. She was petite—under five feet, and quite thin. She had a little girl's voice to match her appearance. Although she always wore the mask of a pleasant smile on her face, I'm sure Ellen endured years of being teased about her appearance. Just as people who are very overweight are often made fun of, people who are very thin are fair game, too. I guess it goes along with the territory. Whatever God gives you in the appearance department, you have to deal with it—just look at my hair! But sometimes other people aren't very compassionate—I learned about that when I was a kid.

I rarely saw Ellen laugh, except when I was at a nearby table and I was clowning around or telling a joke. Ellen would drop her guard and I would see her rare emotions come through. She always came in alone and ordered a small juice. Many times she wouldn't even finish it. She never had a salad. She never exercised.

One day, I asked her what she did. She told me shyly that she made teddy bears. She confessed that she loved making those bears. And for my next birthday, Ellen came in as usual for her juice. When she left, I discovered a beautifully wrapped package at her table. Ellen had made me the most adorable teddy bear. It looked antique, with rusty-brown fur and a happy smile on its face. No one had ever given me anything like that before, a special, handmade present. I was touched by her thoughtfulness.

The next time she came in, I thanked her for the little bear. And she thanked me right back. She told me that she loved coming to Ruffage because it was the one place where she felt like she really belonged.

Over the course of the next year, every so often when I'd open up the studio early in the morning, there'd be a package at the front door. In the package there'd be a note from Ellen, thanking me for something I'd said, or sometimes simply the words, "Hope this makes your day." And, of course, along with that note would be another little bear. I could never guess when one of those packages would show up. But each bear was a detailed work of art.

While Ellen wasn't exactly opening up, I did begin to feel closer to her. And I began to worry. I noticed that she was getting smaller. She started to look frail and sickly. I never saw Ellen eat. I have always had an unwritten rule, which I still go by to this day. I will never walk up to a person and ask what's wrong, even if there appears to be a problem. I am always here to listen, but I do not make it my business to pry. I never say, "Hey, you're overweight, and I'm here to help you lose that weight." It's up to each person to make the first move.

And that's what I said to her. "Ellen, you've been so sweet to me, and now I have this beautiful collection of bears. Is there anything I can do for you?"

Her face immediately closed up, and she said, "No, no. I'm fine." Ellen never complained, and while I was worried, I guess I didn't realize the gravity of her situation. On one level, she seemed content with her work and very much at peace with herself.

Then, one day when I went home, I looked at her teddy bears, which I kept in my living room. I noticed that they seemed to be getting smaller, just like Ellen.

A few days later, when I came to the studio early one morning to open up, there was a teeny little box by the door. Right away, I knew who it was from. I opened it, and inside, wrapped in tissue, there was the tiniest, most detailed teddy bear I'd ever seen. It was no more than the size of a postage stamp—it must have been made under a large magnifying glass. Unlike Ellen's other works, this was not a happy-looking bear. It seemed very lonely sitting in that box, all by itself.

I didn't see Ellen over the next few days. I realized then that I knew so little about her. I didn't know her phone number or where she lived. I had no way to contact her.

A few more days passed, and I remembered that Ellen sold her bears to a boutique down the street from Ruffage. After lunch, I walked down to the store to see if I could find out more about her.

Outside, I noticed Ellen's bears in the window. In the store, I talked with the owner, explaining my relationship with Ellen and asking if she had seen her.

The woman looked at me with sad eyes and said, "I'm sorry. Ellen's no longer with us. She died a few days ago."

"What? What do you mean? She died?" I asked.

"Well, you know, she was anorexic."

I was confused and stunned by the news of Ellen's passing. I thanked the woman and walked out of the shop, in a daze. I'd never really heard the word "anorexic" before. If I had, I certainly hadn't paid attention. I didn't think I knew anyone who was anorexic.

The next day, there were a couple of nurses who took class, and I asked them what it was. They told me that anorexia nervosa is a condition that is thought to be psychological, and that is found mostly in young women. It causes them to have an aversion to food, which in turn can create a severe nutritional deficiency. So, an anorexic is a person who stops eating for no reason and millions of reasons; it's someone who gets smaller and smaller, just like those little teddy bears. That alarmed me, because I had once starved myself to lose weight.

I asked the nurses, "When I starved, was I anorexic?"

"Not necessarily, though it's a fine line," they told me. "You starved to lose weight. Anorexics starve to disappear. There are usually feelings of self-loathing or lack of self-worth connected with anorexia." That really struck me. In Italy, when I'd starved, it was because I finally realized my own self-worth, so I thought. I'd wanted to live, and to look my best so I would fit in, although I'd gone about it in a very harmful way.

I was angry with myself for a long time over Ellen's death. Why hadn't I done something? As I thought about all this, I would always return to my old dilemma. If Ellen didn't want help, what could I have done? Still, I knew I hadn't tried hard enough.

* ⋆ *

Always a Student

I learned so much at the Anatomy Asylum. For me, it was more than just a place to work and a way to earn money. It was my way to maintain my weight and my sanity. Much as with the diet pills, I still had a tendency to overdo things. But I found that I could throw myself into work and working out, and there were no harmful side effects, no physical repercussions. I felt great, I was healthy, and I slept soundly. I was actually building a positive career around my disorder: compulsiveness, which included overeating.

But there was still so much I didn't know. And in those days, there was still so much that wasn't yet known about exercise and weight loss. Remember, this was only the early Seventies. But I did begin to see some patterns develop. And one of the things I noticed when I taught class is that there were other people like Ellen. I saw the signs. There were people who may not have known what anorexia was, they may not have known how to spell it, but all the indications were there.

But with my policy of not approaching people first, I was stuck. And I worried about these Angels I'd come to think of as my family. That's when I came up with an idea: I would talk about these issues, without discussing them individually with people; I would do it in a group. I started holding meetings thirty minutes before each exercise class. We'd get in a circle on the floor in the studio, and we'd talk. In these meetings, we'd discuss anything that came to mind regarding exercise and weight loss. They were motivational meetings. We weren't professionals—we were just people of all different shapes and sizes who were sharing information and our feelings with each other. It made everyone feel closer—those who were stressed had a few moments to unwind before class, and the newcomers could settle in and get comfortable. I also discovered that more new friendships were formed during these thirty-minute sessions. I had started doing these meetings for myself, but they really became good for everyone.

I would overhear weight-loss discussions in Ruffage, or I would read about health issues in the news, and then the next day, I'd turn them into motivational talks. I'd always start by saying, "Look, there's a lot I don't know. But let's discuss this topic and see what we can learn." And because there was often an expert of some sort in the class, inevitably we'd come away from those meetings knowing more than we did when we'd started. After a while, I began to get anonymous letters from people in class, asking me to discuss certain issues.

Back in those days, you didn't discuss your physical or emotional problems unless you went to a therapist. You hid them from your family and friends, and you just didn't talk about them. (Sound familiar?) But over the course of these meetings and through my teaching classes, people began to open up, and I became aware of a broad array of dangerous ways to lose weight that I'd just never thought possible.

One day coming out of the studio, I saw one of the women who'd just taken my class leaning up against the wall, smoking a cigarette. She'd been working hard to get healthier.

I turned to her and said, "What are you doing?"

She said, "God, I just had to have a cigarette."

I tried to explain to her that when you exercise, your lungs become very expanded with all the air going in and out. Right after class is the worst time ever to light up a cigarette. You've done something so nice for your lungs and then you go outside and you do something destructive. (I'd never been a smoker. As a kid, I always wondered why you'd want a Pall Mall when you could have an ice cream float. It made no sense to me.)

She said to me, "Richard, if I did not smoke, I would be a cow."

"I beg your pardon?" I said.

"I smoke to keep my weight down."

Well, that was a surprise. This was another thing to discuss in class. And I found out that an enormous number of people smoked heavily as a method of weight control. They felt that smoking increased their metabolism and burned up calories, and that keeping a cigarette in their mouth didn't leave any room for food. Rather than eating a cookie, they'd smoke a cigarette, and they'd lose weight. This was their philosophy.

Just when I thought I'd heard of everything, a lady came into the salad bar. She was a regular customer and had always been very talkative and sweet. But this day she wasn't talking or smiling as she made her salad. She walked over to me, and with her teeth clenched, she asked me to put her salad in a blender. Her entire mouth was a prison.

"Oh my God, what happened? Were you in an accident?" I asked.

"No, I did this on purpose." With her teeth bound together I could barely understand her as the words forced themselves out.

"Oh, you got braces?"

"No, they're not braces," she managed to say. "I got my jaw wired shut. I have to lose fifty pounds." I couldn't believe it. It was beyond braces. How bizarre—that someone would actually pay to have their teeth locked together. And on top of that, she'd had one back tooth knocked out so a straw could go through it.

I put her salad in the blender. Now, I have to say that I'd come to love salads, but the dark-green glop that I poured into a glass for her was about the most unappetizing thing I'd ever seen. I thought back to my days of powdered drinks. I didn't even think a scoop of ice cream could have helped this concoction. She sat at a table and daintily sipped through her straw. I knew it had to be painful. I remember thinking to myself that there must be one nutty doctor out there performing this sadistic procedure. And then the parade began. All of a sudden it seemed I was blending salads by the dozens.

⋆ ⋆
⋆

One day, I was teaching class and a group of girls came out of the bathroom. They were hip, young girls who definitely wanted to be thin. As a matter of fact, they were already thin—they just wanted to get thinner. Class was about to start. They were sniffling and their noses were rimmed with white powder, like the powdered sugar on the Café du Monde beignets I used to eat as a kid. I went into the bathroom and I saw this white powder on the basin.

One girl, Betsy, returned to the bathroom and saw me staring at the sink. I decided to ask her what was going on.

I said, "I love you, and I'm glad you come here, but I have to ask you something because I don't understand it. What is this?" I pointed to the sink. Betsy got absolutely panicked and didn't want to talk about it. She burst into tears. But I was not ready to let her off the hook.

I said, "Tell me what this is."

"Richard, it's cocaine."

"Cocaine?!" I was shocked. These were young girls.

"Well, my brother told me I could lose weight if I used cocaine," Betsy explained.

I had seen that each generation was trying something different. But I couldn't believe this one.

My studio was right across the street from the Beverly Hills flats, an affluent area of town. This was a young girl trying the latest, most expensive gimmick available to her to lose weight. Betsy told me the best thing was that after snorting cocaine, she had no appetite—none at all. Plus, it was giving her a little bump of energy. She could take the class and run around all day, and she was never hungry.

In fact, Betsy and her friends, unable to expend all the nervous energy they were getting from the cocaine, had begun taking more than one class a day. I had to sit down with one of the girls and tell her she couldn't come to that many classes in one day. She was overexerting herself, putting too much stress on her muscles, and especially on her heart.

As I saw the signs of cocaine use more and more, I decided that this was definitely a subject for my motivation classes. Again, I was surprised at how many people were using cocaine as a method of weight control.

I did my research—back to the Beverly Hills library. And then in class, I talked about the disastrous effects of cocaine. I didn't have to talk long. Within the next few classes, this group of girls began experiencing dizziness, shortness of breath, and bloody noses while they exercised. They began to realize that they were living for this little brown bottle with the black top. Maybe our talks before class had helped them, and now they were thinking a little more about their health.

* ⋆ *

On the Other Side of the Tube

Not everyone who came into the studio took shortcuts or had self-destructive habits. There were many people who were working hard, measuring food, eating healthy, and losing weight slowly—for good!

Phyllis was one of those people. She said very little, but she really put her heart and soul into exercise. The weight began coming off. Before long, she'd lost sixty pounds.

She came up to me one day after class and said, "I have to tell you, I have never, ever felt better."

I told her she'd worked hard and she should be proud of herself.

"There's someone I know who wants to meet you. He can't believe how you've helped me."

"Oh, who's that? Your husband? Your boyfriend?"

"No. My boss." Well, this was a new one. Phyllis explained. She worked for a producer who had a show on television. The segments were all human-interest stories. It was called *Real People.*

The next week, I went to an office on Beverly Boulevard about four blocks away from my studio, and there I met George Schlatter, Phyllis's boss. He was a bearded, jovial man, almost like a young Santa. He said, "I want you to appear on my show because you're a *Real People* person." He scheduled me to come to the studio to tape a segment.

I told him, "I have an idea, if you're interested. I have ten people in my class—they've lost forty, fifty, sixty, seventy, eighty, ninety, and even a hundred pounds. Let's include them." He liked it. So when we taped the show, he let me put them all in the front row. He introduced me and showed a video they had taken of a class in my studio, with the great music and me and my crazy antics. Then Sarah Purcell, the host of the show, had the women in the front row stand up. Each one gave her name and how much weight she had lost. The place went nuts! The show was very inspiring and emotional.

From that small segment, the mail started pouring in, and the phone at the studio started ringing off the hook. People wanted an address where they could write. The *Real People* production office started bringing mail to my studio on a regular basis. This was my first taste of getting letters from people around the country asking for help. As a result, I opened a post-office box in Beverly Hills—Post Office Box 5403—which I still have to this day.

There was one person who had seen the show and was so inspired and touched—she would become the stepping-stone to my next television appearance. Another angel, a person I didn't even know, who would change my life. She was Joy Philbin, the wife of Regis Philbin. At that time, Regis had a local morning television show called *AM Los Angeles.*

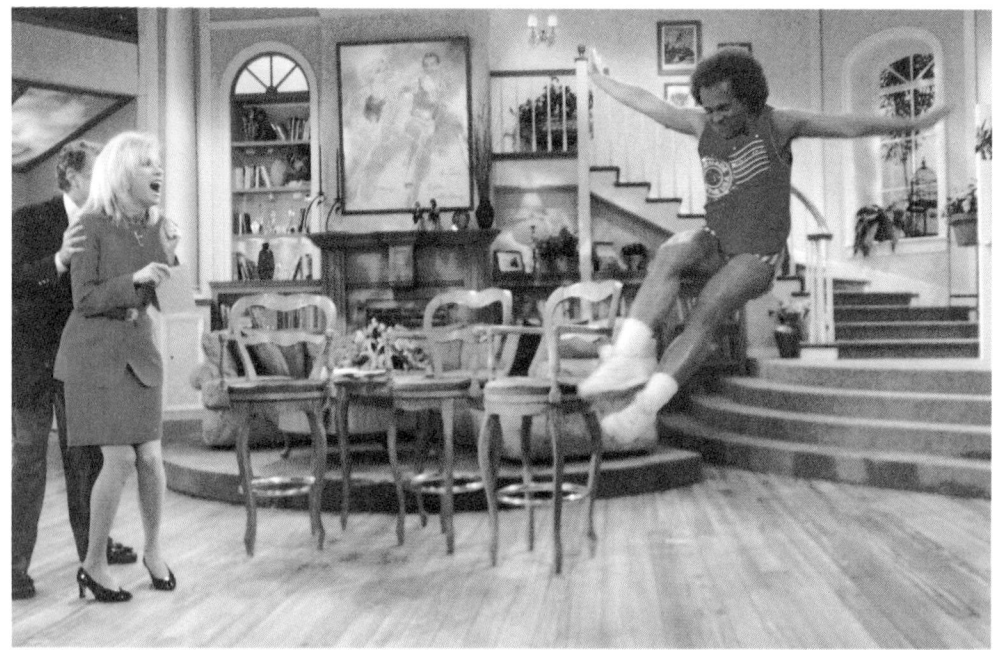

Kathy and Regis, my friends of twenty-five years, who have always believed in me

It   was   a   very   positive   feeling.   I   knew   I   was   helping   people   w

Joy told Regis, "You've gotta book this guy on your show. He's so full of energy, so fun. And he really helps people. I've never met him, but I think he's probably a nice man."

So, I got a call from one of the producers at *AM Los Angeles.* She told me, "Regis wants to surprise his staff. They've been working hard, so he'd like you to come in and hold an exercise class. It's a little present for everyone who works for him. "

And the next thing you know, I was booked on the show. There I was in my leotard and tights, exercising with Regis's staff. The response was overwhelming. It was a very positive feeling. I knew I was helping people who were stuck in the mud just like I once was. I felt good about the message I was spreading.

$$* \,{}_*{}^*$$

Start Spreading the Word

$\mathcal{I}$ have always been the kind of person who talks about something before it's a reality. I've always felt if I talked about it enough, I could make it happen, just with my will. One of my customers at the Anatomy Asylum was an intelligent, no-nonsense woman. She had come in a couple of times, and I always made casual conversation with her. (She was yet another angel waiting to flap her wings in my life.)

One day, I was talking with her about the book I'd begun writing. Of course, I'd always intended to write a book, and I could just picture it. It would be humorous and inspirational and filled with practical advice that anyone could understand. Well, this woman became very curious and asked me all sorts of questions about this book that I had not yet even started. When I answered in an authoritative manner, she reached into her purse and pulled out a business card.

"I'm Chris Conrad, West Coast editor of Warner Books," she told me.

All I can say is, Thank God my mother read me "Cinderella" as a child. I knew dreams could come true. She told me to bring an outline of the book to her office the next day.

"No problem. See you then," I said. Well, that was great, except for one thing. I had no outline. And what's more, I had no idea what an outline even looked like.

After lunch, I rushed to the trusty old library, which was becoming my home away from home, to borrow books on writing. Then I went home and wrote down everything I thought should go in my book. I got the lady across the hall to type it for me, and promptly at noon the next day, I was at Chris Conrad's office door, with my five-page outline of *The Last Diet Book You'll Ever Have To Read.* Chris looked at the outline, and she liked it. But she said to me, "Could the title be a little longer?! Would you like your name on the back?" We changed it to *Never Say Diet.* And then Chris introduced me to Suzy Kalter Gurtzman, who was going to help me write the book—she was one of the most intelligent women I've ever met, so we got right to work. I was starting to write a book.

Mail kept pouring in and the phone continued ringing at the Anatomy Asylum. And people kept signing up for classes, to the point that I was running out of room. Even the fire marshal, who had begun to pay regular visits, was concerned. He said, "There's just way too many people in this place." The time had come to make some changes. And that's when I decided to take the restaurant out.

Up to this point, 1975, I was really in two businesses. I knew I could either be the Colonel Sanders of salads, or I could focus on what I really loved: exercise. So I decided to put all my energy into running this unique, motivational exercise studio, with music and fun, that no one else had.

I took the plunge. I gutted the place and made it into a bigger exercise studio. Once I redid the place, I wanted a new image to go with it. So I took my name and added an "L." And Slimmons was born.

With Slimmons came a new curriculum. Those little motivational meetings became "Project Me" meetings. I called them that because it was a project—to lose weight and to keep it off was a project. For a while now, I'd been in the habit of writing down motivational sayings to remind myself of the things I needed to work on in my life. On my bathroom mirror I'd tape little pieces of paper that I had written them on—like "I will take a daily inventory," "I will be truthful with myself," and "If I didn't do great yesterday, I will try harder today." I'd read these out loud each morning as a reminder of the attitude I should always have and the things I should focus on. One day, I realized that I couldn't see my hair, let alone my face, in the mirror anymore. I pulled the pieces of paper off the mirror and collected the sayings on a card. I had twenty-one of them, and I called them the "Project Me Passport."

We used the Passport as the springboard for our discussions in class. We'd always begin by reading those sentences that got us focused on why we were there and how we were going to achieve our goals. I was using these motivational getting-to-know-you meetings to create an even more positive atmosphere for my exercise classes.

I decided that next I had to give more direction and structure to the eating part of Slimmons. I knew I needed a visual way to keep track of daily dieting. I had been through all the diets I had cut out of magazines—I'd tried them all. I'd been through that anonymous diet sheet Dr. Hallman had provided. I'd been through all the fads. But there had been nothing I'd ever seen on the market that would let you see at a glance what you'd eaten and what you had left to eat during the course of your day.

The Yellow Is for Fat

I had an idea. So, I went to Westwood to an art-supply store called Sam Flax, where I bought construction paper and marking pens. Next, I went to a religious store—which was hard for me to do after all the rosaries I had "recycled"—and I bought a plastic wallet that was made to hold holy cards. I remembered those wallets from my Catholic school days.

I took my supplies home, and here's where all those years of art school paid off. I cut and pasted and drew. I sat for hours and figured it out. The brown cards—they would be starch. The red cards would be meat and protein. The yellow would be fat. The blue would be dairy. The green would be vegetables. And the pink would be fruit. I made a set for myself and then set after set for the students in my Project Me classes. A few hours later I had finished what would later become the first Deal-A-Meal.

I brought my creations to class the next day. I had made about twenty sets of these cards and wallets, and I handed them out. I explained how to use them. You'd pick the amount of calories you wanted for the day: 1,200, 1,400, or 1,600. The wallet had two sides. When you'd eat, you'd move the cards over to the other side. When your cards were all moved over, you were done eating for the day. I began to use the cards along with a lot of my students.

And you know what? Those little cards seemed to work! My students loved them. The only complaint was from me—my poor hand was permanently cramped from cutting out those cards from construction paper!

I began to use the cards to keep myself at my healthy weight, and because I knew they were working for me, I knew they could work for anyone.

I was getting requests for more sets of cards. Students wanted me to make sets for their brothers or sisters, fathers or mothers. I got more new members, and each new person got a set of cards. The cards became part of the program at Slimmons.

In the meantime, when I wasn't cutting and sorting little pieces of paper, I was answering mail, and my popularity as a local celebrity seemed to be growing.

Jerry Lewis was doing a Muscular Dystrophy Telethon in Las Vegas. He asked me to fly there to exercise the crowd—get them moving—and to answer the phones. I had never been to a telethon before, and I thought it would be fun. Little did I know that my next angel was waiting in the wings. They seemed to be coming fast and furious now.

Stop Tape!

I got on a plane headed to Las Vegas. Sitting next to me was a very intense woman—brunette, professional-looking, and well-dressed in a three-piece suit. She was slight and very strict-looking, almost like a principal of a private girls' school. She was reading a script and busily scribbling notes in the margins and making changes. She was so focused, I felt like I was sitting alone, until suddenly she turned and looked over at me.

"Aren't you that guy that jumps around on television?"

"Yes, I guess I am."

She said, "You're very funny. I've never seen anyone like you on T.V."

She said to me, "I want you on General Hospital." "Well, tha

"Well, that's because there isn't anyone on T.V. like me."

She introduced herself. Her name was Jackie Smith, vice president of daytime programming at ABC. She said to me, "I want you on *General Hospital.*"

"Well, that's very nice." Given my past experiences, I was not real keen on any hospital, let alone a general hospital. She explained that she was talking about the soap opera on television.

"Look, I'm not an actor," I said. "I have an exercise studio where I help people lose weight. I'm part comedian, part fitness instructor. And I'm a motivator."

"I think our writers could do a great story line with you, and you could play yourself."

So before you could say "Tracey Quartermaine," I was signing television contracts. This was during the heyday of *General Hospital*—the highly publicized, much-watched romance of Luke and Laura. I was to play myself, Richard Simmons, and teach exercise classes in Luke's disco. They'd hired a young woman, Louise Hoven, to play an overweight friend of Laura. Rather than finding a thin actress and stuffing her clothing so she looked overweight, they'd hired a woman with real-life struggles. Both Louise and her character battled with their weight. Louise also suffered from severe asthma.

Before I began my first day of taping on a Monday, there was a publicity photo shoot scheduled at the studio. The producers asked me to come in on Sunday afternoon and take press photos for the new character and the new season. I was thrilled.

I knew it was time to change my look. I was sure the producers weren't going to want me parading around in leotards and tights. So I had some colorful jogging suits made. I thought I looked a little Jack La Lanne-ish, more athletic and fitness-oriented than the *Swan Lake* dancer look I was used to wearing. I packed my car with all the stuff I thought I'd need for the photo shoot, including makeup and wardrobe. I headed to the studio for an exciting afternoon, where, for the first time, I met the people who would become my co-workers and friends on *General Hospital.* I changed clothes several times and had my photo taken both individually and with other cast members. My first photo session was a blast. I just couldn't believe this was all happening to me.

Four or five hours later, I got back in my car and headed home. I was exhilarated from the photo shoot, so I turned the music way up.

Suddenly, two police cars came out of nowhere, red lights flashing. The officers pulled me over, took me out of my car, and handcuffed me. They never bothered to read me my rights. Instead they sat me in the back seat of one of the squad cars. There I was, with all my possessions, being transported to the Sheriff's Department on Santa Monica Boulevard and San Vicente in West Hollywood.

I couldn't think. All that went through my mind was, Oh my God, this cannot be happening to me. I have to report to work *tomorrow* on *General Hospital.* I'm going to be a star, don't you understand?

These policemen were just like the cops on *Dragnet.* They weren't telling me anything. They were polite, but they weren't making eye contact or giving me any information. And I had no idea what to do or say. I was thinking to myself, "This is it. I'm going to get fired. What did I do? Was I wearing the wrong color jogging suit? Was my radio too loud?"

At the police station, I went through the horrible, intimidating process of being fingerprinted. Then they logged in my possessions. They carefully catalogued every item. How embarrassing!

A big, beefy cop sorted through my things. "Jogging suit—aqua . . . jogging suit—fuschia with pink pinstripe," he said in a monotone, like this was something he saw on a daily basis. I was always one to carry coin change. Ever since I made money at the praline store and my father taught me all about change, with his neat little piles on the dresser, I'd carried lots and lots of coins. The officer counted . . . very . . . slowly. Quarters . . . twenty-four. Dimes . . . sixteen. Nickles . . . forty. Everything I owned was itemized and recorded. It wasn't that they were judgmental about what I had with me. I'm sure they'd seen worse. It was more that they were weary and maybe a little too finicky, itemizing to no end.

And the worst was yet to come. They opened my makeup case. "Max Factor, medium base. Mascara, sable brown. Blush, Revlon raspberry. Lip moisturizer, strawberry-flavored." I can't imagine what they thought. I realized then that I was still in complete makeup and wearing a jogging suit from the photo session.

After my possessions were dissected, they took me to a holding cell. In about a half an hour, I went from the glamour of being at ABC, and having my photos taken, to the lockup cell in West Hollywood. This drab, gray place did not match my outfit at all. I was in a cell with the smallest bed and a pillow the size of a piece of Chiclet's chewing gum. Luckily, I was arrested in West Hollywood, where crime is not rampant, so I was in the cell alone—it was solitary confinement. Or maybe they were afraid to put me in with other criminals. They probably thought I'd do make-overs on the bad guys.

As they waited to get more details on the information they'd taken from me, and as I calmed down a little, I realized that no one had told me anything. I wanted to ask someone, "Did I do something wrong? What am I in for?"

This was the first time in my life where I knew humor was not going to get me out of trouble. "Hey, did you hear the one about the policeman and the nun who were in a lifeboat?" No, this was serious—very serious. There'd be no calling my parents. There was no one to help me. I just sat there. I was in the cell for about fifteen minutes—it seemed like two hours—and all I could think about was, It's over. It's just over. They'll find out about this on *General Hospital.* I could see the headlines: "Richard Simmons in Jail with Jogging Suit—Contract Canceled!"

As I imagined my short-lived career in show business slipping away, the policeman who had put the handcuffs on me earlier came in and told me, "You can go now."

I said, "I can go now? What do you mean I can go now? I mean, a few minutes ago I was a criminal. I was Susan Hayward about to have my last meal! Could I have a little explanation here?" Some of my nerve was coming back.

"Well, someone involved in a crime was driving a car exactly like yours," he said. I'd just bought a brand-new car, a four-door black Mercedes. (Okay, I had leased it.) I had applied for special vanity plates that said YRU-FATT. They hadn't come yet so I was still driving around with no plates on the car. The officer explained that earlier in the evening there had been a robbery and shooting at a convenience store. The car that drove away was a brand-new, four-door black Mercedes, no license plates. So when the call came through, there I was driving on Santa Monica Boulevard in this car. They just assumed I was the person they were looking for. Once they got a look at my things, I'm sure they figured out that I may

gging suit—fuschia with pink pinstripe," he said in a monotone, have been dressed to kill, but I was not the killer. And while I was in the holding cell, they found the right person—well, the right person who did the wrong thing. So they let me go.

All in all, it was a horrifying experience. When I got back in the car, I think I drove home at about four miles an hour. I rivaled my Uncle Milton for the slowest speed record. I even used my blinker and hand signals. And frankly, for at least a week, I didn't even want to drive anywhere if it wasn't absolutely necessary.

The next day, I would be starting on *General Hospital.* After my brush with the law, I was going home to get a good night's sleep.

I was going to be on television. And it was frightening. Inside, I felt the fear that I would fail—this was a big fear. My father had never wanted me to be in show business. He hadn't done well with his show-biz career, and he told me that I would fail, too, if I tried it. That always echoed in the back of my mind.

So why was I pursuing a career in the spotlight? Even as I went to the phone to call my parents to tell them I was going to be on *General Hospital,* I felt the fear that I could fail. They were happy for me, but their reaction seemed to be tempered with a warning. So, I walked around with that little devil on one shoulder, telling me, "Maybe you shouldn't be doing this. You could have the exercise studio and just be happy with that." But there was an angel on my other shoulder, who said, "Wait a minute. You're on a soap opera—a big one! Luke . . . Laura!"

I took a deep breath, and thought, "You know, this is an actual job. I have the contract." I was going to be a soap-opera star. There had already been announcements in *Soap Opera Digest* and *Soaps Alive.* Writers and reporters were calling for interviews, and I hadn't even started yet.

My call time was very early that Monday. The show was shot on a schedule called "block and tape." In the morning, all the scenes were rehearsed and blocked out, showing where the cameras and people would move. We'd take a break for lunch. Then, in the afternoon, we'd actually tape the scenes we'd rehearsed that morning.

I had watched *General Hospital* for the entire week before I was on, so I knew all the characters' names. I had watched as they'd begun working me into the story line, talking about Richard Simmons and his exercise studio.

On my first day, everybody on the set was so nice to me. Many of them had seen clips of me on shows. Some of them had been to Ruffage in the past or had exercised with me at the Anatomy Asylum or at Slimmons. I felt very welcome. I may have been a little scared, a little nervous, but at least I didn't feel fat. I didn't feel different, like I stuck out. This was somewhere where I was finally going to fit in.

That first Monday morning, we blocked my first scene: an introduction of me—I was playing Richard Simmons—and the people who were going to be in my exercise class in Luke's disco. I thought it went well, and I was eager to get it on tape.

After lunch, when we started to tape, all the soap girls, such as Genie Francis and Jackie Zeman, were hanging around the disco, and all I had to do was come in and say my one line. So, with the cameras rolling, I bounced into the room and yelled, "Hi, everybody! Let's start class!" All of the sudden, I heard a woman's voice over the P.A. system.

"STOP TAPE!"

Well, everyone on the set froze. Apparently those were the two most feared words on the set of *General Hospital.* They were followed by the sound of quick-moving high heels heading my way. *Click-click-click.* A woman came out of the director's booth, located in the back of the set, and walked right up to me. Oh my God, it was my first day, and it was turning out to be worse than the day before with the police.

"Mr. Simmons." The imposing woman held her hands in the air, wide apart. "The Broadway stage is this big." Then she brought her hands together, about a foot and a half apart. "The television set is this big. So let's bring it down, shall we?!"

Click-click-click. She stormed off back to her booth. I heard everyone on the set exhale, all at once.

This was Gloria Monty. She was the executive producer of *General Hospital* and a powerhouse—most probably the toughest woman I'd ever met. A dark-haired, serious woman, who pulled no punches, she treated me as she treated everyone else. There would be no allowances and no special welcome for me on my first day.

Gloria was the queen bee of the soap opera. I'd met her briefly once, in her office, after Jackie Smith, the network executive, had pitched to Gloria the idea of using me on the show. Gloria had loved the weight-related story idea, and our meeting was merely a formality. I remember trembling when I had to meet her for the first time. I had heard that she was like the wrath of God. But she had been very courteous to me.

Now, here on the set, I found I was just petrified. I wanted to quit. Tony Geary (who played Luke) and Genie Francis (who played Laura) and Jackie Zeman—all three of them came over to offer words of encouragement. Of course, they did it out of microphone and monitor range, where Gloria Monty wouldn't be able to hear or see them.

We started over with the same scene. When it came time to say my line, I tried to remember that small square that Gloria had made with her hands. I tried to pretend I was in a box that size.

"Hi everybody, let's do our workout," I said again, this time with much less enthusiasm.

"STOP TAPE!!" I heard those dreaded words again.

Click-click-click. It was those high heels again.

"What's the problem here?" she asked. Everybody froze again. But I was tired of being scared.

I said, "Look, Miss Monty, I really don't know what you want. It's my first day and frankly . . . "

"What?" she challenged me.

So in a kidding way—I didn't know there was no kidding with Gloria— I said, "You do this scene. Show me what I'm supposed to do."

I heard another collective gasp, and I think people were running for cover so they wouldn't get hit by my flying body parts when Gloria shredded me to pieces.

But she simply took the script out of my hand. "Okay, let's run this scene."

Well, everybody was shocked. Nobody had ever stood up to this woman. She did the scene for me exactly as she wanted me to do it. I watched her carefully. She handed the script back to me and *click-click-click,* she walked right back to her booth.

Over the P.A. system she said, "Let's try it again."

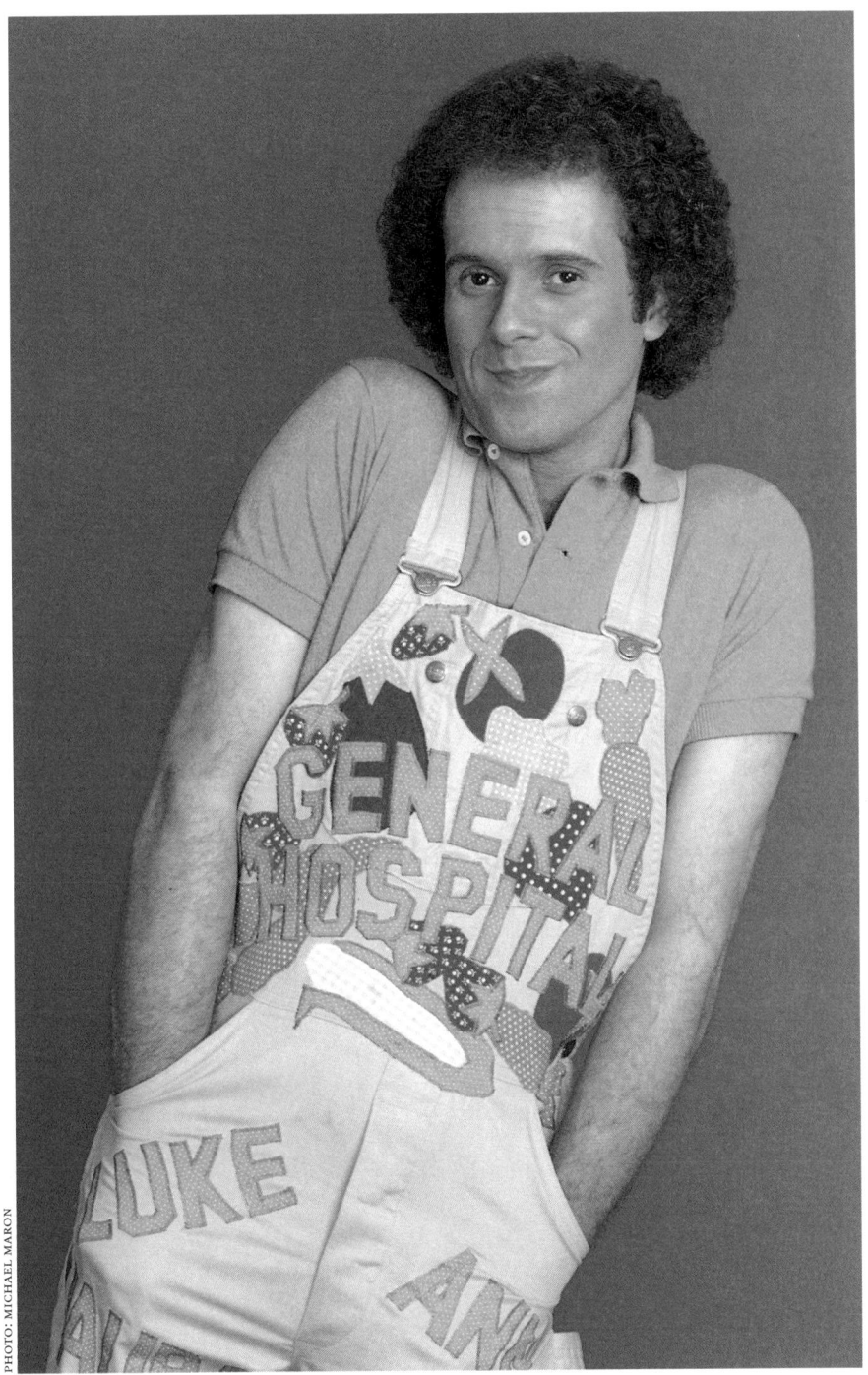

Fans of General Hospital *were always making presents for me—
quilts, stationery, overalls . . .*

We did the scene a third time. When I was done, she announced, "Moving on."

Everybody applauded, and the ice had been forever broken. I knew Gloria Monty was just doing her job, and that as long as I did my best, I had nothing to fear.

That night, she called me into her office. Maybe I had spoken too soon. I thought to myself that this could be it. She was going to say, "Well, that was your first and last day." But I had signed a contract at ABC, and I knew they didn't take those things lightly.

Gloria had something completely different in mind. She called me in for personal reasons. She went from a tyrant of a woman to being very motherly. She told me that if I ever needed any help, she'd be glad to do what she could.

Then she said, "Will you do me a favor?"

"Well, of course," I replied without hesitation.

"Would you have time to exercise me?" she asked. "I've got to get some of this weight off. Would you come to my office a few times a week?"

Well, that was better than getting fired. Like a poodle on a leash, I was there. I began to go to her office during lunch hour with my boom box, and I would work her out. We quickly developed a special bond. We even became sort of chummy. On the set, I'd reached a new level of respect with my co-workers because I had the inside track on Gloria Monty.

Gloria worked hard, and she began to lose weight. And she started to drop dress sizes. My character on the show continued.

* ⋆ *

Soap Success

After the first week, I returned to my dressing room on Monday to find huge, gray postal trays of envelopes. I went out to the receptionist and I said, "Someone left all of these bins of mail in my dressing room."

"They're yours," she replied. "That's your fan mail for the week."

"I have fans?" The producers kept careful track of how much mail each character was getting and then wrote their scripts accordingly. In other words, if you and your character received a lot of mail, you'd spend more

I g o t   l e t t e r s   f r o m   a l l   o v e r   t h e   U n i t e d   S t a t e s ,   f r o m   p e o p l e   w h o

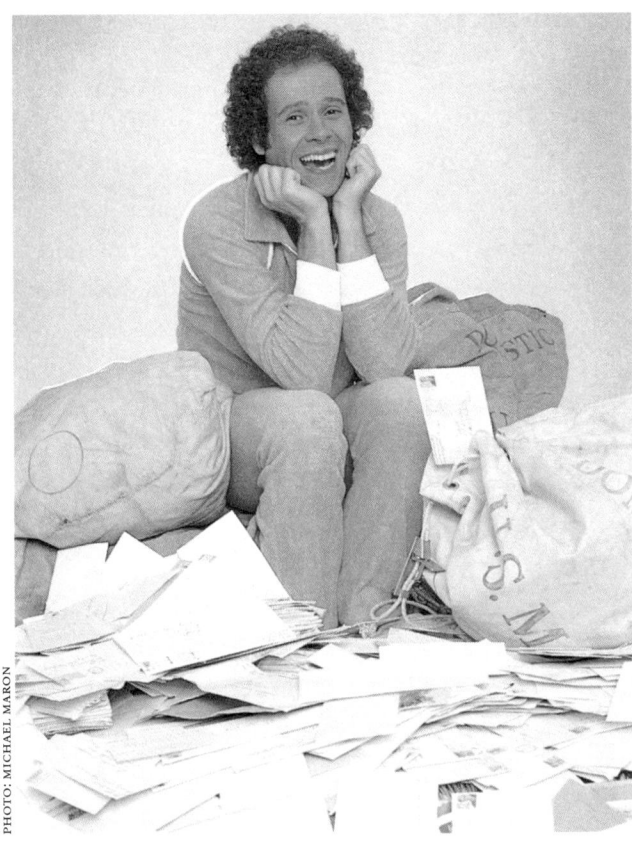

PHOTO: MICHAEL MARON

I got thousands of letters about my story line on General Hospital—*helping an overweight mother and daughter to lose pounds.*

time on-screen. If your mail dropped off, then bye-bye! The Luke and Laura story was so strong that it overshadowed any other story line on the show. But now, people began to respond to the overweight girl, struggling with her self-esteem and her exercise and eating habits. This subject had not been touched upon before on any soap opera. It hit a big, collective, national nerve. I got letters from all over the United States, from people who were avid soap-opera fans and who could relate to this girl's plight.

I read each one of these heart-to-heart letters from people I did not know and had not met. Each one was a cry for help, and they affected me deeply. These were the letters that started me in yet another career direction.

The other soap actors had a 5×7 card with their picture on it. It was stamped with the words "Best wishes" or "Fondly" or "To My Biggest Fan." They would sign them and send them out in response to their fan mail. I would receive very few requests for photos. Instead, I got twelve-page letters telling me about someone's son, mother, daughter, husband, or wife who was dangerously overweight. Or a letter from someone who knew firsthand just what Louise was going through.

In response to the overwhelming amount of mail, Gloria and the writers had the idea to bring in a woman to play Louise's overweight mother. They casted the actress Vanessa Brown. She had been a thin, breathtakingly gorgeous actress in the Forties and Fifties. Though still quite beautiful, in her middle age, she'd become overweight. So the choice was perfect—so true to life. Viewers loved this story of a mother and daughter working out and working together to lose weight.

Through my soap-opera connections, I met a husband and wife team, Joyce Becker and Allan Sugarman, who had a company called Soap Opera Festivals that booked soap-opera stars in malls and theme parks. They were quite successful and had a good reputation. They asked me if I would come with them just to watch one of the events they were having at Knotts Berry Farm. Stuart Damon (who plays Alan Quartermaine on *General Hospital*) was one of the stars scheduled to be there, so I felt fairly secure, since I had worked with him. The theater was jam-packed. Four seats were set up on the stage. As Joyce introduced the stars one by one, and they took their seats, the fans' screams were deafening. During a question-and-answer period, an audience member would hold his or her hand up, and Joyce would bring the microphone over, so the person could ask a question. "Will you ever come out of your coma and marry Bobby?" was the most popular kind of question.

As I was watching from the side, someone spotted me, and the audience started screaming. The Sugarmans put some music on and brought me up onstage. I made everybody get up and stretch. Suddenly, my two worlds had combined. This was what I really did—exercising with people. But I was doing it as my soap character, who was, in reality, exactly who I was. Somehow it all worked. I felt a tremendous rush the minute I was in that amphitheater, doing this exercise–soap-opera thing. Afterwards, I sat with the other scheduled guests and signed pictures. Right away, I noticed something different about the people in line to see me. They weren't just interested in getting a picture. They wanted to talk to me. And I won't flatter myself—it wasn't that they wanted to talk about me. And they didn't want to talk about the characters on *General Hospital.* They wanted to talk about themselves. They wanted to say, "I saw you helping that girl on television, and I have a daughter and we're so worried about her. What can we tell her? What can we do for her?"

While all the other actors' lines filed past, mine was like a mule train. People were crying and getting very emotional. And you know me. I was crying right along with them. I loved the broad scope of people who came to me. And I liked the face-to-face contact, being able to kiss and hug and hold them, to ease their pain, even if only for a moment.

* * *

Malling It Alone

I started going out to the malls with other soap-opera people on the weekends. Before long, Joyce and Allan were sending me out on my own, to do my little traveling exercise show.

Then I got an offer to do a shopping-mall appearance in South Bend, Indiana. It was the dead of winter. It was snowing hard, and since arriving, two feet of new snow had fallen. There were tractors in the road, making paths and salting the streets. It was a winter wonderland, and in the middle of it all was the beautiful gold dome of the University of Notre Dame. I had my *General Hospital* jogging suit on—pants and a little zip-up jacket with my initials on it.

A limo drove me to the mall from the Holiday Inn where I was staying. There were no cars on the road. As we turned into the parking lot, I realized that everyone in town had to be there. It was packed with cars. I turned to the limo driver and I asked, "What's going on here today? Are they having a big fifty-percent-off sale?"

He said, "You. You're here today."

I said, "Well, I know I'm here today. But who else is here?"

"Just you." I didn't understand. I was escorted to the mall office. The fire marshal was there. Security was there.

"What's all this about?" I asked.

"We got a mob out there," they said.

"A mob?! For me? Are you kidding?" I had seen mobs turn out for the soap-opera events when several big stars were onstage. But they were gorgeous men and beautiful women, and everyone screamed for them. They had names like Raven and Dameon. I never had much of a great self-image. But that changed in South Bend, Indiana. As I came down the escalator and got on the stage, the screaming was like a mini-Beatles event. I wanted to put my hands over my ears. I got on that little stage and looked around. All these people had come to see me! They didn't come to make fun of me. They didn't come for a negative reason. They came to see me. For a person who never fit in, now I knew I was in.

Onstage, I didn't waste any time. I put on "It's My Party," "Locomotion," and "Devil in a Blue Dress," and I got the crowd moving. I stayed for hours afterward and signed pictures and heard people's stories. I stayed so long, I almost missed my plane.

The appearance was a great success, and before long I had multiple offers coming in. Every time I'd do a mall appearance, the local press would show up and the word would spread.

I still had the exercise studio in Los Angeles, and I was starting to hire more teachers to fill in for me while I was traveling. I was still on *General Hospital.* I was still working on my book *Never Say Diet.* I was traveling every weekend now to a different city to do a mall appearance or a fitness expo, helping people feel better and look better, just like I had when I was doing make-overs for Coty.

At the malls I would have a stage and my boom box with speakers, and all my dance tapes. It was just like a concert. First, I would say, "Okay, all the little kids come up on the stage here." And three-, four-, and five-year-olds would come up, and I would do a Disney number with them. Then the teenagers came up, and I would do a rock-and-roll number with them. Next, the men came up, and I would do a contest. I talked them into doing a strip. (No, not all the way!) And, you know, they did it. The women loved it, and they'd vote for their favorite performance by clapping. It was better than *The Full Monty.* The mall visits were like a revival, and I was the evangelist of fitness. It was a revival of motivation.

These "concerts" would go on for about an hour. Then the managers of the mall would set up a table for me, and people would line up. I'd sit on the table, signing pictures and autographs, and listening to stories. People

People would talk about their weight. But I learned that the

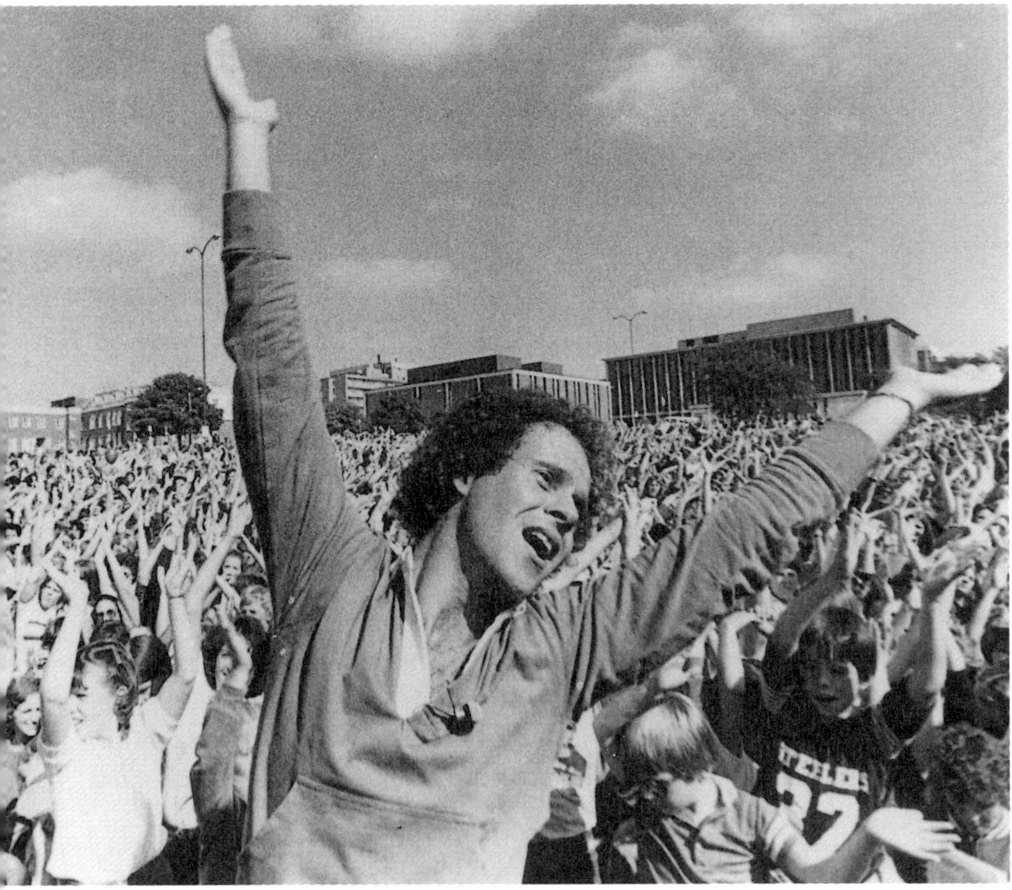

The beginning of . . . travelin' sweat

would talk about their weight. But I learned that their problems were about different kinds of weight: the weight of what you have to go through with family, with friends, with jobs—the weight of the world. And I attacked all that weight with whimsy and exercise. After hours more of meeting these people, it was time to run. By then, I would already be two hours late.

* * *

The more I traveled and the more people got to know about me, the more I would get special requests to talk with certain people. "We're desperate, Richard. We need your help."

On one trip, I got a call in my hotel room. The caller told me she knew a woman who was very overweight and in a wheelchair. Could I meet her in

ems were about different kinds of weight: the weight of what

the back of the mall in one of the offices, before my mall appearance? So I got to the mall a little early, and I went to the manager's office. I sat with this woman in the wheelchair and held her hand, and we talked.

She began crying as she confessed that she was too embarrassed to go out into the mall. She was over four hundred pounds—no longer able to walk or breathe without pain, and she was on oxygen. She told me that she never missed seeing me on *General Hospital.* She loved the way I treated the people in my class on T.V. She said, "You're the first person whom I've ever seen who's treated overweight people with dignity and love. You don't judge them."

I talked with her and gave her some guidance. I tried to make her feel better about herself, to help raise her very low self-esteem. And I asked her if she'd let security bring her out to watch me exercise onstage.

"Maybe this will inspire you," I told her.

She agreed, and they brought her out to watch while I did my mall show. I just loved doing the shows. And way, way in the back, I saw the woman in her wheelchair, lifting her arms and exercising with everyone else. She was moving, she was clapping. And whether or not I ever saw this woman again, I hoped I had changed a life. The scene was repeated many times as I traveled from mall to mall.

I'm like Johnny Appleseed. I go from city to city and plant the seeds. Only instead of apples, my seeds are exercise and eating healthy. I nurture them while I'm there, and then move on to let them grow on their own.

Hey! You Lookin' at Me?

People all over the place began recognizing me. People weren't just noticing me, they were noticing my weight. They were watching what I ate in restaurants. They were watching what I bought in the supermarket. Because of this, I accepted the fact that I was living in a glass bubble. Sometimes, though, things would happen that would just astound me.

On one of my mall appearances, after a strenuous workout in front of a large crowd, I just had to use the rest room. While I was in a stall—trying to have a private moment—there was a knock on the partition next to me. Oh, no. What was this!?

My life had gone from worrying so much about myself and be

I heard a male voice. "Hi! Is that you Richard? Are you in there?"

Why do I always have these conversations in bathroom stalls? And who was this man knocking?

"Yes. This is Richard Simmons."

"Oh, good. I was afraid maybe it was someone else. Are you busy? Can we chat?"

"Well, quite truthfully . . . "

"Great. My name is Al. I'm here with my wife. Oh . . . I don't mean she's in here in the bathroom with me. She's waiting outside. But, Richard, she loves you. You've helped her so much."

"Oh, I'm glad."

"Richard, could you do me a favor? My wife would love an autograph."

"Well, Al, I don't have a pen and paper with me."

"Oh, here. I have a pen—I'll slide it under the wall here. And you can just use a piece of toilet paper—that'll be okay."

No matter where I went, I was literally a walking advertisement. A lot of times when soap stars and movie stars go out, they wear sunglasses or turtlenecks or wigs or mustaches. Not me—I could never do that. I was never comfortable in a baseball hat because I'd never played baseball—and I didn't want hat hair. I was never comfortable wearing sunglasses because I have one ear that's a half an ear lower than the other. So if I wear glasses, it looks like I just came out of a bar. I decided that I would always forgo any kind of disguise. I was fair game; I was on T.V.; I was nationally known. So wherever I went, I went looking like Richard Simmons, because that's who I am. My life had gone from worrying so much about myself and being on diets and trying to improve myself, to being concerned about others. The coin had flipped. I was the worrywart. I was the one who was the nurturer.

The Big Break

So while the *General Hospital* show was going on, I was still teaching classes when I could. And even though the studio no longer had the social element that Ruffage did, I still seemed to meet people there who would have a major effect on my life.

One day before class, I talked with a man who'd come to see me. His name was Woody Fraser and he was a producer. He had a show called *That's Incredible*, and was one of the creators of *Good Morning America*, among other shows. He was a legend in the entertainment industry and a man with a vision. Woody's agent brought him into my studio to take a look for himself and see what it was that I did. At this point, besides Jack La Lanne and Debbie Drake, no other fitness instructors had emerged—so I was almost one-of-a-kind.

Woody came to my studio and watched me perform with one of my classes. He loved what he saw, and he asked me if I'd ever thought about doing my own show.

I said, "Well, I'm on *General Hospital.*"

He said, "What about your own show?"

I told him that if I could, I'd do the same things I did at the studio: exercise, motivation, maybe even a little low-cal cooking—and lots of fun.

Eventually, in 1981, we created *The Richard Simmons Show.* At this point, talk shows were just beginning to emerge. Phil Donahue was the king of daytime. Soaps were still supreme. There were some talk shows, but there was nothing like this idea we came up with. Woody and I pitched the show and sold it very quickly to a syndicator called Golden West.

I called my parents to tell them the news. My father said, "If you've made your mind up to do this, I'm going tell you something right now. You better have something to fall back on."

My mother was a little more supportive. She was excited and cheered me on. But my father, ever cautious about the perils of show business, sounded more like the voice of doom.

We shot a pilot, and we were then scheduled for more shows. These days, to get your program on television, you have to be in at least seventy percent of the television markets across the United States. *The Richard Simmons Show* premiered in five markets. (New Orleans, to my family's disappointment, was not one of them.) The show ran on stations in Los Angeles, New York, Chicago, San Francisco, and Dallas. I did the half-hour show five days a week.

The show always started with an outrageous opening that gave you the theme. Then, we rushed over to the kitchen and cooked up a low-calorie dish. Next, we'd do some exercises, we'd have a success story, and finally, at

If people could watch my show, it might help them feel better

the end, I would sit quietly. I would talk about issues, almost like Project Me, and I'd try to leave people with a message that would inspire and motivate them. It was a daily dose, something to keep people going. If people could watch my show, it might help them feel better about themselves. It was almost like I had turned my exercise studio and salad bar into a television show. My family was now even more huge—it was everybody on the other side of the T.V. screen.

Let me tell you, when you have a show on television, it's always nerve-wracking waiting for the reviews. When *TV Guide* came out after the first show aired, we flipped to the back page, because that's where new shows were critiqued. A very tough critic reviewed our show for *TV Guide,* and he loved it. We received nothing but positive press about the show.

House to House

Right up to the end of the *General Hospital* run, I was still living in apartments. My accountant finally said to me, "You know, Richard, you should probably be thinking about buying a house and getting out of the apartment. I think you're going to need the tax deduction this year."

"A house?"

"Yes, you should buy a house. Take some time and start looking. Come to think of it, there's a house on the market right now designed by a very famous architect for his wife. They just finished it, but they're getting a divorce, so the house is up for sale. And I think they want to sell it fast."

Just the thought of owning a house made me crazy. The memories of 926 St. Louis Street stuffed with furniture and paintings and drapes—I didn't want to deal with all that.

Without much enthusiasm, I said, "Okay. Let's go look at it."

We drove up into the hills above the Beverly Hills Hotel. Finally we turned off and drove through a gate onto a road that was one block long. Richard Chamberlain and Victoria Principal lived nearby. Well, we walked up to the house and it was like, my God, what a house! It was very modern, with fifty-foot ceilings and polished wood, glass, and chrome on six different levels. Outside there was a black pool and a black Jacuzzi. The master bedroom was upstairs, somewhere. And in the bathroom was one of those very Hollywood green marble bathtubs. At least, I thought there was a tub, but I really couldn't be sure, because everything in the bathroom was green marble. The sink blended in with the counters and the counters blended in with the floor and the floor blended in with the tub. It all looked the same to me, like one of those puzzles where you try to find the hidden objects. Where's Waldo? Except if I bought it, it would be, "Where's Richard?"

The house was so sleek, it really wasn't me. But everyone kept telling me how wonderful this house was, how unique. I dreaded the thought of more house-hunting. So I bought it.

At the time, I didn't own enough furniture to fill up a house. I had a couch and two chairs and some stuff from my apartment, and that was it. So, I had an interior designer come in and decorate the whole house.

Since Christmas was fast approaching, I called my parents and my brother and told them to fly out and spend the holidays with me. This was all so exciting. It was my first house, and I wanted to prove to my father I had made it. They couldn't wait to get on the plane and fly to L.A.

I picked them up at the airport in a limo, and we drove to the house.

I opened the front door and my father stepped in. He backed up and gasped, "My God, Richard, what is this? I've never seen so many steps in my whole life." From the front door you saw all six levels, each with its own set of stairs. Nothing had changed between my father and me. I was afraid he was going to send me to my room—except I couldn't find it myself.

"It's so modern! Who ever designed this? Why did you buy it?" He walked through the whole house, room to room, commenting as he went.

In the kitchen, he said, "Richard, this kitchen is stainless steel. You're going to have water marks and fingerprints everywhere."

He walked into the living room. "There are too many windows and too much glass. It's going to be very drafty. And where's the nearest grocery store, fish market, bakery? You have to drive all the way down the side of this mountain. This just doesn't make sense!" Nothing I did seemed to be right.

My father finally picked up his luggage and went to the bedroom he was going to use. A few minutes later, I heard him scream, "Oh, this is great! No hot water!"

It was Christmas Eve. My family was all there. They were tired. My father hated the house. And there I was, so proud of myself: I was on a soap

One weekend, I was driving around and I got lost. I was in the

opera, I was making money, I was driving a Mercedes. (Yes, I know it was leased.) And still, he found things to complain about.

My father said, "We fly all the way out here and now we're in a big mansion, this big modern thing, and there's no hot water? Do something, Richard!"

I called the Beverly Wilshire Hotel and managed to get a string of rooms: one for my mother, one for my father, one for my brother, and one for me. That's how I spent Christmas that year.

The next day, December 26, I put the house up for sale. I didn't want to clean all those windows anyway.

I called my accountant and told him the house was on the market, and that I was temporally moving into the L'Ermitage Hotel on Burton Way. What I thought would be a short stay wound up being six months. After Christmas, I went back to work, a man without a home.

It really wasn't so bad. I loved living in a hotel. I loved that I never had to make my bed and that I didn't have to wash the dishes. But I knew I couldn't stay there forever. I wanted to find a home. So I spent quite a few weekends looking at houses with a realtor. But nothing was quite right for me. Nothing said to me, "This is home." So I kept on looking.

One weekend, I was driving around and I got lost. I was in the hills above Sunset Boulevard when I came around a corner and out of nowhere, there it was in front of me, the house I live in today. I looked at it, and a full orchestra began playing the *Gone with the Wind* movie theme in my head. (Later, one of the neighbors told me that the exterior was actually used in the opening shots of the movie.)

There were columns and a two-foot wall in the front, and these wonderful magnolia trees. The house had seen better days. It was a definite re-do, but it was like a little ink spot of New Orleans, right in the middle of these hills. I was back at 926 St. Louis Street—but this house was bigger and with a little more glamour. There was one tiny problem—the house wasn't for sale. I figured I had nothing to lose, so I walked right up to the front door and I rang the doorbell.

A woman, who was somewhere in her forties, answered. She greeted me like she'd been expecting me. "Well, you're Richard Simmons."

"I sure am," I said cheerfully.

"Oh, my mother watches *General Hospital* every day and she just loves you. Come in. She'll be so excited. What are you doing in the neighborhood? Do you know someone?"

"Well, actually, no. I got lost, and found myself on this street. Where's your mom? I'll say hello."

And then I saw the staircase. It had a wheelchair lift.

We went upstairs, and there the woman introduced me to her mother. They had been playing checkers. I explained how the house had reminded me of New Orleans where I grew up. We talked for quite a while, and I even joined her in a game of checkers.

Her mother said to me, "The way you talk about this house is the way I felt about it when I moved in. You like this house, don't you."

"Yes, I do. Very much. It reminds me of my childhood and my family in the South. I love the columns and the magnolia trees out front."

"If you want this house, it's yours," she said.

So, I bought it, and thirty days later I moved in. It was as easy as that. Another Cinderella story. The year was 1981.

The mother and daughter were happy to move to a smaller place. They were ready to downsize, so much so they insisted I buy the house completely furnished. I got a couple of friends to help me move everything outside, and within a day it was all gone. Somebody else's past wiped clean.

My Father's Blessing

Soon after I bought the house, my father came out to visit again. I wanted my parents, but especially my father, to like it. I really needed his approval on this one. I just couldn't put another house up for sale and move into a hotel again.

Well, off I went to the airport. When the limo stopped in front of the house, Leonard got out. He stood there a moment, looking around. He didn't say a word. Then he opened the front gate, and said, "Now, this is a house!"

My dad began to make trips to L.A., usually on his own, without my mother. Whenever he came, the first thing I would do is to take him shopping for clothes. When I was growing up, all his clothes were stylish, but they had always been secondhand. Now I was able to take him to the finest

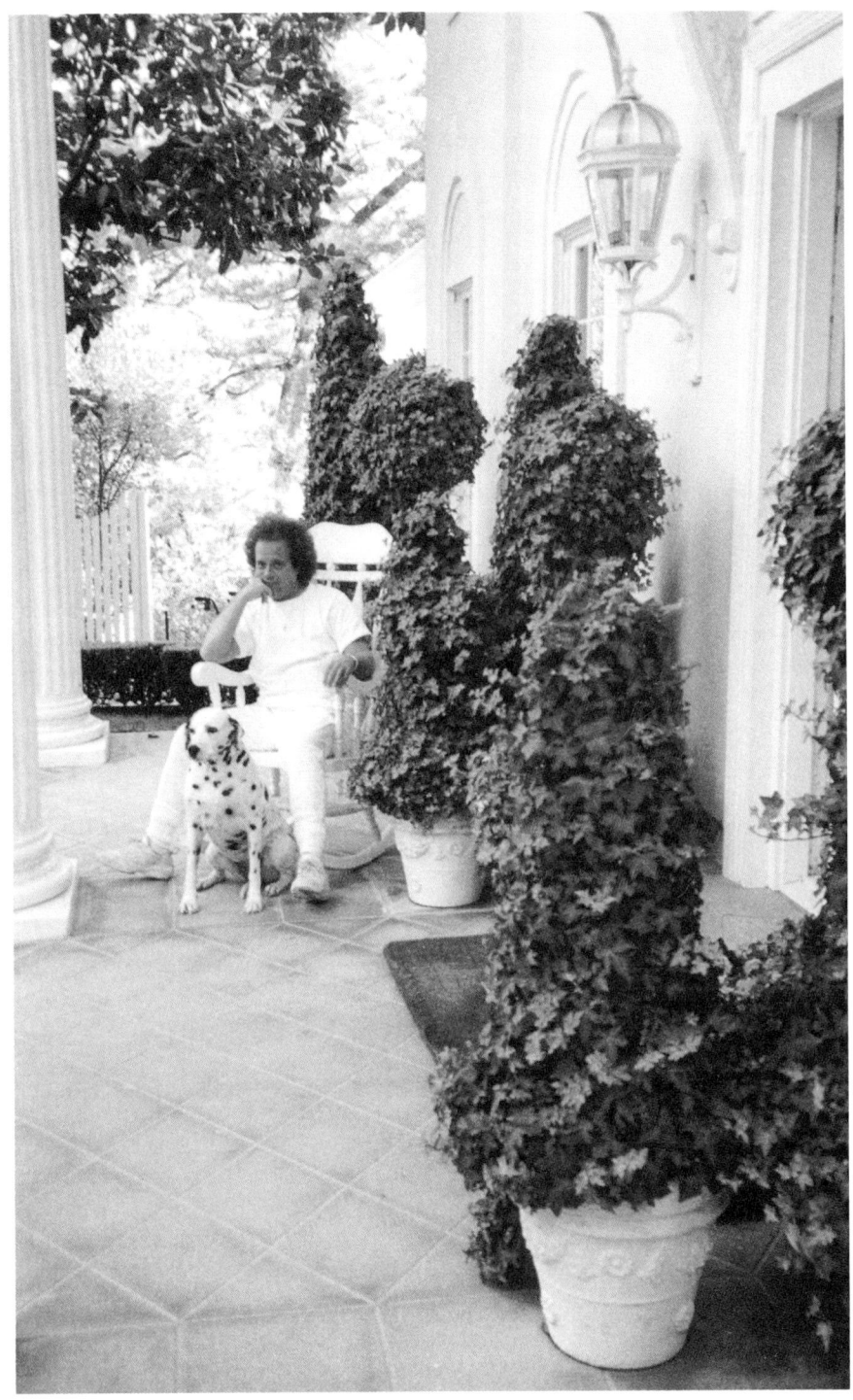

A quiet moment at home with twelve-year-old Melanie

n he opened the front gate, and said, "Now, this is a house!"

stores. I had cashmere coats made for him, and vests and shirts with his initials on them.

I also started to show him a lot of affection. I would hug and kiss him in restaurants, grocery stores, men's shops, in any public place, and he would just go, "Stop it! Leave me alone. Don't do that. People are staring. Stop it!" No matter where we went, he wasn't safe from me. I just drove the man absolutely crazy. Finally he would joke, "When's my plane. When? Can we change the reservation? Can I get an earlier flight?"

I just couldn't stop hugging him and giving him a hard-loving time. One of the last times he came out to L.A., we were sitting in a restaurant, and I said I had to go to the bathroom. Well, I walked away, but I sneaked back and, on hands and knees, I slithered under the table like a snake—and bit his leg! He screamed so loud, people dropped their forks.

Our relationship was beginning to soften. My dad was starting to look at me in a different way. I could see it in his eyes—he knew I was going to make it. I was driven, I didn't have his temper, and I would succeed. Failure was not going to be part of my story, so he could relax a little. He wasn't going to have to protect his little boy anymore. He began to enjoy our relationship, and finally, so did I.

* * *

My Mother's Blessing

Shortly after my father's trip, my mother came out for her blessing of the house. Since I hadn't remodeled or redecorated yet, the large living room held only a couch and a table, and that was it. I picked her up at the airport, as I had done with my dad, and pulled up in front of the house. She liked the outside immediately, and we walked in through the front door together.

"So where's the furniture in this house?" she asked. "Why is it so bare?"

"Mother, this is called post-modern."

She said, "No, honey, it's called empty. Forget about post-modern. This is an empty house. Get a little something for over here. And you need something here. And then get some paintings on the walls."

In the long run, my mother was an easier sell. She was happy that I was happy.

Remodeling

After my father's first visit, I realized that the house was beautiful from the outside, but the inside was a little old-fashioned for me and would need some fixing up.

I was wandering through a bookstore one afternoon, and I picked up a book called *Ornamentalism.* And on the cover was this unbelievable postmodern picture of an office. I looked in the back to see who wrote it. It was a famous architect-interior designer team. I liked their work so much that I flew them out to Los Angeles. We sat in the dining room and worked on a design and master plan for the interior

The wrecking crew arrived and began to gut the entire inside of the house. I moved into the maid's room, and that's where I lived for almost five years while the house was being redone. Why did it take that long? Well, during that time, I was finishing up *General Hospital,* I had *The Richard Simmons Show,* I was doing malls, I was traveling, and I was writing a book. Plus, I knew I would live in this house forever, so I was meticulous about every detail. Once all the construction was done, it took another year to paint, and another year to select the furniture and carpet. And here it's years later, and I'm still working on it.

Gradually, the house became sort of my own little monastery, a haven away from the world. I have such a chaotic existence, I needed a calm house.

Good-bye, *G.H.*

During this time, two very strong people were running my life. Gloria Monty was still calling the shots at *General Hospital,* and Woody Fraser was putting together *The Richard Simmons Show.* These were two people who were used to getting their way, and two strong personalities meant tension.

Gloria was happy for my success with my own T.V. show, but she wasn't thrilled when *General Hospital* began to take a back seat in my life. Gloria was Gloria, and I hadn't forgotten that I really owed a lot of my overall success to *General Hospital.* Although I had talked with her about my show and gotten her blessing for it, I knew she really wasn't happy about it. In addition, I was burning the candle at both ends. I was pushing it, but you know me—I've always pushed it, all through my life.

The day finally came when I had to decide between the two shows—it was all becoming too much. Something had to be sacrificed. But the decision would be made for me.

The change happened very quickly. Gloria and Woody had words—I'm not sure exactly about what. But one day I was on *General Hospital,* and then the next day, I wasn't, just like that. The writers on *G.H.* didn't have me go into a coma, or get lost in the woods, or get abducted by aliens. In 1980, I just quietly left the show. It wasn't so difficult, since I wasn't a major character. But I was so attached to all my friends there that it was a very hard good-bye. The cast threw a little party for me and wished me well.

I packed up my makeup case, my bathrobe and slippers, and a few other odds and ends, and walked the two blocks to Channel 5, the KTLA studios owned by Gene Autry (God bless him, he's in Heaven now). And then I threw myself into *The Richard Simmons Show.*

It had been my dream to do a show where I could be myself and tell my own story, hoping it would inspire others. That's what we tried to do with *The Richard Simmons Show.* Our production team was a young, enthusiastic group. Woody and his wife, Nora, produced the show together. At first we didn't exactly know what we were doing. Every day we would all sit around and have our planning meeting, just like a Project Me discussion. Woody and Nora were my new family, almost like my parents.

On the show, I always felt at home. The set was my own little world, with a kitchen, an exercise area, and a living room with the couch where I could do interviews. It was like inviting people to my house. There was a live audience that started out with about fifty people. Soon, it got to be sixty, and then a hundred. I don't think there were any other shows where the audience showed up in leotards and spandex. You could always pick out the line waiting to get into *The Richard Simmons Show.* The audience would be booked three months ahead. People would sign up to be in the audience, and then they'd stay, not for one or two shows but for all three shows, which were taped in one long day.

The Richard Simmons Show was now my full-time job. The show

I   p a c k e d   u p   m y   m a k e u p   c a s e ,   m y   b a t h r o b e   a n d   s l i p p e r s ,   a n d   a

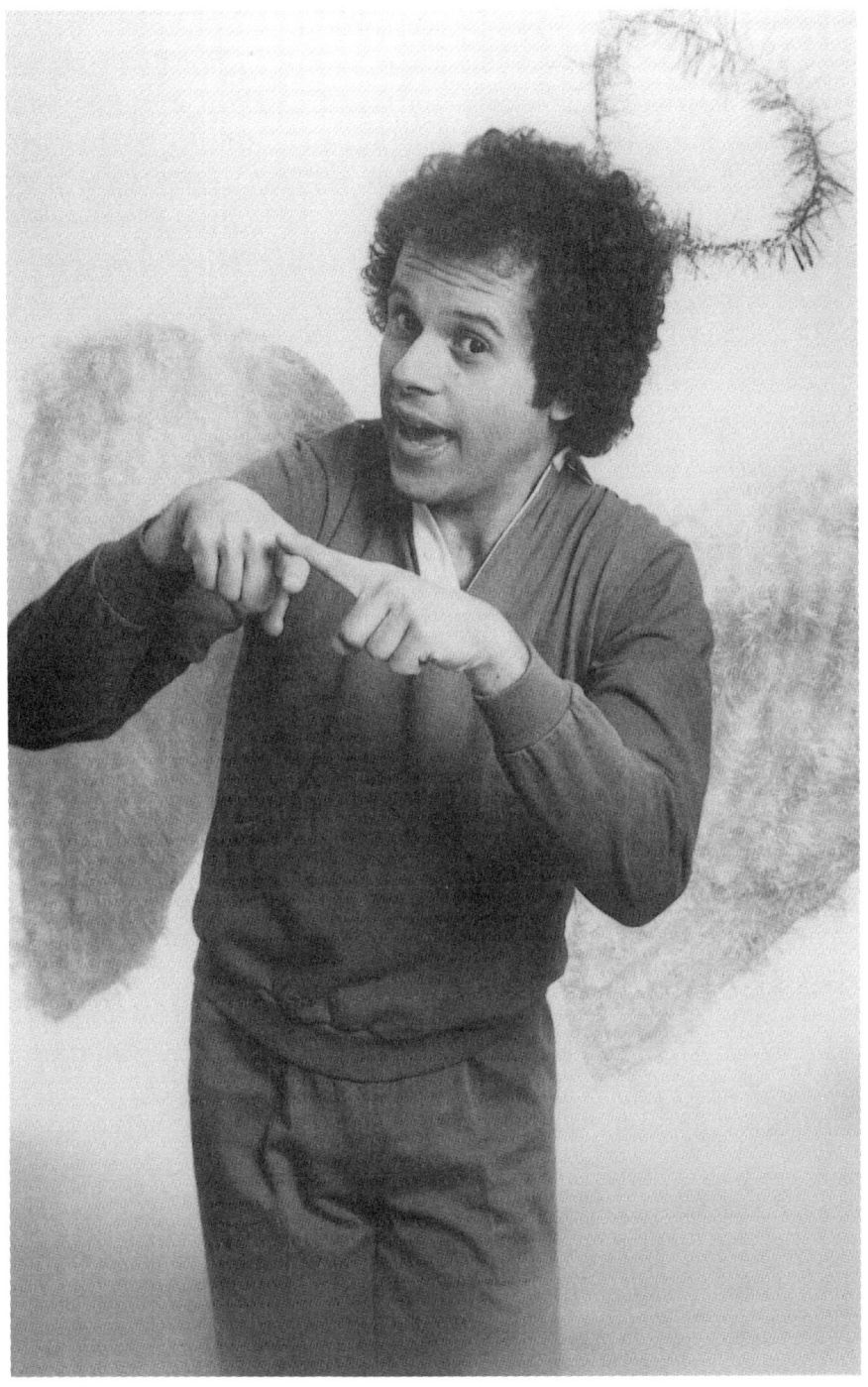

"Just say no!" A press photo of the "Weight Saint" from
The Richard Simmons Show

er odds and ends, and walked the two blocks to Channel 5, the

increased from five stations to forty stations, then to eighty stations, and finally to 196 markets. The response and the mail increased right along with it. The audience had never seen anything like it—a show that was so full of hope. And besides that, it was very interactive: The viewer could send for recipe cards. There were contests. We flew people in who had lost weight so they could tell their stories. We had celebrity guest stars who'd come on and do bits with me. We became sort of a cult show, and I was reaching more people and expanding my message.

I created a family of characters: Sister Mary Lo-Cal, Groana Barett, Anna Maria Spaghetti, and Reverend Pounds—a man of the tablecloth— who would recite things like "Twinkies are my shepherd, I shall not want . . . " It was pretty outrageous. We always got a lot of ideas from our mail, and practically anything could inspire a bit for the show.

And we had lots of celebrity guest stars. Bob Barker from *The Price Is Right* would pop out of a cabinet, or Betty White or Phyllis Diller or Barbara Eden would show up.

There was one guest who came on the show who surprised even me. When Jack La Lanne, the father of fitness, first saw my show, he was interviewed by a reporter who asked, "What do you think of that new, spry, happy show called *The Richard Simmons Show?*" Jack said, "Well, he's too fast for me. He's got a lot of energy." When the article appeared, Nora showed it to me, and it wasn't too flattering. Now there are some people who can read a piece of criticism in a newspaper and it just rolls off their back and that's the end of it. Not me. I have to get to the root of it, and sooner rather than later. I asked Nora to get me Jack La Lanne's telephone number.

I'd never met Jack La Lanne. This was the man I threw stale popcorn at when I was a child. I watched him on T.V. simply because my father wouldn't let me flip the channels. I remembered that he had organ music and a dog, and that he always wore the same powder-blue jumpsuit. It was just so ironic that I was calling him now.

Jack's wife, Elaine La Lanne (I'm not making that up), answered the phone. She had a very bubbly, cheerful voice and was very sweet on the phone. I told her I was Richard Simmons. She said Jack wasn't home, but then she exclaimed, "Oh, I just love your show."

Jack La Lanne was booked on the show, and yes, he was still

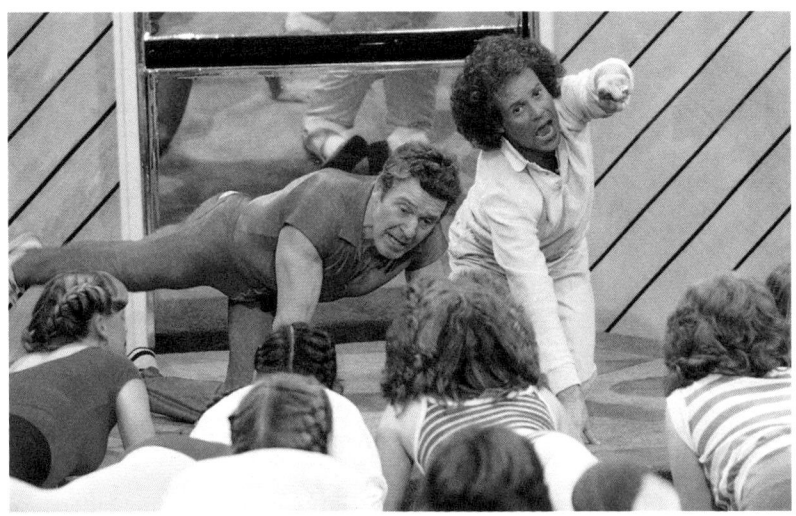

Sweating with a sweet man, Jack La Lanne.
At first he thought I was an alien!

I said, "Well, to tell you the truth, I'm the kind that wears my heart on my sleeve. Your husband was quoted in an article in the newspaper . . . "

"Oh, I know, I know," she said. "Did that hurt your feelings?"

I admitted that it did, and I told her he could make it up to me by being a guest on my show.

The very next day we got a call—Jack La Lanne was booked on the show, and yes, he was still in that powder-blue jumpsuit. We had the best time. When it came to exercise, we were from such different schools of thought. But there was something about him—maybe the military tone of his voice, or the patter of the way he talked—that reminded me of my dad. We became friends, and sometimes we would be booked to do other shows together. With one phone call, I went from throwing popcorn at him to doing jumping jacks with him.

* * *

A Family Affair

Some of my proudest moments were when my mother and father were guests on *The Richard Simmons Show*. My mother did a cooking segment with me. She was hilarious. She would take a low-fat recipe and she'd say, "Now you add a stick of butter."

"Mother, there's no butter in this recipe."

"Oh, Richard." she'd say. "A little butter never hurt. Then, use a cup of sugar . . . "

"Mother, there's only one tablespoon." Everyone loved her.

Once, we took the whole crew to New Orleans and did the show from there. By then, it was being televised on a local channel, and my father had seen it. I called Leonard and asked if he wanted to be on with me.

He said, "Well, that is the silliest show I have ever seen in my life. You are so wacky and crazy on that show."

And I said, "Do you want to be on?"

And he said, "Uh-huh."

My father had always made fun of the way I dressed. When you're overweight, you stay away from sweaters and coats that make you look heavier, and you wear things like overalls to hide certain things. I'd had a whole collection of jogging suits made for *The Richard Simmons Show.*

I always began the show with a little three-minute skit that set the theme. The day my father appeared, the theme was about being an individual: Whoever you are, it's good to be yourself.

We had made a set that looked like my dressing room, with all of my outfits hanging up on a rack. In the skit, my father said, "Well, you really do have your own show now, huh?"

"Yes, I do," I replied.

"You're really doing good. I like it. But when are you going to start dressing like an adult? Look at you."

I was wearing a light-green jogging suit with my name on it. He said, "You dress like a five-year-old child."

"Well, dad. Maybe I'll go shopping and get some adult clothes," and I left. Then Len walked over to my rack of clothes and started sorting through them. With a look around to make sure no one was watching, he unzipped a jogging jacket and tried it on. He checked himself out in the mirror with a satisfied grin on his face. What a ham he was! He was very much into it, a performer at heart.

I began to understand how frustrating it must have been for my father not to have succeeded in show business. I think his appearances on my show helped him to get past some of those regrets. And I discovered that I was getting closer to my dad.

On one show, I talked about how I was always teased in scho

I was extremely involved in *The Richard Simmons Show,* and so were the viewers. There was no other program that encouraged people to write in and tell their stories. The lines of communication were very open. And then something else began to happen. People started sending me things. There were handmade items like needlepoint pillows, dolls, and T-shirts. And there were poems. I began to present these things on the air, and that opened the floodgates. We began to get as many of these things as we did letters.

On one show, I talked about how I was always teased in school about my weight. I told my viewers that for a long time I actually thought my name was "Pig" because that's what the kids had called me in class. Well, I started to get pigs sent to me from all over the place. Before long, I had a room full of them. I've always been a collector—I picked that up from my father.

One afternoon, a huge box arrived at the studio. In it was a life-size stuffed pig that a blind woman had made for me. I put the pig in the front seat of my car, and for three years that pink pig went everywhere with me. Heads certainly would turn as we drove down the street.

I received so many gifts that I no longer had room for them all. When I went to nursing homes or visited hospitals, I'd take some of these things with me to brighten the days of others.

In 1982, about a year after I bought the house, my book *Never Say Diet* hit the bookstores. I did a promotional tour of eight cities. My first stop was Chicago. It was freezing and there was a blizzard, and I'll never forget it. (I always seemed to have these weather problems.) It was snowing heavily as I was on my way to a B. Dalton bookstore. I saw ropes strung from parking meter to parking meter, and people were pulling themselves along the ropes. That's how intense the storm was. At the store, I got a copy of the *The New York Times* and looked in the "Book Review" section. My book was number one. I couldn't believe it. And it stayed on the best-seller list for the next fifty-six weeks.

I found that each stop on my book tour wasn't any different than doing a mall. I still had my boom box. I may not have been exercising the crowd, but I heard their stories as I signed their books.

The Man From Mississippi

Back in Los Angeles on *The Richard Simmons Show,* the mail kept arriving in big bags, like Wells Fargo. We went from two of us to six people on staff who just read letters and organized them. There was a pile of letters from the people who were really desperate, a pile from people who had ideas about shows, and a pile from people who gave us a recipe or an idea for an exercise segment they wanted to see.

Then we had a special pile of letters with stars on them. Those were from the successful people, the people who had lost weight and sent before-and-after photos, and were wishing and hoping that we would fly them out. And we did. Our audience loved the success stories.

Once, one of the staff members said, "Oh listen to this one. It's a guy from Mississippi." And then he paused for a moment and said, "Wow, look at these photos."

The letter was from a man named Elijah Jones, who lived in Hattiesburg, Mississippi, and who had lost about three hundred pounds. He didn't use pills, surgery, or any bizarre diets. He lost weight by eating healthy and exercising. We decided to fly him out, so we called him. After a lot of coaxing—a lot—he got on a plane and flew to Los Angeles. Everyone fell in love with him, instantly. He was such a great storyteller, and his story was something to listen to. Back in Mississippi, when he weighed almost five hundred pounds, he used to work in a convenience store. His friends from college would come into the store from time to time, and over the years he watched them go into business and become successful. Meanwhile, he stayed where he was, working the night shift because no one else would take those hours. Finally, one day after seeing *The Richard Simmons Show,* he just woke up and decided to change his life. He was so inspiring.

After his segment was taped, he stayed in L.A. for a few extra days. The office was getting busier and busier, and I could see Elijah didn't want to leave. So I turned to him one morning and said, "Elijah, move your stuff."

He said, "Whaaaat?"

I said, "You don't have a job in Mississippi. You have a job with us. Go home, and be back in two weeks." Two weeks later, Elijah was back and he's been with me ever since.

* *

And then there's Marilyn Lamas. When she first came into Slimmons eighteen years ago, she was over three hundred pounds and a heavy smoker at three packs a day. I instantly felt a connection with this woman who believed in me and in what I was doing. I watched her as she battled the weight and the cigarettes.

I finally said to her one day, "I don't know what you're doing, but you're gonna work for me." And just like that, she did. Through the years she's helped me with all my mail. I must have dictated thousands and thousands of letters to her, because she could type 140 w.p.m.—a rate slightly faster than mine.

About six years ago, Marilyn was diagnosed with Multiple Sclerosis. Marilyn has always been a fighter, and now she is fighting the most difficult battle of her life. Even though she spends much of her time home these days, she still helps me with the mail. She hasn't given up.

* *

My Father's Emmy

From the very first year of *The Richard Simmons Show* in 1979, we always had daytime Emmy nominations. The first year, Jerry Kupcinet won for best director. (He now directs *Judge Judy*.) That same year, Nancy Simmons (no relation!) won for best costume design. Two years later, we won an Emmy for best daytime talk show. I remember Woody and Nora as executive producers accepted the award, and they called me up onstage. Because I was never competitive and never received trophies as a child, winning had never been important to me. For me, it had always been more about doing the show than winning awards. This award had special meaning for me, however.

Offstage, I found a pay phone and called my family in New Orleans. I was holding my statue as I dialed. My father picked up the phone.

"Hi, daddy," I said. I was already crying.

"I can't understand you. Stop crying. What's wrong?"

"Dad. We won an Emmy. Our show won for best daytime talk show. I wanted to tell you this, because this award is yours. You're the one who taught me so much, and I want you to know that this belongs to you."

My father, never one to show his feelings, got a little emotional. "I'm very proud of you, son," he told me. I felt I had made my peace with him. Leonard knew that his boy had done well. And he knew it was because of all he had taught me.

My father, never one to show his feelings, got a little emotional. "I'm
very proud of you, son," he told me. I felt I had made my peace with him.
Leonard knew that his boy had done well. And he knew it was because of
all he had taught me.

* * *

Because of the success of *The Richard Simmons Show,* Woody decided that I should do a show at night, and *Here's Richard!* was born. On that show, I had bigger-name guests such as Sammy Davis, Jr., Dick Clark, and my friend Tony Geary from *General Hospital.*

And as if that weren't enough, a woman who worked for the largest television station in Australia saw my show during a trip to L.A. and loved it. She bought it for syndication, and *The Richard Simmons Show* was picked up in Australia and New Zealand. It was a big hit. When the show premiered, I flew over to do press appearances. At the same time, it just so happened that a big entertainment center was opening in Sydney. There was a whole series of galas, which included appearances by John Denver, Christopher Cross, and me. My bit was to exercise the Australian Army to the tune of Tschaikovsky's *1812 Overture.* It was an unforgettable aerobic experience!

* * *

I See Spots

When I returned from Australia, I opened the front door of my house, and there on the couch was a basket holding a wiggling eight-week-old Dalmatian puppy. So I became a dog father in 1982.

The dog was a gift from my publicist on *The Richard Simmons Show.* He had wanted to get me a welcome-home present, and when he checked with my friends and co-workers, they thought it would be a great idea for me to have a dog. I had a house; I had a yard. It was time to fill them up with the pitter-patter of little feet, or in this case, little paws.

Because of my attachment to *Gone with the Wind,* I decided to name the little pup Scarlett. I loved her right away, and she loved me too, and followed me everywhere when I was home. But Scarlett seemed a little lonely for the company of other dogs, especially when I was traveling. So I visited the breeder and came home with Ashley. The family was growing. Now I had two dogs, Scarlett and Ashley.

I had started some construction on the house, not only for the renovation but because I was adding a retaining wall so the dogs could have the run of the yard. One of the construction workers didn't know I had dogs and left the door open. Scarlett and Ashley took the opportunity to check out the neighborhood. They wandered off and didn't return.

It was such an empty feeling. I'd become so close to those two dogs, and now they were gone. I searched the neighborhood in my car, I put up posters, and I called the newspaper and the shelters. Five days passed without any word. My house was so quiet. I couldn't sleep at night. I needed some company.

I called the breeder and I got a third dog. Her name was Martha, but we called her Marty, for short (not the breeder, the new pup).

On the fifth day that Scarlett and Ashley were missing, I took the opportunity to go on a local radio talk show. During the course of the conversation, I talked about my missing dogs. I described them, explained how they had left home, and told everybody listening how to get in touch with me. An hour later, the phone started ringing. I drove to meet the people who were positive they had found my babies.

Ashley had gone east and was living with two hippies in Laurel Canyon. When I pulled up to the house, there she was, sitting on the porch under the wind chimes with a man and a woman in tie-dyed clothing. I was surprised Ashley wasn't wearing her own little tie-dyed doggie outfit.

"Ashley, where have you been?" I demanded. "You come here." She popped herself up off the porch, groveled a little, and then, without looking back, she hopped into my car. I thanked the couple, obviously animal lovers, for taking very good care of Ashley, and then we were on our way.

Scarlett, being the lady that she was, was a little more refined in her taste. She went west, to Bel Air.

With Ashley by my side, I drove up to this beautiful mansion. I rang the bell and was escorted into a huge living room. There, I found Scarlett sitting on a couch, and a woman who was painting a portrait of her.

"Scarlett, get off that couch," I said, "and put down that caviar (just kidding)." I thanked the woman, the mistress of the house, who had given my precious little Scarlett such royal treatment.

sket holding a wiggling eight-week-old Dalmatian puppy. So I

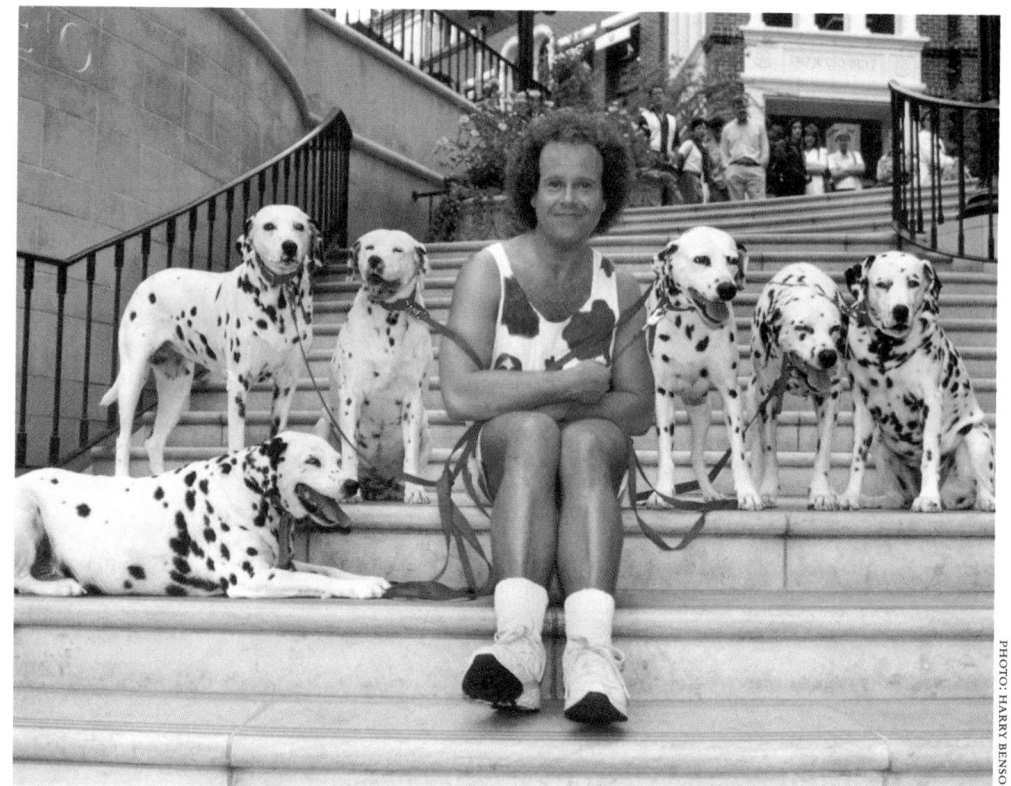

My Family

So now I had three dogs. I loved them so much, I wanted a bigger family. Scarlett was introduced to a nice young male dog at the breeder's, and she gave birth to six puppies. I kept two of the puppies myself, and gave the rest to friends. I named one Pitty-Pat. She was liver-spotted brown instead of black, and so much like chocolate that I knew she had to stay. Originally I was going to keep only the one pup, but when the last was born, the veterinarian told me she was deaf.

"She's the littlest and should be put to sleep," he told me.

"No! I can't kill a dog!" I said. "As far as I'm concerned, that just makes her special."

And that was how I came to have Prissy in my life. Suddenly, I was the owner of five spotted dogs.

A few years later, Marty showed the signs of maternal instincts. You could just tell that she was going to be a motherly dog. She had pups, too. I kept the only female from her litter. I named that dog Melanie.

There I was with a six-pack. I had wanted to fill up my life

So my family was complete. There I was with a six-pack. I had wanted to fill up my life with dogs, and now, somehow, I had gotten a herd. I couldn't go somewhere and take just one of them. You know what a softy I am. So, the six dogs and I went everywhere together. They went in the car with me, they went to the studio with me, and they went on shows with me. My life was full of joy . . . and spots.

The Woman I Live With

Yes, there is a woman in my life—a beautiful woman who looks like a thirty-five-year-old Sophia Loren. Her name is Teresa. I know this is the part of the story you've been waiting for.

Because I had a house full of kids—oops, I mean dogs—and was still doing a lot of traveling, I needed someone to run the house in my absence. Well, in fact, I actually needed someone there when I was home, too.

I'd been through quite a few housekeepers. When someone came in and saw a herd of dogs coming at them, they tended to say, "Oh my God, this is more than a housekeeping job."

Getting a housekeeper is a whole process that I really don't like all that much. When you get a housekeeper, you go to the agency and you sit down. And one by one, these women come in. You sit with them and you talk, you ask them questions, and then you go home and think about it. When you're ready, you call the agency with your answer. I have my rules, and they have their rules. They have days they want off, and preferences such as non-smokers (no problem there) or no pets (uh-oh!).

Well, a man at the agency phoned Teresa and told her she should come in to meet this guy, Richard Simmons. She'd never heard of me (can you believe it?!). She'd been working for the same people for years and years, and she was not a television watcher.

"Well, I don't know," she said.

He said, "Well, if I were you, I would just come in and at least take the interview with him. He's sitting here right now. Just take the interview."

So, she quickly drove to the agency to meet me. It was like love at first sight. Something really clicked, but still, I knew I had to get past the difficult questions.

"Do you like dogs?" I asked, with my fingers crossed.

"Well, when I was a child I had a Dalmatian." And that's all she had to say. I fell to my knees.

"You're hired." I told her.

"I'm hired?"

"Yes," I said. "It's done. Let's get your stuff and you can move in right away." That was twelve years ago. Teresa is the link that makes it possible for me to travel and reach people wherever I go, and still be able to care for all the dogs. She's a very strong woman. People always say, "You help so many people. They talk to you and unburden their sadness on you. Who do you talk to when you feel sad?"

And my answer is Terri. I have had this fantasy life, and Teresa is the one who grounds me. Terri will tell me stories about her family in Mexico, or we'll listen to music together, or we'll play with the dogs. And she's very honest with me. She is the one who brings me back to the reality of it all.

* * *

The Dalmatian Room

In the past, people had sent me pig stuff. Once I got the dogs, it became Dalmatian stuff. Dalmatian pajamas, T-shirts, refrigerator magnets, and figurines started rolling in, and before you knew it, I turned a spare room into a Dalmatian room. My entire office at home was spotted with every conceivable item anyone ever thought of putting spots on. And people made things by hand. They would do wood carvings; they'd ask for photos of my dogs and do paintings of them. People really got into it. Each day the mail arrived, we'd all sit around on the floor and open the gifts people had sent. I cherished every thoughtful item and found a place on the shelves or the wall for each one. The dogs liked them, too, but they were really there to see if anyone had sent homemade biscuits. Every once in a while, they got lucky and found themselves in cookie heaven.

The other great thing about having six dogs is that they're high-spirited and they need a lot of exercise. So I was always going for long walks, sometimes several times a day. The dogs were great for me to have, both emotionally and physically.

By the time my father made what was to be the last of his visits to Los

Angeles, I had five of the six dogs. Leonard was like St. Francis of Assisi. Animals love my father. He'd come into my kitchen and I'd stand back and watch him greet each dog by name, as they cried and ran circles around him.

It wasn't all roses and beef bones with the dogs, however. Scarlett developed epilepsy, and then eventually so did Prissy. By the time the dogs were full-grown, I could have become a veterinarian with all the knowledge I'd attained about dog illnesses. Ashley was sick as a young pup and had to have a hysterectomy. Pitty-Pat had a skin disorder. Prissy was born deaf and then got cancer of the nose. And in between there were ticks and fleas and colds and other assorted illnesses. But we weathered them all. However, there was another storm I wasn't expecting, and my dogs were soon to be a bigger comfort than I could ever imagine.

* * *

A Hard Good-Bye

In November of 1982, my father, at age 85, was supposed to have a minor operation to remove kidney stones. For reasons I couldn't explain, I just didn't have a very good feeling about it. My father and I had become extremely close during the last ten years of his life. He'd been out to L.A. to do *The Richard Simmons Show* several times, and then he had taken vacations out here with me, just to relax. When he was back in New Orleans, we talked every day. In addition, I went back home all the time. We understood and respected each other, and we were pals. We had finally gotten past all the problems and tension from when I was growing up. My attitudes about him had completely changed. And now, with this operation, I was worried.

I said, "Daddy, you're eighty-five years old. Are you sure you want to have surgery?"

My father insisted that it was a very simple operation. He went ahead and scheduled himself for the procedure. I was in Los Angeles, keeping in touch with my mother and my brother while he was operated on.

I got a call from my brother Lenny. He told me something had gone wrong, very wrong, and that I should get on the next flight to New Orleans. I didn't know what had happened.

When I walked into my father's hospital room, I didn't know the man I saw in that bed. There were tubes running everywhere, and he had lost a great deal of weight. This was not my father, dressed in his vest, making his grocery list for the day. It was the hardest thing I'd ever faced.

After a few days, my father came home from the hospital. Once we got him settled in and comfortable, I asked him if there was anything else I could do for him.

He said to me with a serious look, "Yes, Richard. There is one other thing you can do for me. Go to Rome and meet the Pope. And say a prayer with him for me." This was too much—this was the ultimate faux Catholic thing. He said it to me as if he were asking me to run down to the corner deli to get him a ham-and-cheese sandwich. But I was so worried, I would have done anything he asked.

"The Pope? Really? Okay. If that's what you want me to do, daddy, I'll do it. I'll go to Rome." My father would always watch the Pope when he was on television, and he would read every article he found on the Pope. For not being Catholic, my father was very Pope-ish.

I quickly got on the phone and talked with my publicist, and we started working on the arrangements. And before I knew it, I was on an airplane to Rome. A small group of us met with the Pope, and then I moved into a smaller room for a private audience. I told the Pope that my father was ill

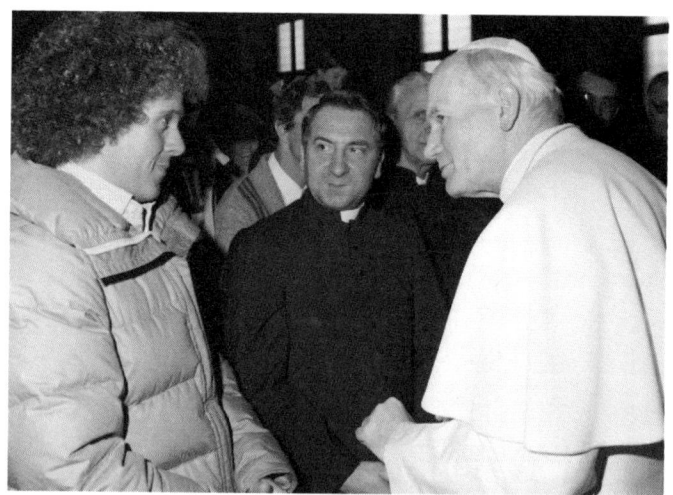

Eye to eye

and that he had sent me to Rome to see His Holiness. We knelt down together and said a prayer for my father.

As soon as I said good-bye to the Pope, I found a pay phone and called home. My mother answered and told me, "Honey, your father is sitting up in bed. I think maybe he's feeling a little better." So, I thought, Maybe my dad's sending me to Rome was not such a bad idea after all. But this sense of hope did not last long.

A few months later, I was scheduled to fly to New Orleans to tape a week of shows there. It was sweeps week on television, the time of year when networks get their ratings, so shows tend to put on sensational or grandiose productions. We were no exception. I was going to Jackson Square in New Orleans to teach an aerobics class of ten thousand people.

The night before my trip, the telephone rang. It was my brother, Lenny.

"Daddy passed," he said. It was Monday, April 18, 1983. I was numb with shock. While my brother was extremely strong, I cried and cried. My father was gone.

I took out my one black suit, packed, and got on the next flight to New Orleans.

My father was to be cremated—that's what he had requested. Lenny carefully planned the wake and the funeral. He wanted it to be perfect, since my father had so many friends, and they would all be there. I was having a very hard time—I was not prepared for any of this. Other than my Uncle Milton, no one close to me had ever died. I had never been to a wake or a funeral or even a cemetery in my entire life.

I was in my room at the Royal Orleans Hotel, and I had laid out all my clothes for the funeral. I got into bed and curled up under the covers, planning to rest for just a few moments. And then I couldn't get out of bed. The phone rang, and it was my brother. I told him I couldn't do it. I couldn't go to the funeral. My mother and brother were so understanding—they said I should do what I felt comfortable with. I was so grief-stricken, I couldn't move. To try and make up for not being at the funeral, I called every florist in town and ordered every white rose they could find in New Orleans and had them delivered to the funeral home. The entire back wall was all white roses. But I wasn't there to see them.

It took me a while to come to terms with this side of myself. Was it cowardice? Was it fear? What was it? I'm not sure I know to this day.

This wasn't all that happened. To add to the pain, there was a robbery. There'd been a big notice in the paper about my father's death, with all the information about the wake and the funeral. So during the funeral, when the house was empty, burglars broke in and took everything. They got my mother's jewelry and many of the sentimental things my dad had given my mother over the years. They got the ring my father always wore, a pinkie ring with a woman's face carved in it—the ring he promised me as a kid that I would some day have. I just felt so empty, just like my mother's jewelry box. My father was gone, along with all the things that reminded me of him. There was a cruel irony here—the slate had been wiped clean again.

Until the recent past, I was unable to deal with my father's passing or, in fact, with the whole issue of death. A few years ago, I was in New Orleans and my brother and I were driving back to my mother's house after attending an event together.

"Oh, I want to take you someplace," Lenny said to me. "I have something to show you." And all of a sudden, he drove into a cemetery.

"Stop the car," I said.

"I want to show you where daddy is."

"*Stop* the car!" I said. I made him back up.

"You know, some day you're going to have to grow up about this."

"Maybe so," I told him. "But it's not going to be today."

When my father passed away, my dogs were an incredible source of comfort. They kept me busy when I could no longer bear to think how sad I was, and when I did feel sad, they were always there for a good hug. Years later, the dogs would still be a link to my father's death, and they would help me repair the shame I'd felt about my inability to attend his wake.

Shirley's Seal-A-Meal

After my father died, I was worried about Shirley, and how she would cope with my dad's death. She had retired from Maison Blanche, and I was worried she wouldn't have enough to do to fill up her time. She grieved, but she held up well.

Shirley began doing a great deal of cooking—it became almost like her hobby. Leonard had always done the cooking. Now Shirley had free reign at the stove, and in addition, I had arranged for a limo and driver for whenever she wanted to do major shopping and needed help with heavy packages. Soon, she was going to all the fancy epicurean food shops that reminded her of Solari's. Just as my father had shopped the French quarter, Shirley became selective, buying her meat in one store and her bread in another. And just like my father, cooking became her absolute passion. But if she was doing all this cooking, who was going to do all the eating? Well, her favorite person to feed—me!

She would make twenty different kinds of soup and gumbos, and crawfish étouffé, and red beans and rice. She would seal them in heavy-duty plastic bags, pack them in ice in boxes, and FedEx them overnight to me. One day I'd be dining on a delicious gumbo, and the next day, broccoli soup with Cheddar cheese. All these unbelievable home-cooked delicacies arrived monthly.

As one chapter in her life closed, another opened. I watched her begin to flourish on her own, showing an independent side I had not seen before. I knew my Shirley was going to be okay.

Pick a Card . . .

Back in L.A., there was a change happening in daytime television. It was the beginning of the talk-show phenomenon. Suddenly my show was put up against a whole lot of shows with people talking endlessly about their problems. The unbelievable ratings for *The Richard Simmons Show* seemed to be leveling off after three and a half years.

I was doing *Here's Richard!* at night and the other show during the day, but I was no longer really happy. I felt pushed in too many different directions. I had been doing this for a long time, and when you're doing five shows a week, week after week, plus doing locations, plus doing the sweeps weeks where you're taking your show on the road—well, I was spreading myself a little too thin. The ratings were dipping, and Woody was moving on to other shows. Everything runs its course, and I began to feel that we were heading toward the end of the line.

as gone, along with all the things that reminded me of him.

During the Christmas break in 1983, we got the news that we would not be coming back to tape more shows. It was like my life had ended. What was I going to do now? People thought, however, that I was still doing the show, because it was repeated for three more years in syndication on Life-Time. *Here's Richard!* was also ending—that lasted only a year. It was a strange period of transition for me, and I found myself slipping into a bit of a slump. There was a void in my life.

* * *

One afternoon, I was walking to my car in the parking lot at Century City in L.A., when I ran into Larry, an attorney—a friend who I had not seen for a while. We first met when he came into Derek's for dinner. After we hugged and exchanged a warm greeting, he asked, "So, what are you doing these days?"

"I'm doing a lot of stuff, but I just feel . . . I don't know."

"What's wrong?" he asked.

"Well, I've done many things, but now I'm sort of at a crossroads. I can't quite figure out what to do next."

"Hmmm. Wait a minute. Well, what do you enjoy? There must be something you really get a kick out of."

"I don't know."

"Wait. I have an idea. Let's try this." He took out his wallet and slipped out three of his business cards and tore them in half. "Here's six pieces of paper. Think a minute, and then write on these pieces of paper what you most enjoy doing and at the same time can make a living from."

I felt like I was on a quiz show. Was a new job going to be the prize? I wrote down six different things and gave the pieces of paper back to Larry. He cupped them in his hands, shook them, and said, "Now, pick one."

I shut my eyes and picked one. I read from the card. "It says 'malls' on it. Malls!"

"Malls?" Larry asked.

"Yeah, I do these exercise events in shopping malls. I travel around and I love it."

"Well, Richard, that's what you should do. Take the other five pieces of paper—keep them. Do this for one year—give it a year. And if that doesn't work out, shake up those five other pieces of paper and go for another one."

If I looked at the bottom line, I guess what I missed most was the personal contact with people. Going to the malls meant meeting people, and being accepted and respected, face-to-face. The crowds were still turning out to talk with me, and they were bigger than ever.

Almost like a touring rock band, I'd go on the road for ten days. I'd do all the local radio and television stations and finish my visit with a show in the mall. Being a living example of how you could take the weight off and keep it off meant that exercising and healthy eating, for me, were now more important than ever.

The Album

After *The Richard Simmons Show* ended, I wanted to try something totally different, and that's when I came up with the idea for an album and a cassette of original songs for exercising. I had met Bruce Roberts, who wrote several songs for Barbra Streisand, including "Enough Is Enough." I was also a big fan of Allee Willis, who had done a lot of work for the Pointer Sisters—and I just love the Pointer Sisters. She agreed to team up with Bruce to work on this album. I gave them some titles that I wanted to have songs for, like "Wake Up" and "Reach" and "Laugh" and "You Can Do It." Well, they took my titles and just ran with them. They did some great work and came up with these amazing songs, very inspirational. The album sold over a million copies and won lots of awards. It made me realize even more how important music is to my whole approach to exercise and fitness.

In the Beginning, There Was Beta

In 1983, I got a phone call from a man named Stuart Karl, a young, creative, energetic man who owned a production company. Stuart was a baby-faced blond from Newport Beach, California. He had a vision that he could sell exercise videos and make a lot of money, and he wanted to sign me up. Since home video players or V.C.R.s were becoming popular, his idea was to put Richard Simmons in everybody's living room so they could

I wrote down six different things and gave the pieces of paper

exercise with him—me. I didn't need to be convinced. I thought it was a fabulous idea. He had one other person in mind for the videos—Jane Fonda.

So it was Dick and Jane, each with our own exercise video. Remember Beta? The cassettes sold for $69.95. I must admit, there was a little competition between Jane and me. Jane was an actress, and she was beautiful. I would see bunches of men lined up in the video stores at night, just staring at her tape. I had fans, too. My Dalmatians loved my video—they would bark and bark.

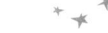

Dick and Jane

ven though Jane and I were two of the first exercise enthusiasts and despite the fact that our work has taken us on parallel tracks over the years, we never really became close friends.

Jane and I first met briefly in Atlanta. We were both there doing separate benefit exercise classes for two different organizations. Well, I must admit, I was a little bit envious that I was not Jane Fonda, that my father had not been Henry Fonda, and that I had not played Barbarella.

I got a call in my hotel room. I picked up the phone and said, "Hello?!"

"Is Richard Simmons there?"

"This is Richard."

"Hi, this is Jane Fonda."

"Barba— Oh, Jane Fonda! What a surprise! Hi! How are you?" Never at a loss for words, I was now stumbling.

"I know you're here in Atlanta, and I thought if you have the time, it might be nice to get together for breakfast." Back then she was married to Tom Hayden and had a couple of kids.

"Yes. I'd love to—what a wonderful idea."

"Good. Why don't you come to my hotel then."

I went over and had breakfast with all of them, but I felt awkward. Our time together was pleasant, but I didn't feel any real connection. And we never bumped into each other again after that breakfast.

Then, a few years ago, *Shape* magazine, based in L.A., called me and said they were having a big event at the House of Blues on Sunset, and they were giving Jane Fonda a lifetime-achievement award. And I said, "You are? Oh, how nice." And then they asked me if I would like to be the presenter.

Now, remember, I didn't really know Jane Fonda. But she had done a lot of good for people, so I said okay. The plan for the show was this: There would be a huge box on stage throughout the whole program. After all the tributes had been paid to Jane, I would jump out of the box, wearing a tank top that said "Dick and Jane," and present the award.

Well, the big night came, and I decided I couldn't go. My dog Prissy was suffering from cancer and had taken a turn for the worse, and I just wasn't in the mood to be funny. I decided I would write a letter of tribute to Jane and drop it off at the House of Blues, which was only a couple of blocks from my house. Somebody could read my letter during the show.

I looked at Prissy and said to her, "I won't be gone long. I'm just walking down the street to drop this letter off, and then I'll be right back." Prissy gave me such a look, as if she were telling me, "Go ahead, Richard. You go and give Jane her award. I'll be here when you get back." And then I realized that all these people were counting on me. I had committed myself to presenting the award, and I couldn't back out now. That was just something I didn't ever do. I looked at Prissy and thought, "Yes, you're right." I kissed her good-bye, put the letter in my pocket, and went down to the House of Blues.

I was so glad I decided to go. When I jumped out of the box, the place went crazy. Jane was crying, I was crying, everybody on stage was crying. I told Jane the whole story about how I wasn't going to come because of my dog Prissy. And then I read the letter to her, talking about what she had contributed to this world and how lucky we were.

The award ceremony was not the end of our paths crossing. In 1997, my cookbook *Farewell to Fat* came out at the same time as her cookbook. Often we'd be side-by-side, sitting at an autograph table, signing our books.

* ⋆ *

The Videos Continue

So in 1983, I did my first exercise video. It was called *Every Day with Richard Simmons,* and that was followed by *The Stomach Formula.* I did a few more videos with Stuart Karl, and then his company was bought out by Lorimar. After that, Stuart faded from the scene. Shortly afterward, Lorimar was bought out by Warner Brothers, and I was contracted to do one more video with Warner. I also began working on a third book, because I still had a book deal at Warner Books, part of a four-book contract. Just when I wondered if things were slowing down, something else would come my way.

* ⋆ *

And then, unexpectedly, I went into a bit of a depression. I woke up one morning and started packing to go to a mall. Trust me, I loved what I did. I loved the traveling—it was in my bones from my parents because they had traveled so much. But I felt that I had had my day in the spotlight and that it was going to be over for me. Here was the simple fact: I did not have the show anymore. People were still talking about it and I still felt so connected to it, but it was a thing of the past.

It didn't help when a producer came to my house for dinner one night and said, "You know you had a good run. You made some money. I hope you've put it away, because I think you were a fad." Needless to say, that man was never invited back for dinner.

I loved the malls, but I missed the show. I didn't want to do a sit-com, though I'd been asked, because I certainly wasn't an actor. I didn't want to do movies. That's not what I did. My home was still Slimmons.

During the following weeks, I found myself watching a lot of television and feeling a little sorry for myself. There was something missing, and I just couldn't put my finger on it.

* ⋆ *

Info-Land

While I was watching television one morning, I saw, for the first time, a two-minute commercial spot. Suddenly, these extended commercials began popping up all the time. One commercial would offer a fishing product, another would be for a pan that fried bacon in the microwave, and another would be a guillotine-like device to chop vegetables with. These two-minute spots would mark the beginning of the next chapter in my life.

At this point in my career, I was really becoming associated with health and fitness. People recognized me as the guy with the big hair who did all that jumping around and who was sympathetic to the concerns of over-weight people. Because of all this, someone was always trying to get me to endorse or promote exercise equipment or anything they thought was healthy.

One day—this was around 1985—a group of men from a company called American Telecast came knocking at my door. They asked if I'd be interested in doing a two-minute spot for them to demonstrate a piece of exercise equipment. When I saw the product, I thought, "My God, it looks like a robot that lost some parts!" You hooked it onto a doorknob, and with a bunch of pulleys and ropes, you could exercise your legs and arms.

I said, "No, thank you. This piece of equipment is not for me. But, you know, I do have something upstairs that I use at my club. It's a whole new approach for managing food portions and tracking the food you eat over the course of a day."

I got it for them—my construction-paper cards and plastic wallet for holy cards. I sat down with these men and I said, "I want to introduce you to Deal-A-Meal."

They thought the name was cute. I explained how it worked, with the six food groups and the cards and the wallet. They said they liked the con-cept, but they would have to think about it and they would get back to me. I thought that was it—I would never hear from them again. They would just go out and find another celebrity who would love to exercise with those pulleys. Well, within a day or two, they called and they said, "Let's shoot a two-minute spot."

So I found myself with this renewed energy because I was now going to be back on television on a regular basis. With Deal-A-Meal, I was back in the saddle again.

Winifred Morice, a registered dietitian whom I'd met at my exercise stu-dio, helped me with the recipes and the menu suggestions that we put on each card. She's a very upbeat platinum blonde from New Zealand, who is almost as crazy I am. I adore her, and we've worked together for almost fourteen years. She's helped me with all my cookbooks and has been on many of my Cruises to Lose (more about that later).

So I watched my little plastic card holder and construction-paper cards being transformed into a refined wallet with different sections and cards that were colorfully printed, and I thought, Oh my God, this is wonderful.

I liked American Telecast. It was owned and run by the Marsh family. One Marsh produced the shows, another Marsh bought the television time—they all did something. Since I didn't have a family of my own in Los Angeles, I was very attracted to them, and I got extremely close to all of them.

They rented a house in Malibu to shoot the two-minute commercial. Everything was clean and white and sunny.

"Hi, I'm Richard Simmons. I've kept my weight off, and now I'm going to teach you how to do the same, the safe way, with Deal-A-Meal."

Then I showed the wallet and all the cards. "Now for breakfast, you could have this." And I would list a healthy balanced breakfast. Then I would move the appropriate cards over. "And when all the cards have been moved to this side, you're done eating for the day. How easy could that be?"

The camera came tightly in on my face and I said, "Don't you want to deal with your life? Don't you want to deal with the things that are happening to you? Then you should Deal-a-Meal."

They put it on the air, and the Deal-A-Meals flew out the window. Then we did another two-minute spot, and the same thing happened. We were selling thousands a day.

* * *

In 1985, President Ronald Reagan deregulated the amount of time that a television commercial could run. This paved the way for the thirty-minute commercial. Someone coined the term "infomercial," and the flow of products began. At first, infomercials ran very late at night and there were only a handful of them.

Because the Deal-A-Meal two-minute spot became so popular, American Telecast approached me and said, "Let's plan a thirty-minute show." At this point, no one was knocking down my door to hand me work. I was doing guest spots on T.V. game shows like *Hollywood Squares* and *The Match Game*. So I said, Yes—I would do the thirty-minute infomercial which they could later test.

Now the question was, what are we going to do for the thirty minutes?

American Telecast sent me Ed Shipley, another angel in my life, who was married to Laurie Marsh, one of the daughters of the Marsh dynasty. He and I were on the same wavelength. He was a young, very thin man who lived off peanut-butter sandwiches, hamburgers, and french fries, and he didn't know anything about health, nutrition, or exercise. But he was creative. He was a Steven Spielberg kind of guy. So we just sat down and began to work.

We put together a wild story called "The History of Dieting." We started with Adam and Eve in the Garden of Eden. Guess who I was? (No, not Eve!) Then I showed wealthy people from the nineteenth century who ate so much that all their buttons popped off. Next was "The Gallery of Dieting," which was several podiums all in a row, with a little plate on each. One had diet pills, another an ugly little dinner, and another was empty, which meant you could starve yourself. This was actually the story of my life—I had done all these things. We also had a lot of success stories with people who were using Deal-A-Meal, and we added those to the show.

We shot the thirty-minute infomercial, and it was ready to go. I learned that this whole process is almost instant. The editing goes very quickly, and at the same time, commercial time is bought in several major markets. Then there's the big test day. For some reason, all the 1-800 numbers you call to place your orders are connected to a telephone center in Omaha. Why Omaha? It's one of the mysteries of life. I even visited there to see what it looked like, and it was amazing: just thousands of people, answering phones. Once the infomercial starts running in the different markets, and the phones begin to ring, and the numbers start rolling in, Omaha decides whether or not you're a success. If I were ever to leave L.A., I'd move to Omaha. I just love telephones.

All I could do was to sit at home and wait for my phone to ring. And finally, it rang. American Telecast called and told me to sit down. We had a hit on our hands. It became the biggest infomercial on television. Because it was seen so many times—it played morning, noon, and night, five days a week—I couldn't go anywhere without someone yelling out, "Hey, it's the guy with the Dial-a-Meal!" I'd say to them, "It's Dial-a-Prayer and Deal-A-Meal." Everyone seemed to be talking about Deal-A-Meal. This was the biggest thing I had ever done. Suddenly it seemed every comedian had a Deal-A-Meal joke in his or her act.

During this time, I was on *Hollywood Squares,* with Roseanne on one side of me and Louie Anderson on the other, and we all had our Deal-A-Meal wallets out. Roseanne leaned over and said, "Can you eat these cards?" Louie hollered, "Can you buy more fat cards?" It was just hysterical. Losing weight had become fun.

⁺ ⋆ ⁺

Putting It Together

*N*ext, American Telecast and I decided to do a major exercise video. I had already done four short ones, but this was going to be a real lavish production. It was 1986 and, up till now, all exercise videos had been done to "elevator music," and they just weren't fun or inspiring. I did have one more video to do for Warner, and I was going to make this one special. I would use music that people knew, so they could sing along with the lyrics and dance their hearts out. I wanted them to forget they were exercising and just have a good time. So, I sat down with my *Billboard* chart, and I put together a list of songs I used to eat to when I played 45s in my room in New Orleans. I called this new exercise tape *Sweatin' to the Oldies,* and it included all my favorites, like "It's My Party," "He's a Rebel," "Personality," "On Broadway," and "Beyond the Sea."

Then there was the big question of what I was going to wear. After I'd lost weight, I went from uniform to uniform. But with this new video, I knew it was time to change again. In the past, I had gone from leotards and tights to jogging suits to the colorful sweats on *The Richard Simmons Show.* Of all these, I liked the leotards and tights the best, because they did show off my best asset, my legs. (You thought I was going to say something else!) Everyone always told me I had good legs. I had inherited their gorgeous shape from my mother, and I strengthened them by being an overweight kid. Let's face it, if you're fifty pounds overweight as a child and you're walking up stairs, you're bound to have muscular legs. My mother had always said, "Dicky, always show them the best thing you've got." And I did. But I knew the tights were no longer right for me. I couldn't wear the jogging suits or sweats because they were too hot and bulky and, truthfully, they made me look fat. I was getting ready to do *Sweatin' to the Oldies,* and I didn't have a thing to wear.

"You've got great legs," she told me. *"You should be wearing s*

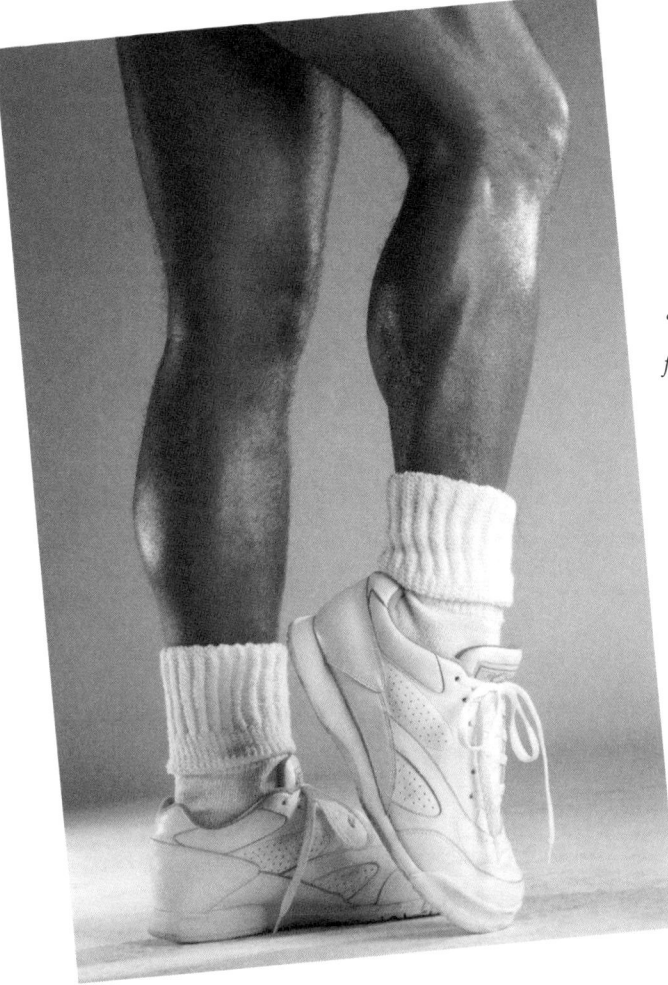

"Pam" is not just for cooking!

Then, I met this magical lady named Leslie Wilshire, my own Edith Head. I say magical because I no longer remember how I came to meet her or when she first started working with me. It seems as though she has always been a part of my life. Leslie was in charge of doing the wardrobe for *Sweatin' to the Oldies*. I told her I didn't know what to wear, but I felt I needed a change. She gave me the once-over, and then said she knew exactly how to change my image.

"You've got great legs," she told me. "You should be wearing shorts."

"Shorts! I don't even own a pair!"

She brought these shorts, Dolphin shorts, and she said, "Here. Try these on." These were the very "in" ones that runners and athletes were wearing.

Then she handed me a tank top.

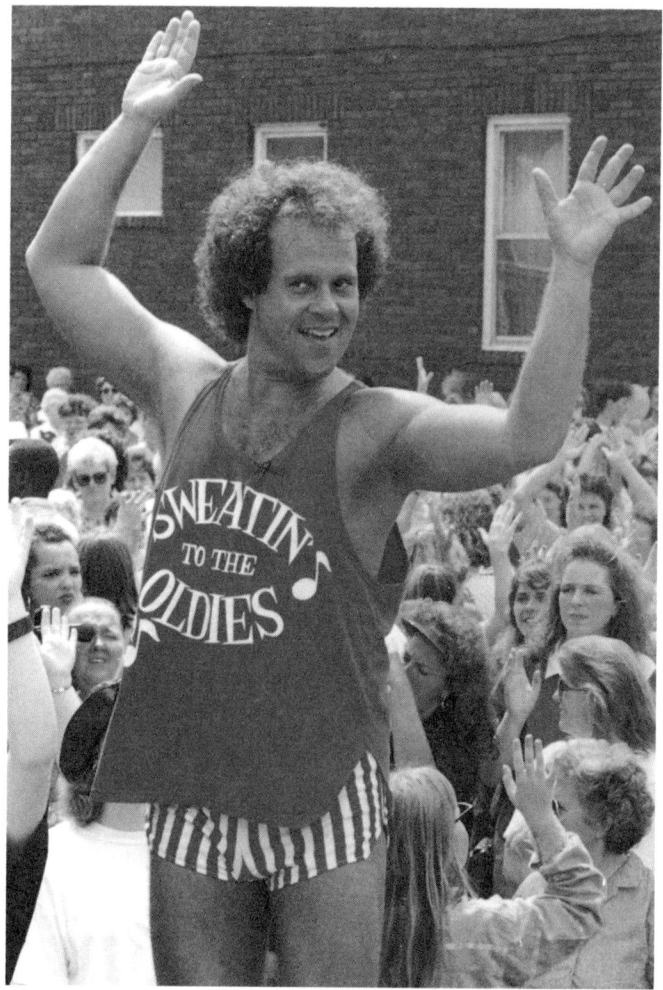

My new uniform!

"A tank top?!!" I asked. I remembered that Marlon Brando had worn a tank top in *A Streetcar Named Desire* and it had looked great. There were only two small problems: I was not Marlon Brando, and there was no streetcar in sight. Never in my life had I shown my arms in public. I had done aerobics. I was not a weight lifter, so there was still a roundness to my shape. After all these years I was still uncomfortable with revealing too much. But Leslie convinced me to at least try it.

The tank top was a little big, so she pinned it up. She said, "Let's put a logo on the front. Then you can walk around in this and see if you're comfortable."

She went home and made the clothes my size. The next day, she came to the house with the outfit and said, "Okay, let's try it on."

And in that tank top and those shorts, I finally knew what Superman must have felt like when he put on the cape for the first time. My legs looked great, and the tank top covered my waist. It camouflaged the area where my underwear made little love-handle dents around my waist. It also gave me an incentive to work a little harder on my chest and my arms. It was the perfect outfit. It looked good on camera, and I felt comfortable in it, and so it became my new uniform. In a matter of weeks, I had several pairs of shorts, red ones and blue ones and pink ones, all with tank tops to match. Over the years, the designs on the fronts of the tops got bigger and they got fancier. This look became my trademark. When people did a parody of me, I was always recognizable because of the tank top and shorts. To this day, people say to me, "You were great in Eddie Murphy's movie *The Nutty Professor.*" I'd say, "Thank you, but actually that wasn't me, it was Eddie Murphy." He played all those characters.

So now I had my new uniform for the video—that was the big hurdle, but there was more to come. I gathered up my team. I had Mary Graves, an instructor who had been working with me for some time, and she was going to help with the exercise group from Slimmons when they performed on camera. And after interviewing a bunch of choreographers, I met Dorain Grusman. I knew instantly she was the right person. Dorain helped me stage all the exercise numbers.

We hired a live band and rented the Santa Monica Women's Gym for the taping, and I had the group from Slimmons who was going to work out with me on-camera. The first number we did was "Dancin' in the Streets." The director showed up with chicken pox—thank goodness we all had been vaccinated. But I should have taken this as a sign. We were taping in one continuous shot, so if anyone made a mistake, we had to start all over again from the beginning. If the band played a wrong note, we started over. If I made a wrong gesture, we started over. Well, none of us had really rehearsed together, and this was the first time we had a live band. You could say we didn't know what we were doing. The whole thing was like a bad, bad rehearsal of the musical *42nd Street.* It took us eight hours to tape that one number. I never wanted to hear "Dancin' in the Streets" again. When we left that night, the dancers would barely talk to me. They just said "Good night," and that was it. I thought I would never see any of these people, ever again—and we still had another eight numbers to do.

Everyone came back the next day, and somehow we got through it all, and it worked. From that video on, Mary and Dorain have been with me for all twenty-one videos.

Next, it was time to put together the cookbook. Again, Winifred Morice stepped in and helped me with this. We tested and tasted all kinds of delicious low-fat recipes. Finally, the *Deal-A-Meal Cookbook* was ready.

You couldn't buy any of this stuff retail—Deal-A-Meal, the exercise video *Sweatin' to the Oldies,* or the cookbook. You had to copy down the 1-800 number from the infomercial and then call that great city of Omaha to place your order. This is how I got my fitness message out.

The dance video really gave a boost to my mall appearances. Many of the people who showed up had the tape, and they already knew all the moves. It was just amazing.

A year later, we shot a second thirty-minute infomercial. It was very emotional, it featured many great success stories, and it gave people a lot of hope. And it was the same thing that I had preached from the very beginning: Make a commitment to yourself. Reduce your portions, exercise to your favorite music, and eat healthy. Above all, you must love yourself.

So one *Sweatin'* tape and one infomercial led to another, and to another. There was *Sweatin' 2, Sweatin' 3,* and then *Sweat N' Shout*—and those led to another cookbook and then to motivational tapes. Every year we would design a new infomercial and then test it. If it worked, we would run it for nine or ten months before a new infomercial was shot. And I continued to support the infomercials by going to meet people in the malls and expos. I knew these places would always be my home away from home.

There I was. I had my own television show again—no matter if it was the same show repeating itself for ten months. And I still had time to go to malls, conventions, and fitness expos; and when I was home in L.A., I always taught classes at Slimmons. I was busier than ever, my plate was full, and I was happy again.

Reaching Out

round the time that my first infomercial came out, in 1986, I wrote my fourth book, called *Reach for Fitness,* which grew out of my work with the Spina Bifida Association.

When you have a national television show, nonprofit organizations request your help to spread the message of their work and to help get funding for their programs. When I was on *General Hospital,* I was approached by the Spina Bifida Association of America. I was immediately impressed with the dedicated people who were a part of the organization, and I was also touched by the courageous children who lived with this debilitating, life-threatening affliction. This is a condition where the spine does not close properly during fetal development, which can result in paralysis, loss of sensation in the lower limbs, and a whole series of other complications.

I became a chairperson and the national spokesperson for the Spina Bifida Association for five years. Even though this was serious work, there were some lighter moments. When I began my spokesperson role, I discovered that people tended to mispronounce the name. Sometimes it came out "Speena Biffada," and people thought it was a Norwegian cereal, because they didn't know anything about it.

While dedicating all my free time to the association, I found myself exercising and working with people in wheelchairs on a regular basis. I saw that there was a great need for exercise programs for the physically challenged. So I decided to write a book and do a video called *Reach for Fitness.* We developed exercises and nutritional guidelines for more than forty different kinds of physical and medical challenges, and we used physically challenged kids to make the video. It was quite an experience for me—these kids were wonderful.

The cover of the book and video depicted children and adults of all ages, some in wheelchairs, some with crutches or leg braces, all raising their arms in victory. When *Reach for Fitness* was published, the book was not widely accepted. People were aghast at the cover. And then the mumbling started, just like it had in grade school.

"This girl is missing a leg. This doesn't look good."

I said, "Hold it. I worked a year on this project. These are real people with real challenges. It's very important that we show them exercising. We need the photographs to make the impact—illustrations just won't cut it."

When I went to book signings, I would bring some of the kids with me. The stores had a hard time with this—they wouldn't promote us, and there were only a handful of books for the display. It was sad for the kids, because they'd worked so hard.

All profits from the book and the video went to the Reach for Fitness Foundation. But because of lack of interest in the publishing and video worlds, and their fear of promoting this project, the foundation closed.

A day does not go by that I don't get a request for the book and video. But there are no more copies.

* * *

Starring Shirley

A short time after *Reach for Fitness* came out in 1986, a man came to me and asked me if I'd be interested in doing a video with my mother. The idea was for me to lead a group of parents of celebrities, including my mother, in a variety of exercises. I felt that my mother's generation had been skipped over when it came to exercise, and I didn't like the words "elderly" or "senior." That's when I thought of "silver foxes"—it was sexy, mysterious, and sleek. So the title became *Richard and the Silver Foxes.* The parents were already lined up: Jackie Stallone, Sylvester Stallone's mother; Harry Hoffman, Dustin Hoffman's father; Pauline Fawcett, Farah Fawcett's mother; and Sal Pacino, Al Pacino's father—and of course, Shirley. We had so much fun working out together, and the video was a huge success as we set out to do a publicity tour.

We went where our audience was: senior day-care centers, retirement communities, recreation centers, clubs. One of our stops was a nursing home. Unlike most of the places we'd visited, this facility was long-term care, and the majority of people who resided there were not active.

My mother was in her seventies and very bubbly, with her makeup and hair impeccably done, as they had been all her life. At the nursing home, the six of us all went in different directions to go say hello to people.

After a while, I couldn't find my mother. I searched several floors and all the common rooms. I couldn't find her anywhere, and no one had seen

In such a short time, she had made such a strong connection w

her. Finally, as I was walking down a corridor, I heard her singing. I followed the sound of her voice to a room near the end of the hall. There was my mother, standing beside a woman's bed, with her back to me. She was braiding the woman's hair. I quietly called to her, and she turned around. All of her makeup had run off and there were tears running down her cheeks. She had been touched by this ninety-year-old woman who no longer knew where she was. As my mother sang to her, the woman nodded her head to the rhythm of my mother's voice. Shirley took a couple of pins out of her own hair and used them to hold up the braid she had made. My mom reached into her pocketbook and pulled out a little rouge, and dabbed it on the woman's thin cheekbones. Then she found a tube of lipstick, and with her pinkie, dabbed a little on the woman's lips. My mother said, "See how pretty you look? Now, when someone comes to visit you, you'll be ready for them."

Once we were outside the room, a nurse told my mother and me that no one had visited the woman in ten years. My mother was devastated by that news. In such a short time, she had made such a strong connection with this woman—just as I had made such a strong connection with my parents and their generation.

Things were starting to make sense to me, and I began to see some connections. Because my parents were older, I had a special place in my heart for the people of their generation. Because I had been overweight, I had such deep feelings for those who were experiencing the battle that I had fought. And because of my work with people who had spina bifida and other physical and mental challenges, I was deeply devoted to helping these people. So I've tried to do whatever I can, to be involved in these three areas I feel so connected to. And this remains my goal, even today.

After I did the tape with my mother, her old show-business genes just started getting active again. She wanted to do more. A couple of years later, we did a Citibank commercial together. It started out with a close-up of my mother saying, "Hi, I'm Shirley Simmons. You know, when you use the Citibank card you get special points to buy presents. And you would think my son would buy me some nice pearls or a long mink coat?" The camera pulls back, and there's Shirley on a stationary exercise bike. And she says,

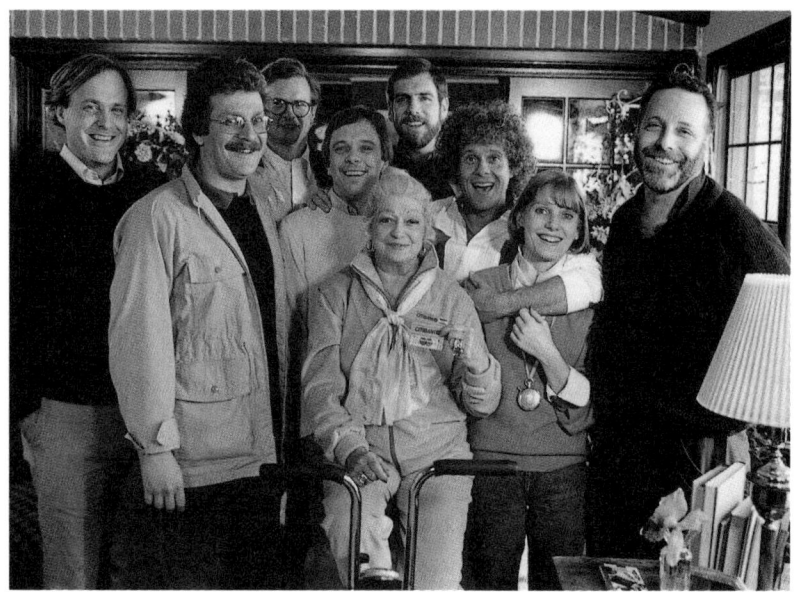

*Once again, Shirley was the star—this time in a Citibank commercial—
and she's always been the leading lady in my life.*

"No! He has to buy me one of these!" And then I pop out and I holler, "Mom, a little faster on that bike. Come on, let's get those miles going. Pedal faster." Then she does this big Lucy Ricardo take, and it's hilarious. Everyone loved it.

The commercial was supposed to run for a year, but it just kept on airing. My mother would telephone me in L.A. and tell me, "Dicky, I got another check in the mail."

"Mother, the commercial is still running."

"Dicky, the check was for fifty-five thousand dollars! Are we doing another?"

Every six months, the sponsor would call and say they wanted to run the commercial again. This went on for about three years. When it finally finished, my mother called. "Hello, Dicky? I'm ready to do another one."

The Forgotten

My first infomercial had been running since early 1986. People across America were watching me in the daytime, they were watching me at night, and in many areas I was on several stations at once. Up until now, I'd dealt with people who were overweight and people who were obese. But because of the infomercial, I began to receive letters from people I knew very little about—the morbidly obese, the homebound.

By this time, I was used to getting long emotional letters. I would spend hours just reading letters and making piles: Call these people; write back to these people; send these people the photo they requested for their refrigerators. Marilyn and Elijah, my assistants, helped me do the sorting. One morning, Elijah urgently handed me a letter as I walked through the door.

"This is the longest letter I've ever seen. You better read it." The letter, thirty pages long on legal-size paper, was about a woman named Rosemarie Carnemolla, and was written by her friend, Diane, from Pleasant Valley, New York. Diane told the sad story of a woman who was currently homebound and weighed over a thousand pounds. I reread parts of the letter several times. I just couldn't believe it.

Then I picked up the phone and I called Rosemarie. The voice that answered was so sad and lifeless. When I told her I was Richard Simmons, she said she'd seen the infomercial and just couldn't believe it was me on the other end of the line. We both cried as she told me of her overwhelming sorrow, her fear of living, and her fear of dying. At that point, I didn't know what to do. I told her I would make some calls to get some professional help for her, and I would call her back the next day.

Rosemarie was in really bad shape. She had an enlarged heart, diabetes, and an array of other serious medical problems. I started dialing. I made calls to hospitals and clinics, including some that specialized in weight-reduction surgery. Through my calls, I found a network of people who were able to help Rosemarie. One of them was Dr. Jim Sapalo in Albion, Michigan. He ran a large clinic, together with his father and brother. They were caring professionals who had performed quite a few weight-loss surgeries, but they recommended that medical procedure only in cases where obesity was life-threatening.

After consulting with a physician who had been to see Rosemarie at her home, Dr. Sapalo suggested she have the surgery in order to increase her chances of living. I am a person who never really believed in surgery as the best solution in cases like this, but Dr. Sapalo said that this was a life-or-death situation.

She had an operation called a gastric exclusion, in which her stomach was reshaped and made smaller, to hold less food. Rosemarie's surgery was a success, and when she was back home and feeling stronger, I just had to get on a plane and meet her. By the time I was able to make the trip, she'd lost nearly two hundred pounds. The town where she lived was an hour and a half drive from New York City. We came up the driveway to a complex of houses. And in one of those houses, I met my friend Rosemarie, who was sitting on a bench somebody had made for her. Above her was a sign that read, "WELCOME ST. RICHARD, I LOVE YOU." At the time, she could walk maybe ten steps, but it took all her effort to do that.

Little by little, Rosemarie continued to drop weight. At six hundred pounds, she got a job in the deli that used to deliver sandwiches to her when she was housebound. With a new attitude and a new will to live, Rosemarie was not tempted by those sandwiches.

Today, after a bout with cancer and an unfortunate car accident, Rosemarie weighs about two hundred and forty pounds. Now she's working and she's going to school. I still hear from her on a regular basis. More than twelve years later, she is among the living. And that makes me truly happy.

* * *

I figure about fifty percent of my letters are from people who are worried about someone else, and who want me to intervene. This can be extremely difficult, because I have to make the first call. And you remember my old rule: Don't offer help unless someone asks for it. But these cases are so extreme, I have to help.

When I make a "cold" call, I just have to play it by ear. I once called Harriet, who a friend wrote me about. She weighed three hundred pounds, she had lost her job, and she had two kids to raise. So I called.

"Hi. Is Harriet there?"

"This is Harriet."

"Hi, Harriet. How are you?"

"I'm fine."

"What are you doing?"

"Oh, nothing." Now I always wonder how someone can be doing nothing. Was she really standing in the middle of the room, just doing absolutely nothing?

So I said, "You're doing nothing? Oh. Well, I'm getting ready to make dinner."

The conversation went on this way for about five minutes, and I still hadn't told her who I was.

Finally Harriet, said, "Can I ask you a question?"

And I said, "Sure. Go ahead."

"Who is this?"

"This is Richard Simmons."

"No, no. Come on, who is this?"

Then I explained that I had received a letter from a friend of hers, and I began to read just a little bit of it to show her that this was for real, and then I stopped.

Harriet asked, "What else did she say about me?"

"Hold it Harriet," I said. "This is a connection *we've* made, even though somebody else started it. So now this is between you and me. Do you want to talk to me? Do you need my help? If so, you talk to me, and you tell me your story. Let's forget about your friend." And then Harriet began to talk to me. I knew she was taking the first step.

⋆ ⋆ ⋆

The Man I Call Every Day

In Canarsie, New York, a man named Michael Hebranko had seen Rosemarie Carnemolla on a new infomercial, heard her story, and had seen how great she did. He, in turn, wrote me a letter and sent a picture: He weighed over a thousand pounds and was sitting on a stoop with a kind of a winter scarf draped over his head. It was a sad picture. As I had done with Rosemarie, I picked up the phone and called him. Then I went to New York to see him, his wife Madeleine, and his son Mikey. I knew he had to get to a hospital for the help he needed. Again, there was press on hand. We did a remote with a plea for help, and we got him into a hospital. Under the guidance of a group of caring doctors, Michael began losing weight. In just nineteen months, without any surgery, I saw him go from over a thousand pounds down to a hundred and ninety-eight—he lost more than eight hundred pounds. This was amazing—such strength. I asked him if he'd like to be in one of my videos, and he said yes. Remember, this was a man who exercised to *Sweatin' to the Oldies* while lying in bed. And now, he was going to be part of the exercise group in the studio for *Sweatin' to the Oldies 2.*

But nothing's for sure. Michael started teaching my Project Me classes in New York. But slowly the weight came back. He began avoiding my calls and making excuses about why he was unable to see me when I was in New York. Eventually Michael stopped teaching classes altogether after gaining back two hundred pounds. He returned to the hospital for a while, but Michael continued to battle.

Watching the news on T.V. a couple of years ago, I saw footage of paramedics removing the side of a house and carrying out an overweight man on a stretcher. It was Michael, cameras shoved in his face, talking about his addiction to food. I called him immediately and then a few days later flew to New York to visit him in the hospital several times. I told him that if he did it once, he could do it again. Despite serious medical complications, Michael is still fighting his battle. I still talk to him every day, and the most important thing is that he's still trying.

I am always losing people who are morbidly obese. This is the greatest pain I go through. Sometimes, I find myself paying for coffins or for burial plots. Many times, people don't write or get in touch until it's way too late for them. They are plagued with the diseases associated with being overweight, such as diabetes, heart disease, and kidney disease. I continue my fight to help these people with their struggles.

With a Little Help from My Friends

 began to realize that the numbers of people I was working with through my daily phone calls, through the mail, through my mall visits, and through Slimmons were rapidly increasing, and I needed to devise a way for dealing with all these people in the best way possible.

I came up with a system in the office for keeping files on people. Many people would say, "I just can't do it alone." So, I would answer, "Let me do it with you." It seemed that when people had a starting point, a file with their name on it, they had a reason to keep trying. This is a system I continue today. Tucked inside each file is a recent head-to-toe "before" picture and a weekly list of what the person is eating, which we call a food sheet. Each person also has to fill out a fact sheet and be truthful about the answers to questions about his or her past, exercise habits, eating habits, and fears and phobias. It's an honest inventory, and there is no hiding.

No matter where I went, radio or television stations would receive hundreds of letters from people requesting to be in the audience to see me.

"I have to see Richard Simmons because he's my last chance." "He's my only hope. I have to see him and touch him."

This made me so uncomfortable! Yes, I know I have cute legs and I'm very huggable, but I am not a miracle worker and I never claimed to be. I never told anyone it was going to be a fast journey. I never said losing weight was easy.

Many of my most public and heartbreaking experiences associated with the morbidly obese have played themselves out on T.V. In the late Eighties, there were plenty of talk shows that were doing segments with themes such as "My wife left me because I was five hundred pounds." I think most of the talk shows are wonderful. But the problem is that they have a schedule to keep and another show to do tomorrow. They may pose the question and discuss it, but the problem isn't really solved in an hour segment. So I'm the one who inherits a person who needs long-term follow-up and support.

* * *

Quality, Value, Convenience

*I*n 1989, American Telecast was still producing my infomercials and videos. They also produced Cher, Pat Boone, and Victoria Principal. One day they got a call from QVC, which stands for Quality, Value, Convenience. This was a cable-T.V. shopping channel, like a twenty-four-hour infomercial, located in huge studios outside Philadelphia. It was live, round-the-clock television where they sold products through their phone banks. I had a few products to sell—Deal-A-Meal, *Sweatin' to the Oldies,* a cookbook, and some motivational tapes—and QVC offered to let me try to sell them on the air.

This was instant, just like the infomercials. I loved it. When you put something on the air at QVC, either the phone rings and you sell, or nothing happens and they say, "Thanks for coming. It's been swell."

Before I made the trip to Philadelphia, I watched QVC and found it to be very conservative. The hosts were very low-key. Well, "low-key" just isn't me. I came in and, oh my God, it was a good thing Gloria Monty wasn't producing QVC. I pretended I was on a Broadway stage! They weren't quite ready for me, but I was a hit. And we sold out all our products. It was just like the instant gratification of selling pralines back in New Orleans.

Now, every seven or eight weeks, I go back to QVC. They've been great to me. They let me bring on people who have lost weight. I call them Cinderella and Cinderfella stories, and they tell their experiences of the amazing changes they've made.

As I'm writing this book, I have just celebrated my eighth anniversary of being on the air at QVC.

* * *

The GoodTimes

At this point, Deal-A-Meal was still selling very well through the infomercial. I had made my own little niche. But none of my products were available through retail, and I was beginning to think that it was time to make that move.

After some talk with the folks at American Telecast and my agents Rick Hersch and Rick Bradley at the William Morris Agency, I was introduced to a family in New York, the Cayres. They were interested in taking all my products retail, and they had a lot of experience in that area, with videos and books. So here was another family. It was three brothers who worked together and lived practically next door to each other. Their company was called GoodTimes.

We all agreed that if I were going to go retail, the Cayres were the ones to help me do it. The next step was the meeting. Joe Cayre and Andy Greenberg, president of GoodTimes Entertainment, flew out to L.A. We gathered around my dining room table, and I knew in five seconds that more angels had appeared. The match was made, and I was passed from one family to another, from the Marshes at American Telecast to the Cayres at GoodTimes.

So I continued to do what I had been doing, and more of it: infomer-

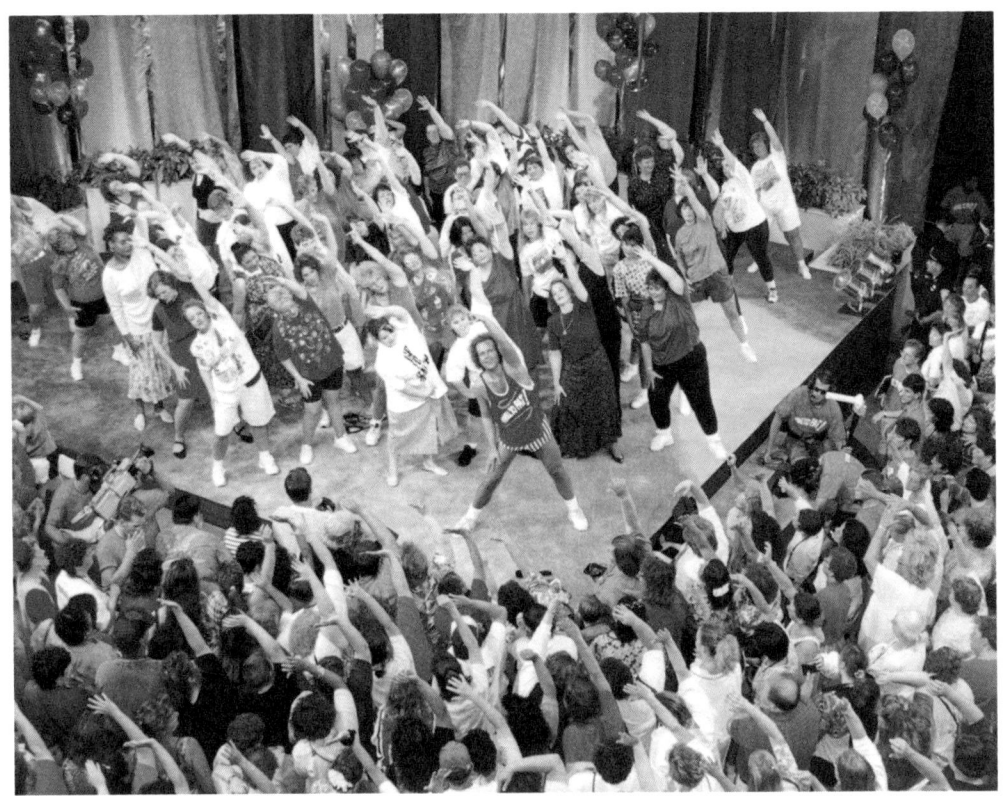

Here's me shooting part of an infomercial at Silver City Galleria,
in Taunton, Massachusetts.

cials, videos, and on and on. We got into a lot more businesses. We got into clothing and aerobics shoes, and it just seemed that retail opened up a whole new world for me. All the superstores were interested in my products. It happened so quickly. One day, there were no Richard Simmons products, and the next day, there were Richard Simmons kiosks in stores across the country.

I got into food products, like fat-free popcorn. So in addition to my mall appearances, I would teach a class in the middle of WalMart and Kmart and Sam's Club, surrounded by merchandise stacked eight feet high.

I was on the road again, and that's what I really loved. (It was that piece of paper in the parking lot with the word "mall" written on it.) I did a lot of personal appearances because I was the traveling salesman—the aerobics traveling salesman—going from city to city.

And finally, after all these years, the taste of cash that had started with pralines on that street corner in New Orleans, was satisfied. Money was important in terms of my always wanting to take care of my family, always wanting to give them whatever they wanted, whatever they needed. That was really my main goal. It's not like I had three homes, five cars, and two boats—that would mess up my hair! I certainly was exuberant, but I wasn't extravagant. I was silly and crazy, but I never was one to party or go out and lavishly spend money. That's just not the way I was raised. My father had started a Christmas Club savings account for me when I was young, and I guess from the very beginning, I just wanted to save.

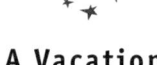

A Vacation?

The first question everyone asks me because I work so hard is, "Do you ever take vacations?" Well, I did try to take a vacation a few years ago, but "vacation" is not exactly the word I would use to describe it. I wanted to go back to Florence where I went to school to see Michelangelo's *David* one more time—and to Rome, to see the Sistine Chapel.

So in the early Nineties, I just picked a summer month and I went. Big mistake. I forgot that summer is the tourist season.

First, I went to Rome, where I visited the Sistine Chapel. Then I went to Florence. You can't get close to Michelangelo's *David,* because a few years ago someone had chipped a piece off of him, so now there's Plexiglas all around him. If you try to get a picture standing next to the statue, the only thing you get are the legs. So, what I figured out was that if someone with a camera lies on the floor next to the statue, you can stand over him and he can shoot upward, so you're in the picture with *David.* Well, I did this, and the place went crazy. Everybody wanted to stand next to me while their husband or mother or Aunt Tillie lay down to snap the photo. Meanwhile, the guards didn't know who I was. They looked at us suspiciously, and finally they gave us a warning. It was just like elementary school. They gave us a second warning, and then we were finally asked to leave. So, my vacation wasn't really a vacation, at all. It was more of a paparazzi moment.

However, I do love traveling. Going to an airport with me is a little like the moment before the parade passes by in *Hello, Dolly!* There are people getting on and getting off planes, people waiting for other people. When I show up, another line forms: These are the people waiting for autographs, or holding their cameras and wanting to take a picture. This year alone, I received eighty Christmas cards with a photo of me and someone else on the front. Inside, the cards read, "Richard and I wish you a very Merry Christmas." All this from a chance encounter in an airport.

As I'm waiting in line to board the plane, I just love meeting all the people I'm going to be flying with for five hours. "Hi, I'm here!" And some of them turn away because they think I'm going to teach a class. "Oh God, trapped for five hours—he's going to be on this plane. Help me!" As I get in line to board, I often say to the person next to me, "Is this the buffet line?" Up to my old tricks, no matter where I go.

I've had my share of canceled flights and emergency landings, which scared me to death. But I've always had a source of comfort—I never travel anywhere without my two pillows. I've had them since I was two years old—you can imagine what they look like! Linus may have his blanket, but I have my pillows.

I travel so many times a year that I've begun to ignore the change of seasons. Especially from November through February, people are bundled against the cold—that's a time of year many people enjoy just because of the clothing. If they've done any overeating around the holidays, people feel that a long coat or a heavy sweater will cover it. Not me. You'll see me in my little red shorts and tank top.

Now when I travel, people always ask, "Where's your coat, where's your sweater?" My mother always wanted to know the same thing. Sometimes I called her from two or three different states in a single day.

"Where are you now?" she'd ask.

"I'm in New York, mother."

"What's the weather like?"

"It's twenty-two degrees."

"Do you have a coat? Do you?!"

"Yes, mother. I'm wearing my coat." I found I had to lie about that, too. It was easier to say I had a coat than to explain that I went from the plane to the airport to the car and then on to the hotel without going outside. "Did you eat?" and "Do you have a coat?" are the things that mothers worry about. At least *my* mother always did.

* * *

The Story of O

As I have said, women have always played an important role in my life, and usually in very positive ways, starting with my mother, Shirley. But there have been a couple of exceptions. The first I call the Story of O.

In the early Eighties, I began doing local T.V. shows throughout the country to promote *General Hospital.* I did one in Baltimore. And the name of the host of that show was Oprah Winfrey. I liked her immediately and thought she was funny, compassionate, and very smart. She was a lot of fun to be around. I continued to do her show from time to time, and always looked forward to going back. After she moved the show to Chicago in 1986, I was on it with my mother and the Silver Foxes to showcase the video we'd made.

When I saw the movie *The Color Purple,* Oprah's performance really knocked me out. I sent her a card and a doll of this beautiful black baby girl. Oprah had always talked about wanting to have a baby, so I wrote to her, saying that this was her baby and to find a special place for it.

I never discussed weight with Oprah, because I could tell she wasn't eager to talk about it. And of course, I wouldn't break my rule of "not approaching people first."

In November 1988, Oprah went on her national television show to tell everyone how she was in the process of losing a considerable amount of weight by using Optifast. She took them on her journey. She got on the scale and showed them week by week how much weight she had lost.

Shortly after Oprah's weight-loss show, I got a call from a reporter in New York—someone I had never heard of before, but she seemed really sweet on the phone. She asked me what I thought of Oprah's incredible transformation. I said that I thought Oprah was a remarkable woman at any weight, and, of course, she looked great. I had heard she lost weight with a doctor's supervision. And I had tried liquid diets years before, and mine were doctor-supervised also. I knew it worked . . . but I knew it worked only for a while. I told her that it was very difficult to keep the weight off once you stopped using the meal-replacement shakes. I told the reporter that for me the most effective weight-loss method is what I've always believed in: a balanced eating plan and lots of exercise.

The next day an article appeared: Richard Simmons, diet guru, says Oprah will probably gain all her weight back. The reporter took our two-minute discussion and twisted it to fit her purposes. She made a huge deal out of it.

The day that article came out, I called Oprah and we chatted. I told her exactly what my conversation had been with the reporter, and that much of what was written in the article did not come from me. I was weeping on the phone with Oprah, because I was really upset about the whole thing and because I cherished Oprah as a friend. Oprah told me not to worry about it, that she understood.

And after that, we all know what happened. Oprah went off the Opti-fast plan and gained all the weight back.

And then a few years later, she found the keys to good health. She met a woman named Rosie, who became her private chef and showed her how to eat healthy, and together they wrote the cookbook *In the Kitchen with Rosie.* Then she met the trainer Bob Greene and started exercising on a regular basis. Oprah finally discovered the right message, following the same path I had. I was so happy for her. That was the good news.

The bad news for me was that her loss of weight was my loss of a friend. A little over ten years has passed, and I've never heard from Oprah since that last phone conversation. I've never been asked on her show again. I discussed this whole episode with my mother. I always turned to her when I felt a little low. And she said to me, "Honey, not everyone is going to love you. Not everyone is going to agree with you. Just accept that." Thanks to my mother's wisdom, I tried to forget the whole thing and just move on.

A few years ago, I saw Oprah being interviewed on another talk show. Someone in the audience mentioned me. And Oprah said, "Oh, Richard Simmons, I just love him." Then she looked straight into the camera and said, "Richard, if you're watching, I just want to tell you that I love you and I respect the work you do, and I still have that little doll sitting on my bed." Those were the last words I heard from Oprah, and I heard them on a television set. But now she looks really wonderful, and I'm happy that she's happy.

eager to talk about it. And of course, I wouldn't break my rule

Hello, Gorgeous!

The story of the next woman is a little longer and a little more complicated, and some of you may already know bits and pieces of this tale. I could write a whole book about her, but here's the condensed version, from my side of the fence.

This one begins back in New Orleans when I was a kid. Growing up, I loved music. Let's face it, New Orleans is a music town. There was a record shop on Royal Street that I would stop in all the time. One afternoon, I heard this song playing there, and I thought, Oh my God, this is beautiful. I asked what it was, and they told me it was from a Broadway show called *Funny Girl,* with a young singer named Barbra Streisand. I bought the album, plus all the 45 r.p.m. singles, and I rushed home. Her voice just knocked me out. When I read the summary of the show's story, I discovered that it was all about Fanny Brice, and both my parents had known Fanny Brice. I listened to the album over and over again.

At this point I was in my early teens, and this is when my parents sent me to visit my Aunt Marion and her kids in New York. I may have forgotten to tell you, but the reason I begged and begged to go to New York was because I wanted to see *Funny Girl.* I just had to—I had to see this woman.

Before I went, I got my hands on every article I could find about Barbra and I started a scrapbook. Some people were Elvis fans, some people were Beatles fans—I was a Streisand fan. But it was more than that. We shared a similar history. She was a thin girl who thought she was ugly and stuck out, and she had a nose that some people made fun of. And here I was, this fat boy with funny hair who thought he was ugly and stuck out. Neither of us had a good self-image. Her father had died when she was young, and I felt I never had a real father in my early years. And now she was famous, with this beautiful voice, and performing on Broadway. If she could do that, then maybe there was hope for me. Maybe I could find something to do in my life that would make me happy, that would make me successful. Even at this early age, Barbra became an inspiration for me, a success story that became my example.

I went to the Winter Garden Theater in New York City, where the show was playing. I didn't have much money. I saw a man going in the back door of the theater, so I went up to him and started one of my soliloquies. "I'm such a fan and I can't afford a ticket . . . " and on and on. Success! He worked in the lighting booth, and he told me I could come with him and watch the show from up there, for free.

That night I saw *Funny Girl.* I loved it. Actually, I *more* than loved it. The lighting man told me stories about Barbra and the show, and he asked me if I wanted to see it again. What could I say? I saw *Funny Girl* five times that week.

When I got back to New Orleans, I had to hear the *Funny Girl* album every day. After a while, both my mother and my father started becoming a little concerned about me. In the middle of dinner, I would just start singing, "A sleeping bee once told me, you can laugh with your feet on the ground . . . " My father would look at me and deliver his famous line, "Go to your room." A Streisand song got me to my room quicker than any of my other antics.

At breakfast, I'd look up from my plate of eggs and sausage and say, "Dad," and then I'd start singing, "Happy days are here . . . "

"Go to your room."

I'm really no different today. I still love to sing. In the middle of a sentence, I'll break into a song. Or I'll leave a song on somebody's answering machine. Or I'll greet someone at my front door with a song. Streisand songs are still among my favorites.

As I moved into my teen years, Streisand became more and more important to me. One afternoon, while I was looking through my Barbra scrapbook, I came across the *Playbill* from *Funny Girl.* Turning the pages, I discovered a notice I hadn't seen before that said if you wanted to know more about Barbra, write a letter to her mother and send it to *Playbill.* Well, to me that was an invitation. So I wrote a letter.

The editor of *Playbill* sent me a letter back telling me that Barbra had a fan club, and because I had spelled a couple of words wrong in my letter, he suggested that I should sign up for remedial spelling. I immediately joined the fan club—and worked on my spelling.

Roz Kind was the president of the club. Barbra's father had passed away when she was young, and her mother, Diane, married Mr. Kind. So Roz is Barbra's half sister.

I started collecting photos of Barbra, and I continued to collect them when I got to L.A. At Derek's, one of my big customers was Ray Stark, the man who had produced *Funny Girl.* And Ray, ironically enough, had married Fanny Brice's daughter.

Late one evening at Derek's, as the crowd was beginning to thin out, I sat down with Mr. Stark and shared my whole story about the woman who had made him so famous. After I finished, he looked at me and said, "Why don't you just meet her?"

"I could never meet her," I said.

All of a sudden, a smile came over his face and he said, "Well, Richard, I'm just going to surprise you. I'm going to bring her into the restaurant sometime, without telling you beforehand."

"Mr. Stark, please don't ever do that. Don't you ever." I explained to him how I didn't want to meet her as a fan. I just wanted to sit down with her, and talk about how each of us had grown up and the similarities between our two lives, and how she had been an inspiration for me. And then I would sing thirty of her best songs, so she'd know I wasn't lying. Mr. Stark laughed, and nothing more was said about it.

One night I was working at Derek's, and the phone rang from downstairs. A valet parker said on the other end of the phone, "You're never going to believe who's in the elevator."

"Who's in the elevator?" I asked.

"Ray Stark and about five people. And, oh—one of them is Barbra Streisand."

"No-o-o-o! You're out of your mind. You're kidding me."

He said, "I swear. They're in the elevator right now. They're coming up."

I quickly put the phone down. I ran right out the back door, leaving my tables to Judy. I just couldn't face seeing Barbra.

You know how sometimes when you've read a book, or you've seen a person, or you've traveled somewhere special, you'll begin to see all these connections and experience all these coincidences? Well, that began to happen with me and Barbra. I seemed to be running into all these people who were connected to her.

There was a bakery called the Butterfly in Westwood in Los Angeles. I walked in and who did I see? Roz Kind. Yes, the very same person who was president of the fan club and who was Barbra's half-sister. She was part-owner of the bakery. So we met, and Roz started coming to Ruffage and the Anatomy Asylum. And where do Roz (Barbra's half sister) and Diane (their mother) live? Three blocks from the Anatomy Asylum. Roz started bringing her mother to my studio, and Diane and I became friendly.

I was in Ruffage one afternoon when someone hollered. "You're not going to believe it! Barbra Streisand is getting out of a car." Maxine Smith, the wife of the producer Dwight Hemion, who had worked on many of Barbra's specials, was coming through the front door of Ruffage with Barbra. Out the back door I went. Twice now, I'd fled and vanished. She was becoming even more my idol, more distant from me on the pedestal I was creating for her.

Then after a long rest from touring, Barbra Streisand decided to return to doing live performances. In December 1993, on New Year's Eve, she opened the brand-new MGM Grand Hotel in Las Vegas with a gala concert. Because Jay Leno knew I was such a Streisand fan, he said he would fly me out to Vegas to cover the opening for *The Tonight Show*. I couldn't believe it. This was a dream come true. Jay called Marty Erlichman, Barbra's manager, and Marty agreed to give Jay the exclusive rights to televise part of the concert, live.

So all the arrangements were made. I was like Peter Jennings, broadcasting live from the MGM Grand. When I got there, I said to one of the producers, "I wonder what Barbra Streisand's suite looks like?" So guess what? They let me into her suite before she arrived. Of course, as I went from room to room, I just began singing songs from *Yentl, On a Clear Day You Can See Forever,* and *Funny Girl.*

The show was so successful, Barbra took it on tour. Eventually she played Madison Square Garden in New York City. I'd seen the show once, but in this case Jacqueline Susann was right, *Once Is Not Enough.* So I went to Madison Square Garden and I sat in the front row. I loved the performance so much, I cried through the whole thing.

The next day I was strolling past Tiffany's on Fifth Avenue (don't you just love those cute little baby-blue shopping bags?). I walked right in and I saw a small, neat, very distinguished-looking woman standing behind the diamond ring counter. I went up to her and we talked for a bit, and she told me that she was the very first woman ever to sell diamonds at Tiffany's. I had an idea. I explained to her that I had admired a certain lady since the

rd, I'm just going to surprise you. I'm going to bring her into

early Sixties. I asked the Tiffany lady, "If I was going to buy a ring for this woman, which one should I get?" She thought for a moment, letting her eyes wander over the rings in front of her. Then she opened a case, reached in, and took out a gorgeous ring. "I'm going to show you my very favorite ring. It was the first ring I ever sold here."

"I'll take it." I never asked the price. Some of the salespeople gathered around and agreed it was very special. This was going to be my friendship ring for Barbra.

That night was Barbra's last performance. And I thought to myself, I've got to get myself prepared here. So I wrote her a note, explaining how she had been part of my life for so long, how we had come from the same place, and how she had been an example of success for me.

Before the concert, her manager said hello to me. I thought, Here's a good way to do this.

"Marty, will you do me a favor?"

"Sure. What, Rich?"

I handed him the blue Tiffany box and the note. "Could you please give these to Barbra before the show?"

"What is it?"

"Oh, it's just a little something I bought for her. Could you just give it to her?"

"Well, don't you want to give it to her yourself?"

"No. Just give it to her before she goes on." I thanked Marty and he walked away.

The concert started, and it was just as amazing as the first time I had seen it. Just amazing.

During the intermission, between my crying and signing autographs for my fans in the audience, Mr. Erlichman walked over to me and said, "Barbra would like you to come backstage after the show."

When Marty came looking for me after Barbra's final bows, my seat was empty. Once again I decided this was not the right time, not the right place to meet Barbra.

I knew Marty had delivered the ring and the note—there was no question about that. So, I just had to wait.

Almost a month went by. Not a word. Then one afternoon while I was out of town, the box and an envelope with my name handwritten on it were delivered to my house. They were sitting on the kitchen counter when I got home. I looked at the Tiffany box, and then opened it. The ring was still in it. To this day, I've never opened the note.

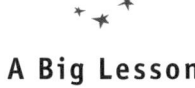

A Big Lesson

There'd been a very difficult struggle in my life that had been unresolved for many years. It's another kind of pain, and it's worse than the pain of rejection or the pain you feel when your body is in trouble. It is the pain of loss.

As you remember, I did not deal well with my father's passing. I had not even visited the place where his ashes were laid to rest. I was always afraid to confront this loss in my life, because it meant I would have to take a harder look at myself. But the death of my dear Dalmatians changed all this. It's hard to believe, but I lost five of my sweet dogs in a year and a half.

In 1996, when Scarlett was fifteen, she went deaf, her epileptic seizures progressed, and then she stopped eating. Sitting on my kitchen floor with her in my lap, I was alone and going through something I'd never been able to face before. I sang to her just like my mother sang to that woman in the nursing home. And Scarlett drifted away right there. She just looked up at me, and I could feel the whole weight of her body in my arms. I sat there and cried while I cradled my sweet Scarlett.

Still, I knew I was very lucky, because everyone always told me Dalmatians don't usually live past ten years old. My dogs were fifteen or sixteen, and they'd had a very full life. But of course the longer you have them, the harder it is. And each time a dog passed, I was there for them. For some reason God wanted me to be home, He wanted me on that kitchen floor, and He wanted me with each dog. And that's how all five of them went.

I learned something very important about myself when the dogs died. I discovered that I could face death, and that I would endure. And I wouldn't have to binge-eat to comfort myself, to escape my own sorrow. It was almost as if their lives went into me, and gave me more courage and strength to work through the terrible phobia that had prevented me from dealing with death in the past, especially my dad's.

I had only Melanie left, and even though I loved her, the house felt so empty. I went from six dogs to one within the span of a year and a half. I was busy as usual with my projects and all the work I had to do, but the house just felt so vacant.

One of the Dalmatian breeders I knew realized that I was suffering. She called and asked if I was going to be home one Sunday. I told her I was. So on Sunday morning, I opened my door and along with my Sunday paper came two litters of puppies barreling into my house. My housekeeper Teresa looked at me and said, "One! Only one."

Well, one caught her eye, and one caught mine—so that makes two. Hers we named Hattie, in keeping with my *Gone with the Wind* theme, and mine, Dolly. My house was full of life again.

This was always a constant in my life, this passion for loving dogs, especially Dalmatians. But I feel they give so much more to me than I do to them. I spend so much time each day with people, either in person or on the phone. Truly, the most relaxing part of my day is getting under the sheets, and having all the dogs get on the bed with me while I read or watch a little T.V.

* ⋆ *

Sail Away

*I*n the early Nineties, I discovered yet another place where I could spread my message. It was a place I had never thought about.

During a sweeps week for television, I was asked to do a segment on a television show where they would be filming live from a ship. It was a local show from Seattle, and they were sailing on the *Princess.* I had never been on a cruise ship before. I thought it would be different and fun. I was surprised to discover that I could essentially do the same things on the cruise ship that I could do at the studio. I had a sound system available to me, so I could put music on and I could get a crowd of people up and moving.

I had continued to make appearances in malls, but I was still troubled with the feeling that these events were too short—that I didn't have enough time to connect with people. Did I do my best? Did people really listen?

Now I started to wonder to myself, What would happen if I had seven days? Not just two or three hours to sign photos. What if I had seven days

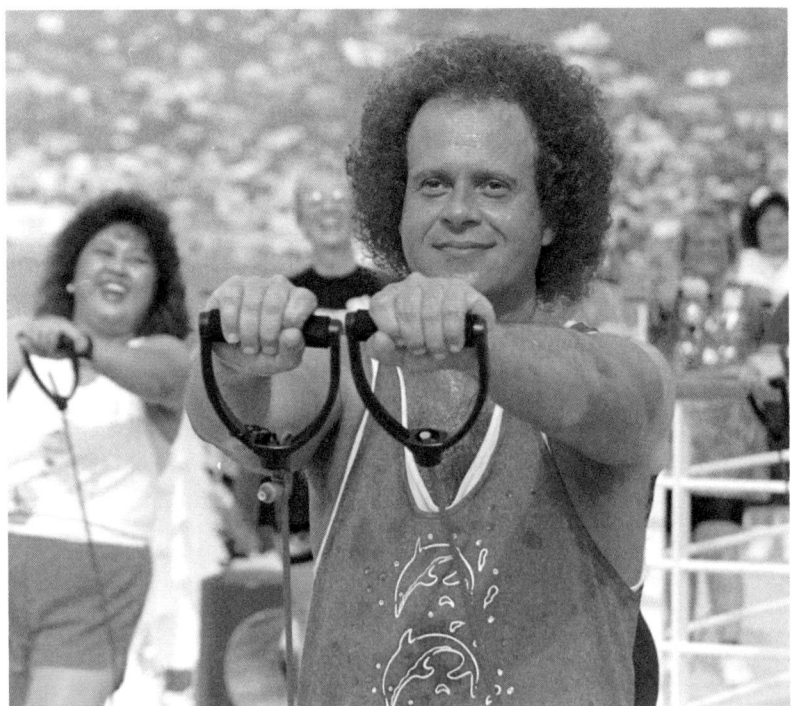

Sweatin' on Water

to really teach nutrition and get people used to the idea of exercising every day? It would be like a spa—a big, floating spa.

I did a little research. I found a really good travel agent, Linda Simmons. No relation, but I liked her already. She told me there was no weight-loss program available aboard any ship that she had ever heard of.

Another travel agent told me, "People don't go on cruises to lose weight. There's too much food and too many buffets."

My response to her was, "Well, you know, it's real life. Life is a buffet. Every place you go there's food. I think I should try putting together a motivational weight-loss program for cruises."

Next, I went down to San Pedro where the cruise ships dock, to see what the accommodations and different ships were like. The exercise rooms connected to the gyms were very small. But the big Vegas-style night clubs were perfect for exercising.

Most people who go on a cruise are celebrating their honeymoon or their anniversary. They go to eat and drink, to stop at a few ports, and to do some shopping.

This idea of mine was going against everything a cruise was meant to be. But now many of the people who go on my cruises feel it's their last chance. They experience seven days of healthy eating, sometimes relearning how to eat in a balanced way and to watch their portions. They wake up to a morning stretch and they exercise with me every day. They meet people who are like them, who weigh what they weigh, and who many times are experiencing the same problems. They can be adventurous and go places and do things, such as swimming or scuba diving, things that overweight people usually don't do.

And so I started Cruise to Lose. And as I'm writing this book, I'm leaving on my fifteenth cruise. I take an average of four hundred people with me. These cruises are fun, they're successful, and they're gratifying. And the strange thing is that no one's ever copied the idea to this day. Who could? No one could do it my way.

⋆⋆⋆

www.richardsimmons.com

There was one more way I discovered to communicate my message to others. In July 1997, I made my Internet debut with my Web page, "At Home with Richard Simmons," at www.richardsimmons.com. (You can go click on it right now, but be sure to come back!)

I had one big stumbling block when I started my Web site—I couldn't type. And to be on the World Wide Web, as many of you know, being able to type is a definite advantage.

When I signed up to take typing as a freshman in high school, Brother Brendan, my typing teacher, told me that I would never be a fast typist. My fingers were just too fat. He was right. Plus, I never got the knack of the shift key. I'd want a period, and I'd wind up with a colon. So, for all these years I've had this terrible typing stigma.

Finally, I came up with a solution for my Web site. I recruited a flock of angels to type for me. I dictate to them what I want to write, and they transform my speech into words on the screen. (I've always had typewriters around, because I think they're pretty and they make me look professional. It gives me that Angela Lansbury feeling.)

My Web site has lots of things going on. When you click on it, you get my daily message, a different one every day, which I write myself. I've written them in blizzards in Chicago, during storms in Texas, and in the hot sun in Florida. I'm always writing them, regardless of where I am. You'll also find recipes, contests, eating and exercise tips, success stories, my schedule (if you want to visit me while I'm on the road), and a whole host of other things. Once a month I do a live auditorium for an hour, where I answer questions online in "real time." When we actually get started, we can have as many as two hundred questions lined up, waiting to be answered.

And we've created chat rooms for groups of people who share specific problems: overweight teens, women who've just had a baby and can't lose the weight, people over fifty who have lost their motivation.

Now I'm getting letters via e-mail from all over the world—from Thailand, Japan, New Zealand, Italy, and from everywhere. Most e-mail runs two or three sentences. Not mine—the e-mail letters I get sometimes go on for two or three pages. And in about fifty percent of them, I'm asked to call other people about their problems, whether they be family or friends. On average there are about ten thousand visits a day to my Web site, and by the time this book comes out, we'll have had more than three million hits. (And it's not all just questions about how I do my hair!)

So besides Slimmons, the cruises and the malls, the Web now gives me access to the world.

* * *

My Telephone

One thing I've always done throughout my career has been my daily telephone calls—talking to people about their weight issues and offering them all the encouragement I can, and helping them to get started on a program of healthy eating and exercising.

I started making these calls after my first appearance on *Real People* back in the middle Seventies. I made more of them with *General Hospital,* in response to all the mail I would receive, and the calls only increased in number with each new appearance or project.

I usually make between forty and fifty telephone calls each day, even when I'm traveling. On a really busy day, I can make as many as one hundred calls.

I first started the calls because I got a few letters from people who really sounded panicky and desperate. I just couldn't bear to make them wait for a reply from me through the mail. So I picked up the phone and made an instant connection. They felt better, I felt better, and everyone was happy. Well, everyone except my accountant.

"Richard! Your long-distance telephone bill—it's outrageous."

"I know, I know. I had a few calls to make."

"A few calls!? This is more than a few. Just who are you calling?"

"I get these letters," I explained. "They're from people who are reaching out."

"That's fine. But why do you have to call?"

"They need someone to talk to, and they just can't wait. So I call. It's good for them, and it's good for me. That's the story."

"Okay, Richard. It's pretty expensive, but if you feel it's necessary, I understand." He never asked me about my phone bill again.

To this very day, and every day, regardless of where I am, I have my letters and my e-mails with me, and I make as many phone calls as I can. I may not be able to type, but I do know how to talk, so I always make the calls myself—no one else does it for me. It's one of the most personal things I do.

The Collector

I've always had this thing about collecting. My father always collected cookbooks, so I must have gotten the collecting bug from him.

During my travels in the early Nineties, I was doing an appearance in Minnesota, and I went to a place called Stillwater, a kind of an artists' colony. While I was there, I fell in love with a glass bowl. Then I took a peek at the bottom to look at the price. (Oh, I'm not supposed to do that?) This was not just a glass bowl. This was the glass bowl that must have dropped from heaven, but it didn't break. I bought it.

Before you know it, I had glass bowls, glass vases, and glass sculptures. Soon my entire house was filled with one-of-a-kind works of art made of hand-blown glass.

And then in January 1994, just after I'd come home from a trip to Missouri, I was in bed at 4:30 in the morning when my entire life started shaking. Things were moving, things were falling, and in just half a minute, every piece of glass that I had in the house turned into glitter! From glass to glitter! The majority of the earthquake damage was done in Northridge, about fifteen miles from my house. I spent the rest of the day sweeping up glass and putting the shards in piles that resembled the sculptures and vases they once were. Luckily, everything was insured and the adjusters were out in force, so they gave me a check to replace my treasures.

To lift my broken spirits, a friend sent me a one-of-a-kind doll. It was a little court-jester doll by Gail Lackey. The pixie jester was holding a chain that led to a small pet snail. It was the cutest thing I'd ever seen. To me, this seemed to be more than a doll. This was a piece of art. And remember, I'd seen a Barbie doll or two in my time. But I'd never really seen a doll like this. Instead of glass, this doll was made of fimo, a type of clay, along with hair and cloth.

I asked around and I started learning a lot about the doll world. I went to doll shows and discovered all these one-of-kind dolls. Some artists are painters, others are sculptors, but the doll creator is both of those things and more. You have to build an armature, you have to sculpt, you have to sew and paint. It was all of the arts applied to one delicate piece of work.

Where every pedestal had once held a piece of art glass, now all through my house are pedestals that display dolls. My home became a doll "museum," with dolls by famous doll artists such as Annie Wahl, Pat and Glen East, Richard and Jody Creager, Akira Blount, and Lisa Lichtenfels.

Most of the doll artists whom I had gotten to know had never created reproductions of their expensive originals to sell at retail. I begged and pleaded with them, explaining that this was a way more people could enjoy their work. Many of them were excited by my idea, and agreed to do it. I signed with L.L. Knickerbocker Toy and Teddy Bear Company, and in two short years we have created one of the most successful lines of beautiful, affordable dolls.

The fact is, my dolls make me happy. They have a very calming effect. And it's not just on me. Sometimes if I walk quietly into a room at home, I catch the dogs sitting and staring at the dolls.

What's It All About?

Now that I've reached my fiftieth year on this earth, you can see that my life has never been boring. And it continues. I'm now working on a television show called *Richard Simmons' Dream Maker*—five days a week from Las Vegas—and it's all about making people's dreams come true. What a perfect fit! I've been rehearsing for this for twenty-five years, beginning with that very first person who walked into the Anatomy Asylum. For an hour each day, I'm Aladdin's genie. I get to fulfill viewers' wishes: Perhaps it's a reunion with a loved one, a thank-you to someone who helped along the way, or a cruise for parents who always gave everything to their family. I might even ask your boss to give you a raise! With hope in such short supply on T.V. these days, *Dream Maker* is a chance to make people feel good about themselves again. I will be the angel to make dreams come true—not bad for a boy who once wanted to be a priest.

I guess that, in a way, I've always been preaching. Mine is the gospel according to Richard. I've made the malls my chapels. I've made convention centers my basilicas. And I've always tried to make my message fun. And that message? Watch what you eat, practice portion control, exercise, and love yourself. It's so logical, but so hard to do. No tricks, no gimmicks, no special pills, no special potions, no special equipment. All it takes is desire and will. This is what I've always preached. And now everybody from the Centers for Disease Control in Atlanta to the Surgeon General are all saying the same thing. In many respects, my Deal-A-Meal as well as the updated version, FoodMover, truly became the United States Government Food Pyramid. That's what my little construction-paper cards in the Catholic holy-card holder were all about: Here's your grain, here's your fruit, here's your vegetables, here's your protein. And there's the fat!

I always wanted to make healthy living into something that's fun, so people wouldn't be scared away, the way I always had been. That's why the Anatomy Asylum and Slimmons have been so popular. I made exercising fun. I do anything that will distract people from knowing they are going to have to exercise or watch their food portions. So, every time I go on a show, I do it with a burst of energy. I run out and explode. I'm sure you've seen me do that somewhere, and you've said, "Oh, there's that crazy nut again."

Well, now you know why I do it. I want to get everybody up: out of their chair and psychologically ready.

My father was fifty when I was conceived. And now, I am the same age my father was when he became a parent. And for that reason, I was really looking forward to my fiftieth birthday. I spent my special day with my mother and my brother in New Orleans. We looked through scrapbooks and spent time laughing, reminiscing, and reliving our memories of what a wonderful man he truly was. My birthday celebration was also a celebration of my father, too.

Being so different—something I've been all my life—is a double-sided coin. Because of who I am, I've been embraced and I've been rejected. Some people think I'm too silly. Others think I'm refreshing and colorful. None of that matters, because what's important is how you feel about yourself.

I always talk about taking personal inventory—making an honest assessment of your good qualities and those things you still have to work on. Some people feel that going to a therapist helps them take inventory. Some people have a good friend they talk to, or they write in a diary. In the past, my personal inventory and, indeed, my self-worth, was based on what other people thought of me, of what other people thought about my weight and my behavior. At fifty, I realized that I am who I am. This is it! It's not like I'm going to change.

For me, turning fifty and feeling as great as I do is proof that if you do the exercise, if you eat healthy, if you do the things that I've been doing, then you can accomplish anything. Remember, I'm the one who never took gym class in my life and was on a first-name basis with all the cafeteria workers. I haven't always lived a charmed life, and it hasn't always been a piece of cake. (Oh, did I say cake?) I was compulsive as a child, I am compulsive at fifty, and I will probably be compulsive until the day I die.

I have said that I built my success around my compulsion—food. So that's something else I've learned. I have to struggle daily and do all the things I do in order to stay at my weight, in order to stay healthy.

At one point, when I was still at Derek's, a very famous celebrity came in. He'd been married quite a few times. On his third martini, he said to me,

"I'll never get married again. You can't have a passion for your work and devote your life to it *and* have a marriage that works." And maybe that's not true for everybody, but I've found it's true for me. By devoting my life to my work, I live an extremely structured, cloistered life. I know what I'm doing every minute of every day because it is so scheduled. It's hard to have a "normal" life when you do the work I do. That's the life I've created, and the life I've chosen. It's like a priest who chooses to be celibate—you choose a calling. I've chosen a public life, rather than a private one. I don't have a traditional family. My family is thousands and thousands of people—those are the people I love.

I've always been a loner. I spent my childhood selling pralines and then going to my room with my 45r.p.m. records. This isn't very different from what I do today. I teach classes, I exercise at the malls, I make my phone calls, and then I go to my room and listen to music or pick out the songs for my next class. It's like nothing has changed. And I think that's good.

There is one big change, though—one thing that's different. When I was growing up, everyone told me that I wouldn't amount to anything, that I'd always be unhappy if I didn't do something about my compulsiveness.

Well, you know what? I'm doing the same thing now that I did when I was a kid. I may not be selling pralines on the street corner, but in many ways, I'm still on that corner. I have built a career out of it, and I think that's a very important parallel. The trick has always been to honestly and truthfully please myself, and not others.

The truth of the matter is, as much as we hate to admit it, we get to be who we are through our parents. I did become Leonard and Shirley, and I'm very proud of that.

* * *

The Premonition

So, yes, at fifty, I'm still doing the malls—it's something I've always loved doing. I guess that little card I picked out of Larry's hands in the parking lot at Century City, the one with the word "malls" written on it, was the best choice I could have made.

There was this one particular mall event I'll never forget, where something very strange happened. It was Saturday afternoon, February 27, 1999, in West Palm Beach at the Uptown-Downtown Mall. After I had finished exercising and motivating the crowd, all of a sudden, while I was signing autographs, a strange feeling came over me—I just couldn't stop thinking about Shirley. I'd just visited my mom the week before—she had been very ill. I was planning to return to Los Angeles after my appearance in Florida, but I couldn't get Shirley out of my mind. I had a premonition. I needed to see Shirley.

So I spoke with Michael Catalano, my manager, who was traveling with me. I asked him to change my plans. Instead of returning to Los Angeles, I would fly from Florida straight to New Orleans.

I boarded the plane and found my seat. I usually try to catch up on my sleep when I fly, to keep my energy up. And I'm one of those lucky people—I can just close my eyes, and off I go. Well, not on this flight. I couldn't sleep. Instead, I found myself staring out the window. The sun had just set, and there was a little orange glow on the horizon. The last two years had been so difficult for Shirley. So much had changed for her. I knew her sun was setting.

Shirley's Angels

The bottom line with Shirley was that she always led a very independent life, even though she was married. After my father died, she didn't slow down at all. She continued to do everything herself. She cleaned the entire house—swept and mopped and did all her own laundry. My mother was such a clean-a-holic, as opposed to my father, who always saved everything. Finally now, her house was her domain. It was her comfort—she had her house and her Dalmatian, Brent. Why have a housekeeper when you can do it better yourself? That had been Shirley's motto.

Then, in the fall of 1997, Lenny, as usual, was very busy with his civic organizations. Among his major interests is his work with the local chapter of Kiwanis. They devote a lot of their time to preventable mental retardation among young children. Lenny also helps feed the hungry, and like our father did, he works with the Volunteers of America.

Anyway, one afternoon while Lenny was gone, Shirley took a fall in the living room. Thank God she didn't break a hip. But after she had fallen, she'd lain there for a couple of hours. I've always wondered what she was thinking while she waited for help—what was going through her mind? When Lenny got home, Brent, who never left Shirley's side, ran to the door, barking, and got Lenny to follow him to where Shirley was laying on the rug, half under the coffee table.

She looked up and said, "Hel-lo, honey . . . "

"Oh my God, what happened?" Lenny frantically asked, as he helped her up.

"Well, I slipped on the rug."

"How long ago?"

"Oh, I don't know. I've just been lying here, looking at the ceiling, and petting Brent."

"Are you all right?"

"I'm fine, but the ceiling could use a new coat of paint."

Lenny immediately took her to the doctor, who took some X rays, checked her over, and said she was fine. That was my Shirley. She just didn't break. She kept going and going—she was the mother of that pink Energizer bunny.

But when she came back from the hospital, Lenny and I noticed that she was grabbing onto furniture to support herself when she walked. She was sleeping a lot, and all of a sudden, dust began to collect in the house, and so did dirty bathroom towels. Lenny started to spend more time keeping an eye on Shirley and trying to take care of the house. But as I've said before, Lenny had never been Mr. Neat. He tried his best, he really did. But one time he'd use too much laundry detergent, and bubbles would pour out of the washer. Or the next time he would forget to use soap at all. Or he'd use too much dust spray on the end tables, and the lamps would practically slide right off when you tried to turn them on.

Things weren't getting done. Lenny and I were concerned about the housework, but we were more worried about Shirley being alone in the house.

Lenny had a full life. He was working and dating and involved in a lot of community activities, so he wasn't always around to keep an eye on things. I was living on the other side of the country, when I wasn't on a plane headed to an appearance somewhere. Shirley had been used to doing everything herself, up to the day she took this fall. But from that day on, we realized that she could no longer handle it. Lenny and I both felt it was time for Shirley to have some regular help. God knows she had earned it.

Through a Kiwanis friend of Lenny's, we met a wonderful lady named Rose, a well-tailored woman in her sixties. Rose is such a special name, so I knew she had to be a special lady. When she came to the house, Brent walked up to her and sniffed her and wagged his tail. Rose had passed the first important test—now there was my mother. Would Shirley like her? Luckily, Rose passed that test too.

Rose began to help my mother, cleaning the house and taking over the chores that Shirley no longer had the strength to do. She became Shirley's first angel.

Rose had a little bit of arthritis. Every time I talked to her on the phone, I would ask, "How's your arthritis, Rose?"

"Well, Richard. The weather here is damp, and you know what that does to my joints."

Rose was very religious. I'm sure her faith kept her going, because the path she had chosen was not an easy one. She was a true caretaker. Like I said, we had hired her to be a housekeeper, but caretaker would be a better description of what she did.

Rose wore her hair in an Afro style, cropped very close to her head. Every once in a while, I would catch her looking at my curls. Rose might have been a little bit jealous—I never asked her!

So my mother began to relax a little more with Rose to help her. Shirley was still as smart as a whip. And she had her baby, Brent, who ate with her, slept with her, and went everywhere with her. Shirley looked after Brent, while Rose looked after Shirley—quite a trio. Shirley spoiled that dog with love, attention, and of course, that same thing she'd spoiled me and Lenny with: food. Brent began to gain weight rapidly, his spots growing larger.

After I had been away for a week or so, I walked through the front door, took one look at Brent, and said, "Mother, just stop feeding Brent. He looks like the coffee table!"

"What? I'm not feeding him."

And of course, I would catch her. We'd be having dinner, and she'd be looking right at me, talking, and her hand would slip under the table with a little something off her plate—and then I'd hear Brent's lapping.

My brother and I talked about this. We tried many different ways to get

Shirley not to overfeed the dog. Then one day, Brent got sick and he had a seizure, exactly in the same spot where Shirley had taken her fall.

Lenny picked up Brent and drove him to the vet. The vet told Lenny, "You've got to stop this. This dog is so overweight, he's just been nominated to be in the Thanksgiving Day parade. He's going to be a float."

I guess when my mother saw Brent lying on the floor, much as she had when she'd fallen, she realized the seriousness of Brent's condition, and she understood that his poor health was due to overeating. So she made up her mind. No more feeding Brent from the table. No more of his favorite snack. Dog biscuits, you think? Not for Shirley's dog. Land-O-Lakes butter cookies.

"Mom? Why do we have nine cans of butter cookies? You don't eat them, Lenny doesn't eat them, and I certainly don't touch them."

"Those are for Brent," she said. "He loves those cookies."

"Mom, dogs eat dog biscuits, not butter cookies." So, the cookies went. Brent went on sort of a FoodMover eating program for animals, and he trimmed down. He became his former healthy self and never had another seizure.

No matter what my schedule was like, I'd always make time to go back every month and give Shirley a manicure and a pedicure. I'd do crazy things, just to break up the routine for her. I'd buy nail polish called Hard Candy—it came in trendy, wild colors with funny names like Trailer Trash and Gold Digger. My mother would be watching television as I'd be painting her toes vivid, metallic blue. Suddenly, she would look down to see what I was up to.

"Oh my God, Dicky, what *is* that?"

And I'd say, "Mother, it's nothing."

She'd say, "Take that off right now and give me my soft pink."

Or I'd paint each toe a different color, and she'd say, "That's *it!* You're not painting my toes anymore."

I never missed a trip home. And I was still calling several times a day to check in. A few months after my mother fell, I got a call from Lenny. My mother had gotten pneumonia, and she needed to go back into the hospital. After a few days, things were under control, and Shirley was home again.

Now each time I went to New Orleans to visit her, and even though her mind was still very much intact, I could see that Shirley was getting weaker.

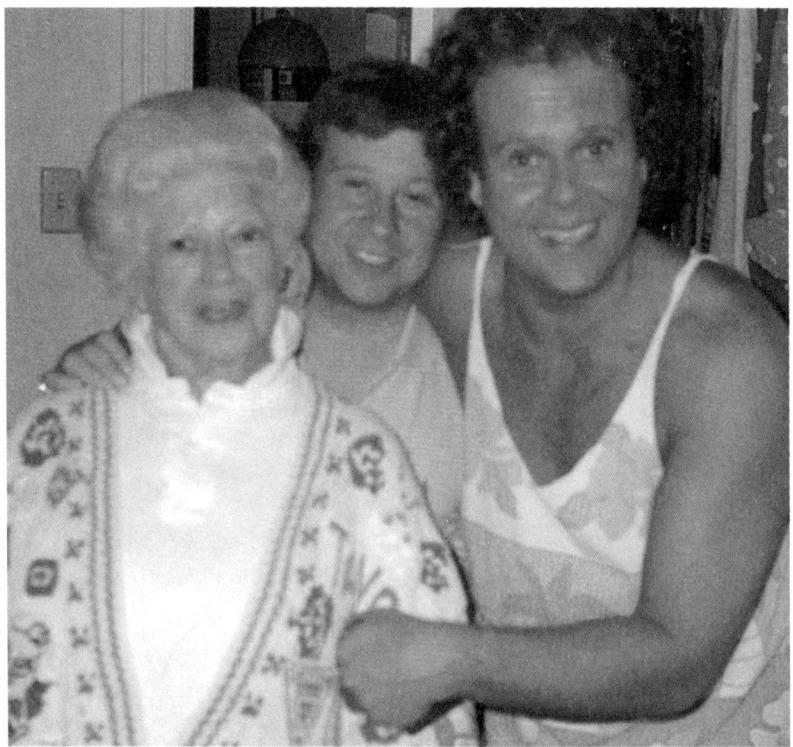

Just the three of us...

Rose could only work a few days a week. As my mother continued to have difficulty doing things, Lenny and I decided to get additional help for her.

We found a place called Kay's Sitting Service. (I've always had good luck with women whose first name begins with "K.") Kay sent us our second angel: Helen. She was thin and in her forties, and she was very much into fashionable hairdos, all different colors and styles, which she changed almost daily. And it was all done with wigs—Diana Ross would have been very jealous.

Helen reminded me in some ways of Hattie, our housekeeper and my black mother from childhood. Maybe that was why my mother bonded with her instantly. Helen was very loving to my mother. She'd comb her hair and sing to her, just as Shirley had done with the woman in the nursing home years before.

The two of them used to watch a lot of television together. "My T.V. pal," Shirley used to call Helen. Helen was always careful about making sure that mom was comfortable. Sometimes Shirley would be sitting there,

vid, metallic blue. Suddenly, she would look down to see what

and her hand would slip off her lap, and she didn't have the strength to get it back up. Helen would quietly lean over, and lift it for her tenderly. Often, Helen would rub Shirley's hands and arms gently with creams and lotions—Shirley just loved that.

Helen had been on a cruise once, and she told Shirley that when she got better, the two of them were going to take a cruise together.

As Shirley got weaker, we found we needed extra help. We still weren't done in the angel department. Shirley's third angel was Joanne, who was also from Kay's Sitting Service. She was a young girl in her late twenties, pretty and with an eye to fashion. She was married, with a family, and she quickly developed a mother-daughter relationship with Shirley. Joanne would often do my mother's makeup when she knew I was coming to visit.

I'd come in and say, "Oh mama, you look so beautiful today."

My mother would beam with pride and say, "Joanne did it for me. It's so gorgeous. I just love Joanne."

Joanne was also very religious and would pray with me when I got upset. She was a very calming person. In fact, all the angels would pray with me from time to time.

One day, when I was really upset, Rose said to me, "Let me tell you something. We all lose people. Yes, I've lost my mom and my dad. But Richard, you don't know what it's like until you've lost a child. That's right, Richard, I lost my daughter. That is the toughest thing I've ever gone through. It is not easy, Richard. But you must be strong." Not a day goes by that I don't think about what she said to me.

Rose, Helen, and Joanne—these were Shirley's angels, and I began to look forward to seeing them each time I visited my mother. Lenny, Brent, and me, and these three women became a team, taking care of Shirley and keeping her spirits up. Sometimes I'd order food from the Rib Room at the Royal Orleans Hotel or from Arnaud's, and we'd all have a fabulous dinner together. There we were, eating all those same delicacies I'd had as a child when I was sitting on Shirley's lap.

The fact that my mother grew so close to these three women was just astonishing to me, because Shirley had never been a woman's woman. I think it had a lot to do with the love and respect that they showed Shirley— it was almost like they were her daughters.

Each time I came home to see Shirley, I saw that the veneer was slowly coming off. I watched her go from a cane to a walker. Then one day, Lenny came home and opened the trunk of the car. I saw something that I thought I would never see. It was a wheelchair. I just cried. From that day on, Shirley was never able to put her feet on the ground again. She went through so much. She lost a lot of weight. She had bouts of illness that landed her in the hospital, and all of a sudden, a virus got into her nervous system and she lost all of her motor skills. She had also suffered several strokes, the doctors told us.

I did what I could to help her. Because she couldn't walk anymore or lift herself, she could no longer get into the bathtub or take showers by herself. We built a beautiful new bathroom for Shirley, all pink, with a huge shower that had a gorgeous seat—throne—so that one of the angels could bathe her as she sat. Lenny went out and bought her all pink accessories: a pink rug, a pink soap dish, and little pink soaps.

As my mother began to have less control over her body, her mental sharpness began to slip away. She had always been used to doing twenty things at the same time. She'd been a firecracker, really smart. Nothing got past this woman, not even me (and you know what a wisecracker I am!).

One day, on one of my visits, we were having dinner. I was sitting next to Shirley and I was feeding her. As I cut up her prime rib into small, bite-size pieces, suddenly I was taken back to a meal at the Rib Room when my mother had cut up my steak for me. Now our roles were reversed. It all became too much for me. I lost it for a second, and I started crying.

Shirley turned to me and gave me a look. "Why are you crying? Oh, you're crying because of me. You're are such a crybaby. Dry those tears. There's no reason for you to cry over me."

I tried to pull myself together. It was important for me to be strong in front of Shirley.

"Oh, mom. I'm crying because I love you and I'm so worried about you," I told her.

"Honey, you see me now this way, and you think that this is not the mother you knew when you were little, and it's upsetting you, and I know it is. But you see, honey, I am eighty-six, and I live in my own house, I have my baby Brent here who takes such good care of me, and I've got you and Lenny, and my angels. I don't have any worries at all. I am so content. Can't you see how content I am? Can you say that about yourself?"

"But mom," I cried. "I'm so scared. Aren't you scared? I just don't know how I can handle all this." My mother took a breath. Every breath was crucial to her at this point.

She said, "I want you to understand something. I don't have any regrets. None, honey. None. My life has been so wonderful. I have no problems. This is your problem. You have to handle this."

That was a major change for me. Shirley had never talked to me like that before. Life, sickness, and death were never discussed in our house. Food was the only thing we talked about. Was there too much red pepper in the stuffed crab? Was there enough ham in the red beans and rice?

But my mother was happy—more than happy. I could see that she was very peaceful. Nothing was getting her down. I knew I would have to find a way to deal with my own fears.

That talk with Shirley really did help. I began to feel a little bit of the peace she'd been talking about. But I still had moments when I was afraid.

* * *

We were getting closer to New Orleans, and there was only about fifteen minutes before we landed. I glanced at the telephone attached to the back of the seat in front of me, and thought of all the calls I had made to Shirley in the last few weeks. I was talking to her two or three times a day.

"You just called two hours ago," she would say to me. "What did you think was going to happen?"

"I just wanted to say hi, mom."

If Shirley was eating or napping, I would telephone back later. She may have thought I was calling too much, but I wanted to take every opportunity to let her know I was thinking about her.

But during the last week of February, the conversations between my mother and me had gotten shorter. Every night before I went to bed, I called to say, "I love you." My mother's "I love you, too," got slower every time I talked to her. At the end of our talk, I would always make her kiss me on the phone—I'd always have to hear those smacking sounds. The last time I'd called before I left for Florida, I hardly got an "I love you" from her, and the kisses were so faint. Shirley seemed to be having trouble breathing, and she could barely finish her sentences.

The plane finally landed in New Orleans. I went directly to my mother's house. My brother was out of town, attending a Kiwanis charity event.

When I arrived at the house and rang the doorbell, I could hear Brent, ever the protector, greeting me with a bark. When Joanne opened the door, I gave her a hug. I walked into that pink bedroom and there was my sweet Shirley, sitting up in bed, surrounded by all the pictures of Lenny and me.

Joanne and Shirley had been watching television together, and Brent had run back into the room and was curled up next to Shirley on the bed. When mom saw me, her eyes sparkled. Although she couldn't say the words, her eyes were still saying, "I love you." And I told her with my words that I loved her. I sat on the bed with her, kissed her, and gently rubbed her hands. She seemed so fragile and translucent. I moved to the end of the bed and knelt down on the Persian rug on the floor. I rubbed her feet—she had tiny little feet. She just loved to have her feet rubbed.

I told her, "I'm going to be here in the morning. We'll spend a couple of hours together over breakfast, then I have to go back to California. But I'll see you in the morning. You sleep well." And then I kissed her and kissed her and kissed her, as I usually did.

My foot rub had made her drowsy, so when she feel asleep, I left quietly and went back to the Omni Royal Orleans Hotel, to my room that was like my second home.

The next morning when I got up, I quickly packed and went back to Shirley's. Joanne had done a double shift and was still with her. I sat very close to my mother on the bed, and I could hear her taking deep breaths, almost like she was asleep. But she was awake. Her eyes were open and fixed on an old movie on the American Movie Classics channel. I kissed her and stroked her forehead.

We watched television together, my mother and I and, of course, Brent, who never left her side. After breakfast, I told her I was going back to California. I held her hand, her fingers intertwined with mine.

"What time will Lenny be home?" she asked weakly.

"He's coming home at two," I told her.

"Two o'clock?" she repeated. "Okay."

very peaceful. Nothing was getting her down. I knew I would

I looked at the clock, and I was already fifteen minutes late getting in the car. So I got out of my chair. As I was leaving, I kissed her and I told her, "I love you."

And I just heard her struggling to breathe. There was no reply.

"*Shirley,*" I said a little louder.

And for a few seconds, her eyes focused. "What?" she asked me.

"I said I love you."

And she got up enough energy to say, "I know you love me." She said it very slowly and quietly. "I've always known you love me."

I wrapped my arms around her and kissed her good-bye, and then I walked out of the room, leaving my mother resting comfortably with her Brent.

In the living room, Joanne could tell I was very upset. Although it was hard not to, I never cried in front of my mother (except, of course, that one slip). I would wait until I got into the living room, and then I'd break down. The angels had all seen me through some very upsetting moments. Each one of them had their own encouraging words for me. Joanne comforted me as best she could.

As I was leaving, that funny feeling came over me again. I stopped at the front door. I had to go back. I turned around and marched right back into Shirley's bedroom.

"Shirley, do you mind if I have one last kiss?" I asked. I don't know why I did that. It wasn't like me. I usually just left, got in the car, and went to the airport. But no—this time was different. I crawled over Brent, who took up most of the bed, and I gave my mother a last kiss on the lips.

"I'll see you next week," I told her. "I'm going to go do some shopping malls and some exercise classes, but then I'll be back." I went to the airport and flew home to Los Angeles.

Now, we've all seen it in the movies—it's that moment when everything is so silent, so quiet, and all of a sudden, the phone rings. I have a lot of phone lines in my house. But there's only one that went directly to my mother and brother. It's the only line I keep on at night.

I had been home for just a couple of hours, and that line rang. It was late Sunday afternoon. I picked up the phone. It was Lenny.

"Dicky, mother has passed," he told me. "Shirley's gone. We've lost our Shirley." He told me that he had returned from his trip at around two o'clock. He had spent some time with Shirley, and then he went into the other room to unpack some clothes. Suddenly he heard Joanne calling out his name. He rushed into Shirley's room. She didn't seem to be breathing. Then he called the paramedics right away, and they were at the house almost immediately. They rushed her to the hospital, but Shirley had already begun her journey. She was gone—she truly was gone.

On the other end of the phone, Lenny began to cry. I thought I was going to break apart. I wasn't in denial about my mother's illness. I knew her quality of life had diminished. That vivacious young woman my father had met at the boardinghouse was no longer there. She had not been herself for a while. So eventually, even though I was grieving, I thought to myself, My God, how lucky. On the last day of her life, Shirley had gotten to see her two sons, and to kiss them both good-bye. I think she had waited for Lenny to return from his trip.

* * *

On Monday, I began making plans to go back home. But even before I got there, I had several conversations with Lenny on the phone about funeral plans. This was completely new territory for me, something I had certainly never done. Lenny, being the older brother, had once again bravely stepped into his role and began making arrangements, just as he had after my father's passing. Like my father, Lenny tended to keep his emotions buried, and he kept himself busy to hide his sorrow. I just knew I couldn't let him do it alone this time, as I had with daddy.

So I said to my brother, "I'm coming to New Orleans, Lenny. I'm going to help you." Lenny had already decided that the wake would be Wednesday, and the funeral would be Thursday.

He said, "Now don't get upset. But a lot of people want to say good-bye to mom, so we're having an open casket."

Oh, it was starting again. My father had wanted a simple funeral, and Lenny had planned a big event. Now he was doing the same thing with my mother's.

"Fine," I said. "I'm just going along with you. Now, since the casket is going to be open, we need to think about what Shirley will be wearing. What shall we dress her in, Lenny?" I couldn't believe I was saying this.

Lenny replied, "You know that purple-and-blue-and-green dress?"

ed at the front door. I had to go back. I turned around and

Uh-oh. I didn't want to tell him, but my brother is sort of color-blind. But I knew my mother would never rest in peace in a loud outfit like that— it was something you would wear to Mardi Gras.

"Lenny, I'm asking you. No, I'm begging you. Please. I know you're in charge here, but let me help in the wardrobe department. I wasn't around to help with daddy, so please, let me help with mom. I need to do this for myself. I need to be part of this with you."

I think my brother sort of understood.

"Lenny," I said, "go get that pink suit with the beautiful beaded camisole." I had bought it for her at Lillie Rubin and it was one of her favorites. When we'd go out to eat, she'd always say, "Get me that pink dress." I knew that's what she should wear.

I told Lenny, "When I get home, I'll get all her makeup, clothing, and jewelry together." In my mind, I began to organize how she should look. There I was. I started out as someone who is terrorized about the whole idea of a funeral, and now I was doing a make-over.

Just before I got on the plane to fly to New Orleans, I had to call my brother one more time.

"Lenny, it's me," I said, "I'm on my way. But I have to tell you, I'm not sure if I can take this. I'm getting ready to get on the plane. I'm bringing a black suit like I did with dad, but I don't know how much of this I can attend. I hope you won't be angry or disappointed or scream at me." Now that I didn't have my father yelling at me, my brother was there to take over. It was pretty similar sometimes. (Although Lenny could never send me to my room—thank God!)

Lenny said, "I don't want you to do anything that will make you feel uncomfortable." In the back of my mind, I heard my mother's words as clearly as if she were standing right in front of me. She'd say to me, "Don't aggravate your brother. Please."

Meanwhile, back in Los Angeles, news of my mother's passing made all the papers, and it was even on television. Regis and Kathie Lee and all the other hosts of all the shows I'd ever been on knew I had this close relationship with my mom. I even got a letter from Paul Harvey, and he did a tribute to my mother on his radio program. It was such an overwhelming thing to me that people would remember this love and dedication I had toward my mother.

With thunder crashing all around us, I looked down onto the

And I also had arrangements of my own to make. There were no flights that would get me to New Orleans fast enough. And so I did something that I've never done before—another first for me—I rented a jet. I had to get there—there was no question about it. I had to be there for both Shirley and Lenny.

As we were flying into New Orleans on Tuesday, we were caught in a terrible thunderstorm. With thunder crashing all around us, I looked down onto the bolts of lightning below, and an inner strength came over me. Even though I'd always been fearful on planes when there was lightning, and I had been a white-knuckled flyer at one time, I knew I was going home, and I had responsibilities. So a little lightning—okay, a lot of lightning—was not about to stop me.

Delayed by the storm, I got in rather late. But the first thing I did was run to the phone and call my brother. I told him I'd landed safely and asked if he wanted me to come over. He said he'd had a really long day and would see me in the morning.

As the storm moved into the Vieux Carré, I found myself back at the Royal Orleans Hotel once again. I was alone at the window as the wind and rain battered against the massive windows, straining to find a way in. Looking down the street, I saw the praline store where I'd spent so many happy hours and ate so many pralines. And farther down, there was the house where I spent my childhood. With the rain pouring down in sheets, it seemed as if my old neighborhood was awash in tears. All of my feelings started to surface, and my inner strength began to crumble. The whole experience was just a replay of my father's death. I was in the same place—the exact same room in the Royal Orleans—where I had stayed for my father's funeral.

I sat down on the bed. Was I going to have the strength to go to my mother's funeral? Or were my fears going to overwhelm me again? I knew Lenny really needed me. And I wanted to be there. But could I do it?

I knew I had to get some sleep, so I went to bed. I was so tired from the flight, but my mind kept going, thinking of Shirley. I was so restless. I tossed and turned. And then, all of a sudden, I fell out of bed. No—actually it was more like I was *flung* out of bed. I'm not kidding!

I hit my head, my knee, and my shoulder, and I knocked over a lamp. I swear, it was as if I had been kicked out of bed. I've told you about all those angels I had? Well, I must have forgotten to mention my kicking angel. Maybe it was my own conscience. Or, maybe it was my sweet Shirley. Whatever it had been, I certainly knew it was a wake-up call. But it wasn't time to get up. I went back to bed and slept.

* * *

I woke up very early to see the sun come up. The storm had passed and washed the streets clean. It was going to be a clear, beautiful day for Shirley.

I met Lenny at the house, and we hugged each other and cried. Slowly, we began talking about the jewelry, the makeup, the clothes—filling in all the details. Lenny had arranged to have the wake from six to nine that evening. The family's viewing would be beforehand, at five.

As he was telling me about the casket, something came to mind. My father had been cremated. Why wasn't my mother going to be cremated? This hadn't occurred to me when Lenny and I had talked on the phone the day before.

"Lenny, I hope you won't be angry with me," I started. "But I just want to know why mother isn't going to be cremated."

"Jews can't be cremated," he said to me.

I said, "Wait a minute, hold it. Jews can't be cremated? We didn't live a Jewish life. So what does that have to do with anything?"

"That's true," Lenny said. "But mother was a Jew."

"So, after all these years of not following a religion, now Shirley can't be cremated and we have to bury her because she's a Jew?" If I remembered correctly, in the Orthodox Jewish religion, burial must come the day after a death. So we had already missed that deadline and broken the rules. But it seemed that Lenny was making up his own rules. It was a whole new religion, a Catholic-and-Jewish mix.

"Now, about the mass . . ." Lenny continued.

"Mass? What mass? Shirley's never been to a mass in her life." I remembered that she'd escorted us to mass a couple of times, but that was it.

"Lenny, I don't get it. First she's a Jew and we can't cremate her, and then she's not Catholic and has never been to mass . . . "

Out of the clear blue, my brother interrupted me, "Should we put shoes on mom?"

"Are you kidding? Of course she has to have shoes. Because when you roll that casket into that Catholic mass, that Jewish lady is going to get up and walk right out."

But this was just the beginning. Lenny's bewildering funeral arrangements weren't through yet.

Next he said to me, "Now, I have to explain something to you and it's a little unusual, but I think that you'll understand. We have to go to the mortuary and get Daddy's urn out of the crypt, and we're going to place it at the bottom of Shirley's coffin."

I just stood there. Now this was a couple who slept in separate bedrooms. I could just picture my mother, in her coffin, tapping her foot against daddy's urn. "What the heck is that?" she'd wonder. "Dicky! Was this your idea of a joke?"

"How is Shirley going to get any rest if she's squeezed in with daddy?" I asked Lenny.

"Well, we've got a new vault to put mother in."

"You got her a new vault?"

He explained that the vault where my father's urn was kept was only large enough to hold the urn—a casket wouldn't fit. Lenny had already purchased a crypt for six in another mausoleum.

"Lenny! We don't even know six people!"

"Well, six—but you can actually fit twelve if you don't mind disturbing your loved ones."

"Twelve! Where are you going to get twelve people?!" Lenny actually looked around the room, as if he were searching for a few more people. But it was just the two of us. Room for twelve people! Leave it to Lenny to get a good deal. At the same time, I was thinking to myself, I can't believe all of this is happening. We're talking about this stuff like it happens every day. It was so strange.

Next, we discussed the jewelry that Shirley should wear. Lenny was very stern.

"I don't want mother to be wearing a great deal of jewelry," he told me. "I want it simple and plain."

Well, I had to speak up, because I knew Shirley wouldn't want that. I said to Lenny, "I want Shirley to look like herself, and Shirley wore jewelry. I want her to look as beautiful as she did when she walked out of the house every day."

d and washed the streets clean. It was going to be a clear,

Lenny and I began looking through the ornate jewelry cabinet where my mother had kept her jewelry. We'd already settled on the pink beaded suit, and I selected a beautiful amethyst ring surrounded by diamonds to go with it. I also picked a gorgeous handmade diamond-heart necklace that I had gotten her in Italy. As we searched through the cabinet, we discovered we couldn't get one of the drawers back in. It was stuck. I pulled the drawer all the way out and there, behind it, I discovered my father's pinky ring, with the woman's face carved in it.

My father's ring! The ring he'd promised me before he'd died. So the robbers hadn't gotten it after all. I knew, at that moment, that my father was there with Lenny and me. It was a sign. I took that ring and I put it in my pocket. When I went to the funeral, a part of my father would be there with me the whole time.

With every moment, I got more strength. This was an event to honor the memory of my mother, after all. And it was almost as if she were speaking to me and helping me through it.

While Lenny and I were at the house, the phone was constantly ringing. Because news of Shirley's passing had appeared in *USA Today*, and there had been a lengthy write-up about her in the *Times-Picayune*, my brother kept being interrupted and having to answer the phone. I began to notice that his conversations were all the same. It went something like this: "Hello . . . Thank you. I know, I know. Oh, I'm so glad you're coming. And by the way, we're serving the artichoke balls. Uh-huh. Do you remember Mrs. Louis's wake? The artichoke balls, do you remember those? Well, the caterer made them for us, so we're serving those, and we have chicken sandwiches. Do you remember those chicken sandwiches, too?" Then along with the menu, he'd give the times and the address and any other information the caller would need. He'd hang up, and the phone would ring again. "Hello . . . Oh, thank you. I know how much you loved her. I'm so glad you're coming. Say, did you have the artichoke balls at Mrs. Louis's funeral?"

I listened from the couch. When he hung up, I said to Lenny, "What is wrong with you? We're talking about Shirley's funeral and you're pushing artichoke balls!"

I could just picture him bringing a whole platter of them and setting them up next to the coffin along with some little toothpicks so people

As I looked around, to the left was a pair of glass doors. They

could come by, pay their respects, and get an artichoke ball. Even in times of sadness, food was still the priority. Some things just never do change.

Lenny and I said our good-byes, and I went back to the hotel to rest. All the while, I worried if I would have the strength to go to Shirley's wake. After my nap, I got dressed in a pair of black pants, a white shirt, and a vest, still unsure of myself. I drove down Canal Street until the car passed in front of a beautiful castlelike building. It was Schoen's Funeral Home. Once it had been an old home owned by a wealthy family. I must have ridden by it a thousand times in my youth, but I had never noticed it before. Maybe that was because any time I saw anything related to death, I just turned the other way. Now I was actually turning into the driveway. As the car stopped, I stayed in the car. I just couldn't go in.

But then Lenny came out, so I opened the door and got out to meet him. I hugged my brother and I kissed him. I held him very tight.

He said, "She looks so beautiful, Dicky. Really, she does. Don't be afraid. She looks so beautiful."

So I squeezed his hand and I took a couple of deep breaths, then I moved toward the entrance. I felt wobbly, so I grabbed the ornate handrail that led toward the front door. I don't know how long it took for me to get up those steps. Inside the entry room, there were two men. They silently opened the doors and led me into a parlor, which looked like a very pretty, old-fashioned living room. Off the main room, there were six parlors, and to my amazement, they were all filled with flowers. There were flowers from Kiwanis people and community leaders, flowers from people from the neighborhood and from our past, flowers from celebrities and from Slimmons and from fans. Each arrangement was bigger than the next, and they were everywhere. The room was drenched with the perfume of these beautiful bouquets. I felt like I was about to do a 1-800-FLOWERS commercial.

As I looked around, to the left was a pair of glass doors. They reminded me of the glass doors in our old house on St. Louis Street. They had lace curtains on them. When I saw those doors, my fear returned. I just knew what was behind them. My brother and everyone else stood still as I walked over to those French doors. I opened them and stepped into the viewing room. In the corner was a woman with long brown hair swept to one side, wearing a cream-colored dress and playing a harp. I walked a little further and I saw it—I saw the casket. It was the first casket I'd ever seen in my entire life.

The day before, I'd told the florist that my mother's favorite color was pink and that all the flowers everywhere had to be pink roses. He had to search every flower shop—I wanted Shirley to have her pink roses. And I saw this coffin cradled in beautiful pink roses. Slowly, I walked over to the coffin, and there she was. My sweet, dear, wonderful Shirley. Just as Lenny had said, she was so beautiful. And she was so peaceful-looking. It looked like she was taking a nap before she was going out to the ball. In her hands was a bouquet of beautiful pink and white orchids.

It was not what I had imagined a funeral would be. I was so shocked at how gorgeous she looked. It was overwhelming. I started to cry. And then I stopped myself. I walked closer and closer. And then I knelt down and I just talked to her.

"Well, Shirley, here I am," I said. "Didn't think I'd make it, did you? I know it was you who kicked me out of bed. Well, I'm here. And no, I'm not going to aggravate my brother. I promise. I love you so much."

Like that moment in her room, I had to have one last kiss. Without a second thought, I bent over and I kissed her. Then I gave her ten kisses on her forehead, like I always had when I'd visited her.

There was nothing more to say. I turned around and opened all the doors. I went to the front of the funeral home, where there was a line of people waiting outside. I opened the front door and I greeted everyone that walked in.

Each person would come in with a really sad face. Some of them were already crying. They'd hug me.

"I'm so sorry, Richard," they'd say.

And then I would answer, "About what?"

"Oh, about your mother."

"Why? What happened to my mother?"

They'd look at me, shocked for a moment, and they'd say, "Oh Dicky, now stop it." And they'd smile, their sorrow forgotten for the moment. I had to have a little mischievousness or I don't think I could have gotten through it. There I was, still using my humor as a shield. It was still there for me.

Each person I greeted told me a story about my mother. In the few short hours of the wake, I heard stories from women whom she'd sold cosmetics to, and stories of people who knew her from the 500 Club. I heard stories from people who had seen her do the dance of the Devil and the Lady, and people who knew her long before I was even born. I collected all these stories and committed them to memory. Each one was so special, and they reinforced what a wonderful lady Shirley had been.

Marie and Marguerite (the sisters from the praline store) and their sister, Betty, came, and so did all the girls who used to protect me when the bully was going to beat me up—Linda Jolly and Gloria Smyra and Joanne Ferarra. They were all there. So was just about anyone whom my mother had sold a lipstick to, and people from Kiwanis, people from the Volunteers of America, and people from the Junior League.

Rose, my mother's first angel, came up to me and said, "Didn't I tell you that you were going to have the strength? Didn't I tell you that the Lord would help you get through this and that your brother needed you and you were going to be here? Well, you're here. I knew you could do it." I gave her a big hug and a kiss as she melted into my arms and began to cry.

Helen walked in next. She looked so beautiful. She must have spent all day at the beauty parlor. She was crying from the very first moment she walked in. I held her and led her over to Shirley's side, and she knelt down and prayed.

I turned around, and Joanne and her husband walked in. Joanne was dressed in a beautiful lace outfit. And there we were, all together, to say good-bye to Shirley.

It had been really rough for Joanne because she had been there, holding Shirley's hand when she passed away. They were all crying. This time, I was the strong one. *I* was the one who comforted *them*.

The next day, I found myself at a Catholic mass. The church was all filled up, and the pallbearers brought in the coffin, and of course my father's urn was already tucked safely inside, like an *I Dream of Jeannie* episode.

The mass was beautiful. Before long, we found ourselves in this stately brown-and-red marble mausoleum. After the priest said a final blessing, we hugged and kissed our friends.

That's when Lenny said, "Come with me. I want to show you where mom and dad will be." We went around a corner to an alcove, where there was a beautiful stained-glass window with a heavenly image of St. Anne. Near the window was the place where Shirley and Leonard would be laid to rest (along with the other ten people we were going to have to find).

Now, I've always thought "big" for my parents. If I wanted to buy them something, even if they didn't want it, I'd force it on them. If my brother didn't want a new car, I'd go and buy him the biggest one they made. They had never asked for anything—never. But that didn't mean they weren't going to get something—something big.

So I looked for a massive tribute to my parents. I looked . . . and I looked . . . Finally, I looked down and I saw a green curtain on the last row on the bottom. It looked like a little Punch and Judy set.

"Lenny, what are we doing—hiding them?"

"This is just temporary," he told me. "They're building a new mausoleum, then we're going to move them over."

"Well, why don't we just move them every year? Or, better yet, why don't we take them around the world? One year they can be buried in Italy, and the next year they can be buried in France. Daddy always dreamed of going on the Orient Express, and you know how much Shirley loved England." Then I heard Shirley's voice just as if she were standing next to me. "All right, enough. You're aggravating your brother."

After a meal at one of my mother and father's favorite restaurants (you didn't think we'd have a funeral without a meal, did you?!), I went back to the hotel, changed my clothes, and packed to leave New Orleans.

I went to say good-bye to my brother. I walked into the house, and there was Brent. He was lying on Shirley's bed, keeping it warm for her. And around him were all the pictures of my brother and me. And the blades of the fan were still spinning, cooling off Brent's face.

A week later, I received a phone call from Shirley's three angels. The four of us were all on the phone together, and we all cried. I told them that my mother had left something to each of them. When I came home, I had written a letter to each one as if I were Shirley. "Dear Rose, You'll never know

Shirley's voice is always still there and I hear her. I really d

how much you meant to me the last several months of my life. You were always so good to me in every way." And I signed it "Love, Shirley Simmons." I enclosed a check with each of the notes. It wasn't about money. I wanted them to go out and buy something special and think of Shirley. I knew it was what my mother would have wanted for them.

I may have lost Shirley on this earth, but I still have my three angels.

Things always have a way of coming full circle. Lenny spent days and hours going through the furniture and clothes. Many of the beautiful things that I had bought for Shirley went to the Junior League and to the Volunteers of America. At one time we had gotten everything secondhand, and now we were giving back, so someone else could have a turn.

Shirley's voice is always still there and I hear her. I really do. You may have a loved one who has moved on but who watches over you and follows you around. Shirley still talks to me, guiding and advising me just as she had done all her life.

After Shirley passed away, I was asked to do several national television shows. Even though I was so proud of myself for being so strong, I had lost my enthusiasm. Remember the saying, "The show must go on"? Well, I just didn't feel that way. I just didn't feel like being funny.

Two weeks after Shirley's funeral, my friend Stephanie Ross, a high mucky-muck who worked for Jay Leno, called and asked if I'd do *The Tonight Show.*

"I don't know," I said. "I've said no to all these other shows. I don't know if I really want to do a show so soon. It hasn't been all that long, and I'm not feeling so happy right now."

Jay Leno's parents had both died recently, and he had done a moving tribute to them on his show. I remembered that I had been a guest during the time he'd returned from his father's funeral. I was there for him, and now I guess he was going to be there for me. I still had my doubts, but I knew I couldn't hide forever. Eventually I said, "Yes, of course. I'll go on."

"He knows that your mother passed away, and he wants to talk about her on the show," Stephanie said.

"Oh my God, I'm just going to go out there and cry," I told her. "I'm going to be in my bedazzled top—one with rhinestones in the shape of a broken heart—and I'm just going to be weeping. It's not going to be pretty. This is supposed to be a comedy show."

But she assured me that everything would be handled with dignity.

I drove onto the NBC lot and headed to my dressing room. In the hallways, people were stopping me and giving me hugs and telling me how sorry they were.

In the dressing room, I sat in front of the mirror, on a little round ottoman with wheels. I began putting on my makeup, still not ready to go out and entertain.

I fluffed my hair and considered finding the producer to tell her that I just wasn't up to it, that I couldn't go on. Then, I heard a voice behind me. "Honey, blend that blush in just a little more. Bring it up toward your temples and blend, blend, blend."

I looked in the mirror. There, behind me, was Shirley in her pink suit. She was sitting on the couch, holding a small bouquet of pink and white orchids.

"Mom. I can't do it," I told her. "I'm here, but I don't know if I can pull this one off."

"Pull this one off? You pulled off so many things in your entire life— what do you mean you can't do this? Look how great you were at my funeral. You were fabulous. I wouldn't be surprised if you'll be booked for other funerals, you were so good."

"Mother, I'm still in mourning. I feel so sad."

"Look at me. Do I look sad? Just like your father and me, you're an entertainer. The show's got to go on, and that's the bottom line. You're doing great for others, and they need you. So clear up those eyes, then get out there and be with Jay. He'll take good care of you."

"Oh mom, I really do miss you."

"I know you do, honey, but I'll always be here for you. Just like you always say, I'm with you every step of the way."

I knew Shirley was right. I was feeling stronger already. I turned back to finish my makeup.

"Oh, Dicky?"

"Yes, mother?"

"Don't say anything to Jay that's going to aggravate your brother."

"I'll try really hard not to, mom."

"And remember—just be yourself. I always told you, never

"And remember—just be yourself. I always told you, never change. Now scoot over a little. I want to touch up my lipstick."

I made a little room on the stool for her and watched her apply her makeup, just as I had watched her so many times before.

"Mom?"

"Yes, son?"

"I love you."

"I know you love me," she said, quietly. "I've always known you love me. And I love you, too, Dicky."

My Storybook Angels

From my very beginning at the Touro Infirmary, to now, my fiftieth year, there are many, many, many people who helped me to become who I am, after all these years.

And now that I've told my tale, I thank my lucky stars for my storybook angels:

God, who gave me my curly locks and my spirit;

Shirley, my mom, who always encouraged me to follow my own path and to do my best, no matter what others might say;

Leonard, my father, the Renaissance man, who when he wasn't sending me to my room, was teaching me by his example to treat everyone the same, regardless of who they are, since we're all related in some way;

Lenny, the Simmons family historian, who from day one has been the best brother—he's always been my rock;

My uncle Milton, who gave me all my first names—and cured my rash;

Jimmy Grote, who helps keep me sane (I really am) and reminds me every day what's important;

Jenifer Catalano, who with loving hugs gently squeezed from me all my tales;

David Ricketts, who helped breathe life into every word you just read;

Barbara Marks, a brilliant book designer, who took the puzzle of my story and beautifully organized its pieces in these happy pages;

My energizer angels who have been by my side through thick and thin—*Marilyn Lamas* for 18 years, *Elijah Jones* for 15 years, and *Mary Graves* for 13 years . . . but they're up for parole;

And all my Dalmatians, who have taught me so much about loyalty and love.

—RICHARD